Infections in Pregnancy

Infections in Pregnancy

An Evidence-Based Approach

Edited by

Adel Elkady
Police Force Hospital, Cairo, Egypt

Prabha Sinha
College of Medical and Health Sciences, National University of Science and Technology, Oman

Soad Ali Zaki Hassan
Alexandria University, Alexandria Governorate, Egypt

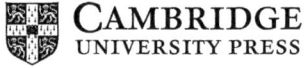
CAMBRIDGE
UNIVERSITY PRESS

CAMBRIDGE
UNIVERSITY PRESS

University Printing House, Cambridge CB2 8BS, United Kingdom

One Liberty Plaza, 20th Floor, New York, NY 10006, USA

477 Williamstown Road, Port Melbourne, VIC 3207, Australia

314–321, 3rd Floor, Plot 3, Splendor Forum, Jasola District Centre, New Delhi – 110025, India

79 Anson Road, #06–04/06, Singapore 079906

Cambridge University Press is part of the University of Cambridge.

It furthers the University's mission by disseminating knowledge in the pursuit of education, learning, and research at the highest international levels of excellence.

www.cambridge.org
Information on this title: www.cambridge.org/9781108716635
DOI: 10.1017/9781108650434

First published 2020

Printed and bound in Great Britain by Clays Ltd, Elcograf S.p.A.

A catalogue record for this publication is available from the British Library.

Library of Congress Cataloging-in-Publication Data
Names: Elkady, Adel, editor. | Sinha, P. (Prabha), editor. | Hassan, Soad Ali Zaki, editor.
Title: Infections in pregnancy: an evidence-based approach / edited by Adel Elkady, Prabha Sinha, Soad Ali Zaki Hassan.
Other titles: Infections in pregnancy (Elkady)
Description: Cambridge, United Kingdom ; New York, NY : Cambridge University Press, 2020. | Includes bibliographical
references and index.
Identifiers: LCCN 2018042769 | ISBN 9781108716635 (pbk.)
Subjects: | MESH: Pregnancy Complications, Infectious
Classification: LCC RG571 | NLM WQ 256 | DDC 618.3–dc23
LC record available at https://lccn.loc.gov/2018042769

ISBN 978-1-108-71663-5 Paperback

Contents

Section 3. Postpartum Infections

Contributors

Maimoona Ahmed MS-FNB (High-Risk Pregnancy and Perinatology)
Maternal–Fetal Medicine Department, Cloudnine Hospital, Mumbai, India

Rania Hassan Mostafa Ahmed MD
Department of Obstetrics and Gynaecology, Ain Shams University, Cairo, Egypt

Christine Helmy Samuel Azer MRCOG FEOG-EBCOG
Department of Obstetrics and Gynaecology, Dr Sulaiman Al Habib Medical Centre, Dubai, United Arab Emirates

Bhavya Balasubramanya MD (Community Medicine)
Rural Unit for Health and Social Affairs, Department of Community Health, Christian Medical College, Vellore, Tamil Nadu, India

Rachana Dwivedi FRCOG FICOG PGC (USS) DFFP
Department of Obstetrics and Gynaecology, Royal Bournemouth & Christchurch Hospitals NHS Trust, Bournemouth, UK

Adel Elkady DGO FRCOG FICS
Boulak El Dakror Hospital, Cairo, Egypt

Youssef Abo Elwan MD MRCOG
Department of Obstetrics and Gynaecology, Zagazig University, Zagazig City, Egypt

Mohammed Hamed Khedr MSc
Police Force Hospital, Giza, Egypt

Professor Soad Ali Zaki Hassan
Professor of Microbiology, Alexandria University, Egypt

Rashda Imran FCPS MRCOG
St Mary's Hospital, Manchester, UK

Ahmed Khalil MSc MD MRCOG
Department of Obstetrics and Gynaecology, Benha University, Benha, Egypt and Department of Obstetrics and Gynaecology, Medway Maritime Hospital, Gillingham, UK

Ashok Kumar FRCSI FRCS (Glas)
Locum Consultant General Surgeon, UK

Nutan Mishra MD FRCOG
Department of Obstetrics and Gynaecology, Buckinghamshire Healthcare NHS Trust, Aylesbury, UK

Mithila B. Prasad DGO MRCOG
Department of Obstetrics and Gynaecology, North-West Deanery, Wythenshawe Hospital, Manchester, UK

Varsha S. Puranik MD Microbiology
Department of Microbiology, Cauvery Hospital and College of Allied Health Sciences, Mysuru, Karnataka, India

Tarek El Shamy MSc MRCOG PGCert (Ultrasound)
Obstetrics and Gynaecology Department, West Middlesex University Hospital, London, UK

Shabnum Sibtain FRCOG
Department of Obstetrics and Gynaecology, Azra Naheed Medical College, Lahore, Pakistan

Prabha Sinha DGO FRCOG MRCPI
Department of Obstetrics and Gynaecology, Oman Medical College, Sultanate of Oman

Akanksha Sood MS (ObGyn) DNB MRCOG FACOG
Department of Reproductive Medicine, St Mary's Hospital, Manchester, UK

Foreword

This book is particularly welcome, as pregnant women are exceptionally vulnerable to infection, due to an increased immune tolerance which is a protective mechanism for the fetus; physiological changes in the mother which make them more susceptible to infection; and the addition of a placenta which can house pathogens. Therefore as an obstetrician, infection is a problem that we all find challenging at some stage. To date we have not had access to a book such as this.

This book gives a comprehensive coverage of infection in pregnancy, from simple everyday infections to severe life-threatening infections. The authors commence by addressing vaccination in pregnancy, and then provide extensive coverage of a diverse range of infections not only during pregnancy but postpartum.

The book has been directed by an internationally renowned obstetrician who has been practising for over 40 years. He has marshalled an international group of obstetricians and gynaecologists who are familiar with diseases that many of us will have never come across, but with our increasing immigrant and nomadic populations we need to be aware of them as their incidence in the UK and globally is rising.

This book should be read by every obstetrician, from trainee to senior consultant, to understand about infections in pregnancy, both how they present and how they are managed, and then it will serve as a valuable reference book on the shelf for any challenging infection problems one might come across in one's everyday future clinical practice.

Janice Rymer, Professor of Obstetrics and Gynaecology, King's College London

Preface

We the editors, Adel, Prabha and Souad, are pleased and honoured to offer this book to our dear readers.

Infections during pregnancy are major causes of maternal and fetal morbidity and mortality. Infections can be transmitted to the fetus transplacentally and during birth, which becomes apparent during the early days of life. Postnatal infection can occur through breastfeeding or direct contact.

The clinical manifestations of fetal/neonatal infections vary depending on the infective agent and gestational age at exposure. The risk of infection is higher during earlier gestation age at exposure, resulting in a severe congenital malformation syndrome.

Infections in pregnancy can have serious maternal and fetal implications; even death can result if infection is severe and is not immediately diagnosed and properly managed, particularly during epidemics.

We felt the medical literature was lacking an up-to-date book to help and guide health care providers and health authorities in the diagnosis, management and prevention of these serious conditions.

We have aimed to present the latest information, knowledge and different national and international guidelines to offer our readers a useful, comprehensive and handy guide. We have tried to cover all possible infections.

We welcome any contact or criticisms from our readers.

Adel Elkady
Prabha Sinha
Soad Hassan

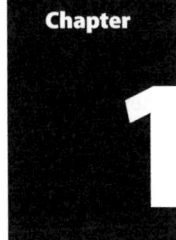

Chapter

Vaccination in Pregnancy

Akanksha Sood

Introduction

Vaccination is one of the most cost-effective successful public health interventions. Maternal vaccination protects both mother and baby from the morbidity of certain preventable diseases.

Basics of Immunology

Immune response is the ability of the body to identify, recognise and defend against harmful toxins, infections or disease by making specific antibodies or sensitised white blood cells.[1,2]

The different antibodies produced by plasma cells as classified by isotype are five major isotypes (IgA, IgD, IgE, IgG and IgM).[3]

Immunity is produced by one of two body reactions:

- **Active immunity** is the ability to produce immunity either by exposure to the disease, infection, organism or by vaccination (killed or weakened form of organism).[4] The protection is provided by a person's own immune system, is natural and often lasts for life.
- **Passive immunity** involves administration of immunoglobulins which provides a quick but short-term immunity that wanes with time. These include varicella zoster hepatitis B immunoglobulin or transplacental transfer of antibodies from the mother.

Vaccination

Vaccination stimulates immune response against a specific antigen and provides protection from contracting the disease by forming antibodies.[5]

Types of Vaccines

Live Attenuated Vaccines

These vaccines contain pathogens, which have been weakened to diminish their infectivity and pathogenicity by repeated culturing. They do not cause illness, but retain their ability to replicate and stimulate production of antibodies. The immune response is virtually identical to the naturally produced long-term immunity with one dose, except oral vaccines which need repeating.[6]

Side effects of live vaccines are:

- The organisms might revert to a virulent form resulting in infection although of milder form
- Contraindicated in pregnancy as they have the potential to infect the fetus
- In immunocompromised individuals they cause uncontrolled replication of organisms, which may cause fatal reaction
- Vaccine can become ineffective by heat, light, presence of antibodies from other sources (transplacental or blood transfusion)[6]

Examples of a live attenuated vaccine are measles–mumps–rubella vaccine (MMR combined vaccine), varicella, measles, rotavirus, smallpox, chickenpox, yellow fever or the antibacterial vaccines, Bacillus Calmette-Guérin (BCG) vaccine and oral polio vaccine.

Live Inactivated Vaccines

These vaccines are produced by growing bacteria or the virus in culture media and then inactivating it with heat or chemicals. They are not alive and cannot replicate, and are therefore unable to cause disease even in an immune-deficient person.

Unlike live vaccines, these are not affected by circulating antibodies and hence can be given when antibodies are present in the blood, e.g. in infancy or following receipt of antibody-containing blood products. They require multiple doses. The first dose only primes the immune system. A protective immune response develops after the second or third dose.

Antibody titres diminish with time and, as a result, may require to be boosted with periodic supplemental doses.

Examples of inactivated vaccines: hepatitis A, flu, polio, rabies.

Recombinant Vaccines

Recombinant vaccines are produced by genetic engineering technology. Currently eight such vaccines are available:

- Hepatitis B vaccine
- HPV (human papillomavirus) vaccine
- Live typhoid vaccine
- Live attenuated influenza vaccine (LAIV)
- Whooping cough (part of the diphtheria, tetanus and pertussis (DTaP) combined vaccine)
- Pneumococcal vaccine
- Meningococcal vaccine
- Shingles vaccine

Toxoid Vaccines

Toxoid vaccines implies administration of the toxin produced by certain bacteria (tetanus or diphtheria) after making them harmless.

Vaccination in Pregnancy

Vaccination during pregnancy is not a routine event, and attenuated live virus vaccinations are generally contraindicated. A woman should be up to date with her routine immunisation before pregnancy against preventable diseases.

Vaccination during pregnancy is warranted when:

- The risk of exposure is high
- Infection poses risk to mother/fetus
- Vaccine is unlikely to be harmful

The benefits to mother and fetus should outweigh the risk of vaccination. It is preferable to delay immunisation until the second trimester to avoid the period of organogenesis unless medically indicated; however, no evidence exists of risk to fetus from inactivated vaccines or toxoids.[7,8] [evidence levels EL 2 & 3]

In the clinical context, vaccines can be broadly divided into three groups.

1. Vaccines contraindicated during pregnancy: live attenuated vaccines could cross the placenta and result in viral infection of the fetus, e.g. MMR and the varicella vaccines.

2. Vaccinations specially recommended during pregnancy, e.g. the trivalent inactivated influenza vaccine during the influenza season.

3. Vaccinations recommended for women at risk of exposure (hepatitis B).[8]

Rubella

Vaccine against rubella is routinely given to all as part of childhood immunisation, and 97 per cent of women in the UK are immune.

Rubella vaccine is contraindicated during pregnancy as it is presumed to cause fetal anomalies; however, if the vaccine is inadvertently administered to a pregnant woman, or pregnancy occurs within 28 days of vaccination, it should not be the reason for termination of pregnancy. She should be counselled about the theoretical risks to the fetus and the need for close follow-up.[9]

At the preconception counselling, a non-immune woman (immunoglobin (IgG) levels <10 IU/mL) should be offered MMR vaccine as a single dose and counselled to avoid pregnancy for 28 days after vaccination.

A pregnant non-immune woman should be offered vaccination during the postpartum period even if she is breastfeeding. Rubella virus is secreted in breastmilk; seroconversion without serious infection is reported in breastfed infants.

Varicella Zoster (VZV)

Approximately 90 per cent of women are immune because of childhood vaccination or exposure.

Universal screening to check immune status is not recommended; however, in certain situations the immune status should be checked.[10]

- Women with an uncertain or no previous chickenpox infection
- Those who come from tropical or subtropical countries
- Those who had an exposure to the infection

Varicella vaccine contains live attenuated virus derived from the Oka strain of VZV and is contraindicated in pregnancy due to theoretical risks of fetal infection.

If a woman is sero-negative, she should be offered postpartum immunisation of two separate doses four to eight weeks apart and advised to avoid pregnancy for four weeks after the second dose. She should be reassured about its safety during breastfeeding.

Women are advised to avoid contact with chickenpox or shingles and to inform a health care worker in case of significant contact. Contact with pregnant women should be avoided if a post-vaccination rash occurs. [EL 2]

If the pregnant woman is not immune to VZV and she has had a significant exposure, she should be offered varicella zoster immunoglobulin (VZIG) as soon as possible.[10]

Inadvertent exposure to vaccine in pregnancy is not an indication for termination as there has been no increase in the risk of fetal abnormality above the background risk.

A review of the Pregnancy Registry for VARIVAX following 362 pregnancies inadvertently exposed to varicella vaccine showed there was no case of congenital varicella syndrome and no abnormal features or birth defects in the infants. [EL 2]

Whooping Cough (Pertussis)

This is an acute bacterial infection. It is highly contagious, caused by *Bordetella pertussis* spreading through droplets (coughing and sneezing).

Vaccinating pregnant women against whooping cough has been highly effective in protecting newborn babies. It offers immediate protection to cover the newborn until they can have their first vaccination at two months of age.

Babies born to women vaccinated at least a week before birth had a 91 per cent reduced risk of becoming ill with whooping cough in their first weeks of life, compared with babies whose mothers were not vaccinated.[11]

In 2012, the UK experienced a nationwide epidemic of pertussis, resulting in serious complications (pneumonia, encephalitis, seizures, brain damage) including death, especially in young babies. A programme for the vaccination of pregnant women between 28 and 32 weeks against pertussis was introduced in October 2012.[11]

However, it can be given at any time until the start of labour, although after 38 weeks the fetus is less likely to be protected by maternal immunity.

The Joint Committee on Vaccination and Immunisation (JCVI) of the Royal College of Obstetricians and Gynaecologists (RCOG) recommended that from April 2016 the vaccination should be offered from 20 weeks (after the anomaly scan).[12]

Many countries including the United States, Spain, Australia, New Zealand, Belgium and Argentina currently recommend vaccination against whooping cough in pregnancy.

Pregnant women need to be vaccinated even if they have been vaccinated in childhood or in a previous pregnancy. Both randomised clinical trials and cohort studies support its safety (no increase in pregnancy complications, preterm birth, low birthweight, congenital anomalies, spontaneous abortion, or stillbirth).[13] [EL 1]

Vaccination of the close contacts of the neonate (mother's partner) is recommended as a strategy for newborn prevention, when the mother has not been timely vaccinated.[13]

Tetanus

Worldwide, each year, tetanus kills an estimated 180 000 neonates (about 5 per cent of all neonatal deaths, 2002 data) and up to 30 000 women (about 5 per cent of all maternal deaths).

Tetanus vaccine is a toxoid vaccine and protects against both maternal and neonatal tetanus.

All pregnant women should receive a tetanus toxoid vaccine during each pregnancy, irrespective of any previous history of immunisation.

The optimum time for passive antibody transfer is from the 27th until the 36th week. A booster dose is indicated if a pregnant woman is exposed to the risk of tetanus infection during or immediately after delivery.

Diphtheria

Diphtheria can lead to breathing problems, heart failure, paralysis and death. The Tdap vaccine has a dose of tetanus toxoid, reduced diphtheria toxoid and acellular pertussis.

All pregnant women should get a Tdap vaccination in each pregnancy.

Influenza

'The flu', as is it commonly known, is a highly contagious disease caused by an influenza virus which occurs in all parts of the world. It spreads by coughing and sneezing of an infected person.

There are three types of Influenza virus, type A (H1N1), type B (H3N2) and type C.

Type C generally causes mild respiratory illness and does not usually cause epidemics.[14]

Influenza A and B viruses cause outbreaks or epidemics and therefore should be included in seasonal influenza vaccine.

Pregnant women are particularly vulnerable to influenza. Strong evidence shows that pregnant and postpartum women are at higher risk of severe illness and complications than women who are not pregnant.

Due to reduced immunity during pregnancy, influenza increases the risk for both mother and fetus with resulting preterm and low birthweight babies.

Influenza vaccine is an integral element of pre-conception, prenatal and postpartum care.

Studies have shown that vaccination reduces the risk of serious maternal medical complications and provides passive protection to the neonate from influenza in the first six months before the baby is eligible for vaccination.

Recent systematic review has confirmed that decreased risk of laboratory-confirmed influenza infection in infants is associated with uptake of influenza vaccine during pregnancy.[15] [EL 1]

There are two types of vaccine: the inactivated (injection) and the live attenuated (intra-nasal spray).

The live attenuated nasal spray is not recommended for pregnant women.

Pregnant women should be counselled about the benefits of the single influenza vaccine for themselves and their unborn child. According to the Mothers and Babies Reducing Risk through Audits and Confidential Enquiries, UK (MBRRACE-UK) report 2010–12, 1 in 11 pregnant women died from flu, and more than half of these deaths could have been prevented by a flu vaccination.[16] Increasing immunisation rates in pregnancy therefore remain important.

Increasing immunisation rates in pregnancy against seasonal influenza must remain a public health priority.

It is recommended that all pregnant women have influenza vaccine at whatever stage of pregnancy when the pandemic starts. The vaccine protects against three of the most likely strains. It is important to have the vaccine every year as flu virus is very variable and strains change over time.

It is strongly recommended by RCOG that flu vaccine be offered[17]

- To all pregnant women
- In each pregnancy
- At any stage of pregnancy (first, second or third trimester)
- To have the vaccine in autumn before the outbreak of flu starts

The vaccine offered is given as intramuscular injection; it takes up to two weeks after vaccination to give protection and is 50 per cent effective.

Human Papillomavirus (HPV)

Human papillomavirus (HPV) infection during pregnancy is not well studied. There has not been any association with an increased risk of birth defects. A link between HPV infection and preterm birth was shown in a case control study.[18]

Currently there are two inactive recombinant HPV vaccines, the quadrivalent vaccine, which protects against HPV types 6, 11, 16 and 18, and a bivalent vaccine, which provides protection against HPV types 16 and 18.

The Centers for Disease Control and Prevention (CDC) do not recommend HPV vaccination during pregnancy, nor do they recommend testing for pregnancy before the routine HPV vaccination.[19,20]

If the vaccine has been inadvertently given to a pregnant woman, there is no need for termination of pregnancy, but the second dose should be postponed until after the pregnancy. If a woman has received an HPV vaccine and then plans to become pregnant, there is no need to delay pregnancy, as the HPV vaccines are inactive.

In a recent retrospective observational cohort study, quadrivalent HPV vaccine inadvertently administered in pregnancy or during the periconceptional period was not associated with adverse pregnancy or birth outcomes [EL 1].

Hepatitis A

This is a formalin inactivated vaccine. The theoretical risk to the developing fetus is expected to be low.

The safety during pregnancy has not been determined. The risk associated with vaccination should be weighed against the risk of hepatitis A in pregnant women. It is recommended for pregnant women who are at high risk due to travel or pre-existing high-risk condition, e.g.

- Long-term liver disease
- Haemophilia
- Intravenous drug users
- Occupational risk – working with or near sewage, working in institutions where levels of personal hygiene may be poor
- Working with primates (monkeys, apes, gorillas etc.)[20]

Hepatitis B (HBV)

Hepatitis B is spread by blood-to-blood contact and may also be present in other body fluids, e.g. semen, vaginal fluid and saliva. Hepatitis B infection in pregnancy may result in severe hepatic disease for the mother and chronic infection for the baby. If the mother is hepatitis B 'e antigen' positive, vertical transmission occurs in 90 per cent of pregnancies, and if she is hepatitis B 'e antigen' negative it occurs in only 10 per cent.

Most infected infants (90 per cent) become chronic carriers, with possible long-term effects (liver cirrhosis and hepatocellular carcinoma). Vaccination will not cure chronic hepatitis but it is 95 per cent effective in preventing chronic infections from developing.

Pregnancy is not a contraindication to vaccination, it is an inactivated hepatitis B surface antigen (HBsAg) subunit vaccine.

The risk to the fetus is negligible. Hence, pregnant women who are identified as being high risk for HBV infection during pregnancy should be vaccinated, e.g.

- Women with multiple sexual partners during the previous six months
- Women who have been treated for a sexually transmitted infection
- Recent or current injection drug use
- HBsAg-positive sexual partner
- Received regular blood or blood product transfusion
- Travelling to high-risk countries
- Female sex workers
- Working in settings that place women at high risk of contact with body fluids, such as doctors, nurses, dentists and laboratory staff
- Women who started immunisation series before becoming pregnant[20]

Infants born to infectious mothers are vaccinated both by HBsAg vaccine and hepatitis B immunoglobulin (HBIG) (200 IU i.m.) preferably within 12 hours. This reduces the vertical transmission by 90 per cent.[21]

Meningococcal

The CDC advice is that this vaccination should be deferred in pregnancy and lactating women unless the mother is at high risk of disease:

- Women with sickle cell disease or thalassemia
- Immunosuppressed

- Travel to high-risk endemic areas
- Contact with infected individuals

The two available vaccines are meningococcal group C conjugated vaccine (Men C) and meningococcal quadrivalent polysaccharide vaccine (Men ACWY).

The UK Department of Health recommends that the conjugated vaccine be used in preference to polysaccharide vaccine because it provides better and long-lasting protection.[20]

Pneumococcal

Ideally the vaccine should be given prior to conception, but indications for administration (patients with asplenia, sickle cell disease, HIV or splenectomy) are not altered by pregnancy. The pneumococcal conjugated vaccine is preferred over polysaccharide vaccine.

The use of this vaccine is limited among women of childbearing age, although no adverse consequences have been reported among newborns whose mothers were inadvertently vaccinated during pregnancy.[20]

Polio

Polio is caused by a virus that can lead to permanent paralysis. It has been eradicated from most countries.

There are two types of polio vaccines, the inactivated poliovirus vaccine (IPV) and oral poliovirus vaccine (OPV). A pregnant woman should avoid travel to polio-endemic areas, but if travel is unavoidable and she requires immediate protection against polio, IPV can be administered.

In a cohort study in Finland, it was concluded that oral polio vaccination is safe for pregnant women.

Inclusion of pregnant women in programmes of mass vaccination with OPV appears to be safe.[21] [EL 2]

Typhoid

No data have been reported on the use of typhoid vaccine in pregnant women. Live vaccines like Ty21a are contraindicated in pregnancy. Vi polysaccharide vaccine should be given to pregnant women only if required.

Pregnant women are advised to avoid travel to typhoid-endemic areas but if such exposure is unavoidable, inactivated typhoid vaccine can be given if clearly needed.[20]

Rabies

Because of the potentially fatal consequences of inadequately managed rabies exposure, pregnancy is not considered a contraindication to post-exposure prophylaxis.

Pre-exposure prophylaxes may be indicated in pregnancy. Rabies exposure or diagnosis should not be regarded as reasons to terminate the pregnancy. It is an inactivated viral vaccine, and studies have indicated no increased incidence of abortion, premature births or fetal abnormalities.[20]

Yellow Fever

Yellow fever is a mosquito-borne viral infection endemic to rural areas of sub-Saharan Africa and tropical regions of South America. The infection varies in severity, but can be associated with significant morbidity and mortality. It is prudent to advise pregnant women not to travel to yellow fever-endemic areas.

Yellow fever vaccines are contraindicated as they are attenuated live vaccines. If travel is unavoidable and the risk of yellow fever exposure is high, vaccination may be justified (due to high mortality associated) after discussion with an infectious disease specialist.

Although no specific data are available, a woman should wait four weeks after receiving yellow fever vaccine before conceiving.[20]

Anti-Tuberculosis Bacilli Calmette-Guérin (BCG) Vaccination

This is a live vaccine, and falls into FDA category C (potential benefits may warrant use of the drug in pregnant women despite potential risks).

It is usually not given during pregnancy even though no harmful effects of vaccination on the fetus have been observed. Further studies are needed to prove its safety.[20]

BCG immunisation causes some pain and keloid scarring at the site of injection. The injection is either given in the deltoid or the buttocks, because it provides better cosmetic outcomes.

Vaccinia (Smallpox)

Smallpox is a viral infection and has been eradicated from most countries. Pregnant women who have had a definite exposure to smallpox virus should be vaccinated, as the risks to the mother and fetus from clinical smallpox infection substantially outweigh any potential risks.

The vaccine has not been documented to be teratogenic; the incidence of fetal vaccinia is low.

If a woman is inadvertently vaccinated or if she becomes pregnant within four weeks after vaccination, it should not be a reason to terminate pregnancy. [20,21]

Anthrax

The vaccine is a cell-free vaccine (developed from mammalian cell lines rather than embryonic chicken eggs).[21,22]

In a pre-event setting in which the risk for exposure is low, vaccination of pregnant women is not recommended and should be deferred until after pregnancy. During pregnancy in a post-event setting, pregnancy is not a precaution nor a contraindication to post-exposure prophylaxis.

Antenatal and Prenatal Screening for Infectious Diseases

In the United Kingdom, all pregnant women should be evaluated for immunity to rubella and varicella, hepatitis B, HIV and syphilis.

Women susceptible to rubella and varicella should be vaccinated immediately after delivery.

A woman found to be HBsAg-positive should be monitored carefully to ensure that the infant receives HBIG and begins the hepatitis B vaccine series no later than 12 hours after birth and the infant completes the recommended hepatitis B vaccine series on schedule.[22]

Breastfeeding and Vaccination

Neither inactivated nor live vaccines administered to the lactating woman affect the safety of breastfeeding women or their infants. Live viruses in vaccines can replicate in the mother, but most live viruses in vaccines have not been demonstrated in breastmilk.

Rubella vaccine virus might be excreted in breast milk, but the virus usually does not infect the infant. Even if infection does occur, it is well tolerated as the virus is attenuated.

Inactivated, recombinant, subunit, conjugated polysaccharide vaccines, as well as toxoids, pose no risk for mothers who are breastfeeding their infants.

Yellow fever vaccine should be avoided in breastfeeding women. However, when nursing mothers cannot avoid or postpone travel to areas endemic for yellow fever in which the risk for acquisition is high, these women should be vaccinated.

Postpartum Vaccination

The two vaccines that should be specifically administered before discharge of postpartum women to protect both mother and neonate are MMR vaccine and varicella vaccine. The woman should be counselled to avoid pregnancy for four weeks after vaccination.

Yellow fever and smallpox are the only vaccines contraindicated postpartum or when breastfeeding.

Conclusion

Maternal vaccination should be carried out with clear understanding, and mothers should be made aware of the implications (benefits vs risks). It can prevent/reduce maternal, fetal and neonatal infection and reduce disease burden.

- Most of the vaccines during pregnancy should be given according to risk/benefit ratios.
- Clearly indicated vaccine recommendations include inactivated influenza vaccine, the Tdap pertussis, diphtheria and tetanus vaccine, and smallpox for post-exposure prophylaxis if there is a definite history of exposure.
- The clearly contraindicated vaccines include the live attenuated influenza vaccine (LAIV), the BCG, the MMR (measles, mumps, rubella), the varicella and the zoster vaccines.

References

1. Dubé E, Laberge C, Guay M, Bramadat P, Roy R, Bettinger J. Vaccine hesitancy: an overview. *Hum Vaccin Immunother.* 2013; **9**(8): 1763–73.

2. Oxford Living Dictionary. https://en .oxforddictionaries.com/definition/immunity.

3. Thermo Fisher Scientific. Introduction to Immunoglobulins. thermofisher.com/antibodies/antibo dies-learning-center/antibodies-resource-library/.

4. Centers for Disease Control and Prevention. Immunity types. www.cdc.gov/vaccines/vac-gen/immunity-types .htm.

5. Biology Online. www.biology-online.org/dictionary/ Vaccination.

6. World Health Organization. Module 2: Types of vaccine and adverse reactions. www.who.int/vaccine_safety/ini tiative/tech_support/Part-2.pdf.

7. ACOG Committee on Obstetric Practice. Influenza vaccination and treatment during pregnancy. ACOG Committee Opinion No. 305. *Obstet Gynecol.* 2004; **104** (5 Pt 1): 1125–6.

8. Centers for Disease Control and Prevention. Vaccination in pregnancy. www.cdc.gov/vaccines/preg nancy/hcp/guidelines.html.

9. Sukumaran L, McNeil MM, Moro PL, Lewis PW, Winiecki SK, Shimabukuro TT. Adverse events following measles, mumps, and rubella vaccine in adults reported to the Vaccine Adverse Event Reporting System (VAERS), 2003–2013. *Clin Infect Dis.* 2015; **60**(10): e58–65.

10. Royal College of Obstetricians and Gynaecologists. Chickenpox in Pregnancy. Green-top Guideline No. 13. www.rcog.orguk/en/guidelines-research-services/g uidelines/gtg13/. January 2015.

11. NHS Choices. Whooping cough vaccination in pregnancy. nhs.uk/conditions/pregnancy-and-baby /pages/whooping-cough-vaccination- pregnant.aspx.

12. Public Health England. Vaccination against pertussis (Whooping cough) for pregnant women. 2016.

13. Amirthalingam G, Campbell H, Ribeiro S, Fry NK, Ramsay M, Miller E, Andrews, N. Sustained effectiveness of the maternal pertussis immunization program in England 3 years following introduction. *Clin Infect Dis.* 2016; **63** (suppl 4): S236–43.

14. Centers for Disease Control and Prevention. Types of Influenza Viruses. www.cdc.gov/flu/about/viruses/typ es.htm.

15. American College of Obstetricians and Gynecologists. Influenza Vaccination during Pregnancy, 2014.

16. MBBRACE-UK. Saving Lives, Improving Mothers' Care: surveillance of maternal deaths in the UK 2012–14 and lessons learned to inform maternity care from the UK and Ireland. Confidential Enquiries into Maternal Deaths and Morbidity. 2009–14. www .npeu.ox.ac.uk/mbbrace-uk/.

17. Royal College of Obstetricians and Gynaecologists. Flu vaccination in pregnancy protects both mothers and babies say doctors and midwives. www.rcog.org.uk/.

18. Gomez LM, Ma Y, Ho C, McGrath CM, Nelson DB, Parry S. Placental infection with human papillomavirus is associated with spontaneous preterm delivery. *Hum Reprod.* 2008; **23**(3): 709–15.

19. Narducci A, Einarson A, Bozzo P. Human papillomavirus vaccine and pregnancy. *Can Fam Physician.* 2012; **58**(3): 268–9.

20. Centers for Disease Control and Prevention. Guidelines for Vaccinating Pregnant Women. www.cdc.gov/vac cines/pregnancy/hcp/guidelines.html. 2016.

21. World Health Organization. WHO/UNICEF immunization summary: the 2007 edition. Geneva: World Health Organization. //whqlibdoc.who.int/hq/ 2007/who_ivb_2007_eng.pdf. 2007.

22. Audsley JM, Tannock GA. Cell-based influenza vaccines: progress to date. *Drugs.* 2008; **68**(11): 1483–91.

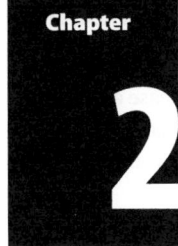

Viral Hepatitis

Rashda Imran

Virology[1]

Viruses are small, non-living parasites, which cannot replicate outside a host cell.

Viruses are grouped according to their genetic material: DNA or RNA.

DNA viruses are mostly double-stranded while RNA viruses are single-stranded.

A virus injects its genetic information into a host cell and then takes control of the cell's machinery. This process enables the virus to make copies of its DNA or RNA and make the viral proteins inside the host cell. A virus can quickly make multiple copies of itself in one cell, release these copies to infect new host cells and make even more copies. In this way, a virus can replicate very quickly inside a host.

DNA Viruses (Deoxyribonucleic Acid)

DNA is a molecule that contains the instructions it needs to develop, live and reproduce. DNA viruses use DNA as their genetic material. Some common examples of DNA viruses are parvovirus, papillomavirus and herpes virus. DNA viruses can affect both humans and animals and can range from causing benign symptoms to posing a very serious health risk.

DNA looks like a double helix and a twisted ladder.

RNA (Ribonucleic Acid)

Unlike DNA, RNA comes in a variety of shapes and types.

Common examples of RNA viruses: hepatitis C virus (HCV), Ebola, SARS, influenza, polio, measles and retrovirus human immunodeficiency virus (HIV).

Introduction

Viral hepatitis in pregnancy is the commonest cause of hepatic dysfunction and jaundice. The viruses resulting in hepatitis are hepatotoxic and include hepatitis A virus (HAV), hepatitis B virus (HBV), hepatitis C virus (HCV), hepatitis D virus (HDV) and hepatitis E virus (HEV).

Epstein–Barr virus and cytomegalovirus could also be the causative agents for hepatitis in rare cases.

Viral hepatitis caused 1.34 million deaths in 2015, a number comparable to deaths caused by tuberculosis and higher than those caused by HIV.[2]

In May 2016, the World Health Assembly endorsed Global Health Sector Strategy (GHSS) on viral hepatitis 2016–21. The GHSS calls for elimination of viral hepatitis as a public health threat by 2030 (reducing new infections by 90 per cent and mortality by 65 per cent).[2]

The hepatoviruses are quite divergent in their structures, epidemiology and routes of transmission, incubation period, clinical presentation, natural history and diagnosis. Prevention and treatment options are also different.

Hepatitis A (HAV)

Hepatitis A is an acute self-limiting illness and does not cause chronic infection. Hepatitis A virus can cause mild to severe disease. A very small proportion of people infected with hepatitis A could die from fulminant hepatitis.[3] It is the second most common form of viral hepatitis in the United States.[4] It is rarely life-threatening, with an estimated mortality of 0.3–0.6 per cent.[5] Approximately 1.5 million new cases are reported annually. The true incidence might be higher as mild cases are not reported.[5]

Virology and Epidemiology

Hepatitis A virus is a non-enveloped RNA virus. The lack of lipid envelope makes it relatively hard and acid-resistant. It can remain infectious for weeks. Human beings are the important reservoir. Hepatitis A virus is highly prevalent in areas with poor sanitary conditions. High endemic areas include Africa, central Asian countries and South America, and low endemic areas include Europe, Canada and the USA.

Pathogenesis and Transmission

The oral route is the primary mode of transmission, usually through ingestion of contaminated foods, especially raw and undercooked shellfish and person-to-person contact. Hepatitis A virus replicates in the small bowel and liver after ingestion, and is excreted via bile through feces. It has a short viraemia period, with peak infectivity during the two weeks before onset of symptoms.

Fetal Implications of Hepatitis A

The incidence of acute hepatitis A infection in pregnancy was quoted as less than 1:1000 prior to the introduction of HAV vaccine.[6]

Mother-to-child transmission (MTCT) of hepatitis A is very rare.

Only few cases of intrauterine transmission following maternal infection in the first trimester have been reported. The transmission resulted in fetal peritonitis and was confirmed by the presence of hepatitis A immunoglobulin M in fetal blood obtained by trans-abdominal blood sampling of the fetal umbilical cord, performed under ultrasound guidance (cordocentesis).[7]

There is increased risk of miscarriage and preterm labour.

Neonatal Implications

- Maternal infection in the third trimester of pregnancy may result in self-limiting neonatal cholestasis or asymptomatic neonatal infection.[8]
- Most viral infections are not affected by pregnancy.
- There have not been any reported maternal or fetal mortalities due to hepatitis A.
- Breastfeeding should not be discouraged, and the child should be protected through administration of immunoglobulin or the inactivated vaccine.[9]

Prevention

Safe water supply, food safety, improved sanitation and hand washing, especially before handling food, are important for its prevention.

Vaccination and Passive Immunisation

- The hepatitis A vaccine (HAVRIX, VAQTA) is the most effective way to combat the disease and should be considered for pregnant women and women of reproductive age before visiting HAV-endemic areas.
- Hepatitis A vaccination (an inactivated (killed) vaccine). **Two doses** are needed for long-lasting protection. It is prepared from inactive virus and is considered safe during pregnancy.[10]
- If a pregnant woman is exposed to hepatitis infection, passive immunisation with immunoglobulins within two weeks of exposure is safe in pregnancy.
- 0.02 mg/mL of immunoglobulin by single intramuscular injection provides protection for three months in 80–90 per cent of people.[7]

Clinical Presentation

The presentation in pregnant and non-pregnant women is the same:

- Fever and chills
- Anorexia, nausea and vomiting
- Dark urine and pale stool
- Jaundice and hepatomegaly

Most signs and symptoms resolve in three weeks.

Complications

- About 7 per cent of patients can have complications like cholestasis, prolonged jaundice, pruritus and fever.
- Fulminating hepatitis occurs in less than 1 per cent of cases.

Diagnosis

The specific diagnosis of acute hepatitis A is made by serology testing of the patient's blood; anti-HAV immunoglobulin M (IgM) is diagnostic. Detection of IgG anti-HAV alone indicates past infection.

The liver enzymes like transaminases are classically elevated by 10–100 times the normal range.[11]

Treatment

- The treatment of hepatitis A is supportive to maintain comfort and adequate nutrition.

- Hospitalisation is indicated if patients develop severe disease with coagulopathy, encephalopathy or severe malaise and asthenia. Liver transplantation may be required in rare cases.

Hepatitis A is not an indication for caesarean section delivery. Delivery should be based on the obstetric conditions of the mother and baby.

Hepatitis B (HBV)

Hepatitis B is an infectious disease caused by hepatitis B virus. The infection can result in acute or chronic course. HBV accounts for 3.5 million chronic infections worldwide and approximately 1 million deaths due to hepatocellular carcinoma and cirrhosis.[12]

Virology and Epidemiology

Hepatitis B virus is a double-stranded DNA virus which infects the liver cells and belongs to the *Hepadnaviridae* family. It has a lipid envelope with antigen protein called hepatitis B surface antigen.

Hepatitis B has three antigens:

1. Hepatitis B s **surface antigen (HBsAg)** is detected in high levels during acute or chronic infection. The presence of HBsAg indicates that the person is infective. As a part of immune response, the body normally produces the anti-HBs antibodies. HBsAg is the antigen used to make hepatitis B vaccine.
2. The total hepatitis B **core antigen (HBcAg)** appears at the onset of symptoms in acute hepatitis B and persists for life.
3. Hepatitis B e-antigen **or pre-core (HBeAg)** is generally detectable in patients with a new acute infection; the presence of HBeAg is associated with higher HBV DNA levels and increased infectivity.

Serologic testing and measurement of several hepatitis B virus antibodies or a combination of markers are used to identify different phases of the individual:

- Acutely infected: **IgM anti-HBc positive, HBsAg positive anti-HBc positive**
- Chronically infected: **IgM anti-HBc negative, HBsAg positive**
- Immune: **HBsAg negative, anti-HBc IgG positive, anti-HBs IgG positive**[13]

HBV is prevalent in areas of sub-Saharan Africa and East Asia where 5–10 per cent of the adult population are chronically infected. In the USA acute hepatitis B occurs in approximately 1 in 1000 pregnancies.[13]

Pathogenesis and Transmission

Transmission of HBV is through different routes: sexual contact, parenteral routes (intravenous (IV) drug users or exposure to blood products), or close personal contact with open cuts and wounds from an infected person.

The highest concentration of the virus is found in blood, but other body fluids like semen, saliva and cervical secretions also contain high viral titres.

In the newborn, it occurs through placental transmission.

It has a 30–180 day incubation period.

Presentation of Acute Infection

Most people do not experience any symptoms during acute infection; however, some people have acute illness with symptoms that last several weeks, including, fever, nausea, vomiting, anorexia, extreme fatigue, dark urine and abdominal pain.

On examination jaundice and hepatomegaly may be detected.[13]

Maternal Implications of HBV Infection in Pregnancy

The course of acute hepatitis in pregnancy:

- Over 90 per cent of immune-competent pregnant women clear the infection and experience complete resolution after acute illness.
- About 5 per cent of adults would develop chronic hepatitis B (persistence of HBsAg for more than six months).
- Fulminant hepatitis might develop in 0.1–0.5 per cent of patients after acute HBV infection.
- The long-term risks of chronic HBV infection are hepatocellular carcinoma and cirrhosis with liver failure.[14]
- Acute viral hepatitis is the most common cause of jaundice in pregnancy.[15] It is usually mild and not associated with increased mortality.[15]
- Women with liver cirrhosis are at a higher risk of maternal complications including gestational

hypertension, placental abruption and peripartum haemorrhage.

Fetal Implications of Acute Hepatitis

Because of its size, HBV does not cross the placenta. Most vertical transmission occurs during delivery.

- The newborn baby's chance of getting infection is 90 per cent if the pregnant woman is an HBV carrier and is also positive for HBeAg.
- Approximately 25 per cent of infected infants will become asymptomatic and potentially infective chronic carriers.
- Consequently, unless adequate prophylaxis is provided, the newborn is at high risk of developing a chronic HBV infection, with its known long-term complications.[16]
- Acute or chronic infection with HBV is not associated with increased risk of congenital malformations or stillbirth.
- However, the fetal prognosis is poor if the woman has liver cirrhosis:
  o Intrauterine growth restriction
  o Intrauterine infection
  o Premature delivery
  o Intrauterine fetal demise

Diagnosis

Acute HBV infection is characterised by presence of HBsAg immunoglobulin M (IgM) and antibody to the core antigen, HBcAg.

Treatment

Treatment of hepatitis B in pregnancy is supportive.

Indications of Antiviral Therapy

Consideration of antiviral therapy depends on high serum HBV DNA levels:

- If the levels near delivery are persistently greater than 10 000 copies/mL
- If a woman develops acute liver failure or protracted severe hepatitis[17]

If antiviral therapy is required, both tenofovir and lamvudine have been used safely in pregnancy.

The World Health Organization (WHO) recommends the use of oral treatment tenofovir and entecavir, because these are the most potent drugs to suppress HBV. The infant should receive HBV immunoglobulin in addition to HBV vaccine first dose at birth.

Safety of exposure to antiviral therapy comes from the Antiretroviral Pregnancy Registry (APR) and the Development of Antiretroviral Therapy Study (DART). Results of both studies seem to be assuring as the birth defects rate was 2.7 per cent, which compares favourably with the Centers for Disease Control (CDC) birth surveillance system.[18,19] [EL 1]

Antiviral therapy with lamivudine, tenofovir or telbivudine in the third trimester can decrease MTCT to less than 5 per cent.[20]

Vaccinating non-infected pregnant women is safe, but is generally recommended for women with high risk of exposure.

Chronic HBV Infection in Pregnancy

In the UK, all pregnant women are offered screening for HBsAg infection to allow effective postnatal interventions to reduce the risk of MTCT.

Effect of Pregnancy on Maternal Disease

Pregnancy is usually well tolerated in women with chronic HBV infection; however, the immunologic change during pregnancy and the postpartum period has been associated with:

- Hepatitis flare with severe clinical sequel. This is uncommon.
- Progression of liver disease. This is difficult to assess during pregnancy because of normal physiologic changes that can mimic clinical features of chronic liver disease.
- HBV DNA. Most studies have found that HBV DNA levels remain stable in pregnancy.

Mode of Delivery

Routine caesarean section is not recommended, as the benefits of caesarean delivery in protecting against HBV transmission have not been clearly established in well-conducted controlled trials. Although two meta-analyses carried out in 2014 and 2017 showed that caesarean section delivery may reduce the vertical MTCT, they still concluded that further trials should be carried out because of heterogeneity and other variables.[21,22,23]

Neither study included statistical analyses of the possible effects of newborn immunisation and vaccination on the reduction of vertical transmission.

If vaginal delivery is performed, it is important to prevent transmission by leaving the membranes intact for as long as possible and avoid invasive procedures (fetal scalp electrodes and fetal blood sampling).

Children born to mothers with chronic HBV infection should receive HBV vaccine at birth, preferably within 24 hours and then at 1 and 6–12 months of age.

HBV immunoglobulin is given to those children where the mother has highly infective status.

Breastfeeding

Breastfeeding should be encouraged. If the mother develops cracked nipples or mastitis, it may be temporarily suspended.

Hepatitis C (HCV)

Hepatitis C virus (HCV) is a major cause of chronic hepatitis, cirrhosis and hepatocellular carcinoma around the world.[24] This virus was first identified in 1989. The prevalence of HCV in pregnant women is approximately 1 per cent (0.1–2.4 per cent), and the rate of MTCT is 4–7 per cent per pregnancy among women with detectable viraemia.[24]

Virology and Epidemiology

HCV is an RNA virus and belongs to the *Flaviviridae* family. There are 11 major genotypes of HCV, with 15 different subtypes, which may be prevalent in different regions of the world.[25]

These types differ in their mutation and replication rates and the severity of disease they can cause.

This virus frequently mutates secondary to change in the structural protein of the viral envelope. This is the reason antibodies developed against HCV do not produce immunity against disease. After infection, HCV replicates with rates up to 1 trillion copies per day. Chronically infected individuals with HCV progress to chronic disease in 75–85 per cent of cases.[26]

Pathogenesis and Transmission

Transmission of HCV is primarily through blood-to-blood contact, e.g. sharing drug injection equipment, non-sterile tattooing, body piercing or acupuncture, non-sterile medical and dental procedures.

Antenatal Screening for the Infection

Currently the National Institute for Health and Care Excellence (NICE) and the National Screening Committee in the UK do not support universal screening of all pregnant women, as the prevalence of infection in England is low, varying from 0.4 to 0.8 per cent with regional variation.[27] Similarly CDC does not recommend testing all pregnant women for HCV infection, only those who are at high risk, and care during pregnancy is not modified by HCV infection.

Screening could be offered to women because of their medical history or women with behavioural risk factors. In the UK, 92 per cent of HCV is acquired in people with a history of past or current IV drug abuse.

Acute Infection

The acute infection is usually mild and undiagnosed, and many women remain unaware of their infection. In about 20–25 per cent of acute infections, immunity takes over with spontaneous resolution.[28]

Chronic HCV in Pregnancy

Women with chronic HCV infection often have uneventful pregnancies without worsening of liver disease or other maternal or infant adverse effects.

In many women, immunity fails, with ensuing chronic lifelong infection. Affected individuals are often asymptomatic or have only non-specific findings such as fatigue. The chronic phase is characterised by stable high-level viraemia, and normal or elevated alanine aminotransferase (ALT).

Fetal Implications

Infants born to HCV carrier women were found to be more likely to:

- Have low birthweight
- Be small for gestational age
- Require neonatal intensive care and assisted ventilation

A study by Riddick et al. found an increased risk of gestational diabetes and non-significant increase in preterm birth and caesarean delivery.

Risk of Perinatal Transmission

Transfer of HCV infection in pregnancy occurs as a result of vertical transmission (from mother to baby during the period immediately before and after birth). Vertical transmission might occur across the placenta, in the breastmilk, or through direct contact during or after birth. The prevalence of HCV is 1 per cent in pregnant women and the rate of MTCT is 2–8 per cent per pregnancy among women with detectable viraemia.

Vertical perinatal transmission occurs in women who are HCV-RNA positive at the time of delivery and appear to be highly dependent on viral load and HIV status which are independent of each other. High viral load of more than 100 000 copies/mL is associated with an increased risk of vertical transmission. Average rate of infection is approximately 4/100 and it is two to three times higher if a woman is co-infected with HIV, probably due to a higher viral load.[29]

Factors for MTCT are not well understood, nor is the natural history of the illness in pregnant women and their offspring. There do not seem to be clear practice guidelines for any evidence-based intervention in pregnant women with HCV.

Mode of Delivery

Currently there is no evidence to suggest caesarean section for prevention of mother-to-child transmission of HCV in pregnancy. The usual precautions to keep the membranes intact and avoid invasive intrapartum interventions are still required to reduce vertical transmission. An elective caesarean section is suggested for an HIV co-infected pregnant mother to reduce the transmission rate to the child by 60 per cent.

Postnatal Care

It is safe to breastfeed, as the transfer of the virus through breastmilk is negligible. There is a theoretical risk that if there is broken skin on the nipples from incorrect positioning, the virus could be transmitted via micro abrasions in the infant mouth. The option of expressing milk and discarding it until skin heals should be considered. Women should not be advised to discontinue breastfeeding.[30]

Diagnosis of Hepatitis C Infection

Initially, testing for HCV infection begins with blood testing for the presence of HCV antibody by either a rapid or a laboratory-conducted assay.

A positive nucleic acid amplification test (NAAT) for HCV RNA result indicates either current or past HCV infection.[31]

Treatment and Vaccination during Pregnancy

Peginterferon and ribavirin are FDA category X and are contraindicated during pregnancy.

Recently the US Food and Drug Administration (FDA) approved Harvoni, Viekira and sofaldi for genotype 1 patients. They are all pregnancy category B (animal reproduction studies have failed to demonstrate a risk to the fetus and there are no adequate and well-controlled studies in pregnant women).[32]

However, the general recommendation is to use these expensive medications on a risk–benefit ratio.

Indications for Selective Treatment

Patients with elevated serum ALT levels who meet the following criteria:

- Age older than 18 years
- Positive HCV antibody and serum HCV RNA test results
- Compensated liver disease (e.g. no hepatic encephalopathy or ascites)
- Acceptable haematologic and biochemical indices (haemoglobin at least 13 g/dL for men and 12 g/dL for women; neutrophil count >1500/mm^3, serum creatinine <1.5 mg/dL)

Currently there are no vaccines for hepatitis C.

Hepatitis D (HDV)

Hepatitis D delta virus (HDV) is a defective, single-stranded RNA virus which is responsible for hepatitis D infection in individuals who are infected with HBV. HBsAg is essential for its transmission, which it uses as envelope protein.

HDV infection can occur as a super-infection on chronic HBV infection or as a co-infection with HBV.[33,34]

Virology and Epidemiology

HDV has six reported genotypes. The most common is type 1 and is associated with both severe and mild disease.[35]

Pathogenesis and Transmission

The transmission of HDV is by exposure to infected blood and blood products. It can be transmitted percutaneously or through sexual contact.

Perinatal transmission is rare.

HBsAg is essential for viral assembly and transmission.

Blood is infectious during all phases of active hepatitis D infection especially before the onset of acute infection. HDV replication is not cytopathic.

Diagnosis

The diagnosis is made by presence of HDV antigen antibodies. Anti-HDV antibodies are detected by commercially available tests. If diagnosis is confirmed, real-time PCR assay of infected serum should be obtained to confirm and document ongoing infection.

Early acute markers of HDV infection clear within a few months after recovery.

During chronic HDV infection, HBV markers such as HBV DNA and HBsAg are suppressed.

HBV viraemia in a co-infected patient is a marker of disease progression.

Treatment

Hepatitis D is not curable; it will eventually lead to liver cirrhosis, liver disease and liver cancer.

There is no specific treatment for acute or chronic HDV infection.

Persistent HDV replication is the most important predictor of mortality and need for antiviral treatment.

Current treatment includes PEGylated interferon alpha and liver transplantation which can be curative.

Optimum duration of treatment is not well defined. Treatment is supportive as in other hepatitis in acute infection. Cases of co-infection are found to resolve spontaneously, whereas super-infection frequently leads to chronic HDV infection and active disease.

Hepatitis E (HEV)

Hepatitis E (HEV) is a liver disease caused by hepatitis E virus. The WHO estimates around 20 million HEV infections worldwide each year, out of which 3.3 million are with symptomatic infection.[36]

Virology and Epidemiology

HEV is a non-enveloped, spherical, positive-sense single-stranded RNA virus. It is composed of viral protein and RNA. The virus has four different genotypes: genotypes 1, 2, 3 and 4. The genotypes found in humans are of type 1, 2 while 3, 4 circulate in animals including pigs, white boars and deer.

Genotypes 3, 4 cause disease in humans also and the main reservoir is pigs. Hepatitis E infection is usually mild to moderate in severity, and the risk of mortality is 0.4–4 per cent, although disease could be severe in pregnancy, with frequent fulminant hepatitis.[37]

Pathogenesis and Transmission

The route of transmission is the faecal oral route due to faecal contamination of drinking water. Other routes have been identified in a much smaller number of cases and include ingestion of meat products from infected animals, especially if meat is undercooked.

Transmission could occur through infected blood and vertically from mother to fetus.

Presentation

Mild fever, reduced appetite, nausea, vomiting and abdominal pain are the presenting symptoms. Jaundice and a slightly enlarged liver may be found on examination. In rare cases, acute hepatitis E could be severe and results in fulminant hepatitis.[38]

Pregnant women are at increased risk of acute liver failure, fetal loss and mortality. Case fatality in pregnancy ranges from 20 to 25 per cent.

Diagnosis

Diagnosis is based on presence of hepatitis E IgM antibodies in the infected person's blood. Additional tests include reverse transcriptase–polymerase chain reaction (RT-PCR) to detect the hepatitis E virus RNA in blood and/or stool.

Previous infection is diagnosed by IgG antibodies. The infection should be suspected during water-borne hepatitis outbreaks occurring in developing countries.

Treatment

Therapy is directed at providing supportive care. No known therapy is available to alter the course of the disease. HEV infection is self-limiting and hospitalisation is not usually required.

During pregnancy the risk of fulminant hepatitis and maternal mortality occurs in approximately 20 per cent of patients, especially if infection is acquired in the third trimester.

Premature deliveries with high infant mortality are also observed. Hospitalisation should be considered for symptomatic pregnant women.

Prevention

Prevention is the most important effective approach against the disease. It is achieved at population level by monitoring quality standards of public water supplies and establishing proper disposal system for human waste.

Individually, hand washing, especially prior to eating or handling food, and avoiding consumption of water/ice of unknown purity are advised.

In 2011 a vaccine to prevent hepatitis E was registered in China but it has not yet been registered in other countries.

References

1. Thompson N. Differentiating RNA & DNA Viruses. Sciencing. sciencing.com/differentiating-rna-dna-viruses-4853.html.

2. World Health Organization. WHO Global Hepatitis Report 2017. www.who.int/hepatitis/publications/global-hepatitis-report2017/en/.

3. World Health Organization. WHO Hepatitis A Fact Sheet July 2017. www.who.int/topics/hepatitis/factsheets/en/.

4. Lemon SM. Type A viral hepatitis: epidemiology, diagnosis, and prevention. *Clin Chem.* 1997; **43**(8 Pt 2): 1494–9.

5. World Health Organization. Hepatitis A. *Wkly Epidemiol Rec.* 2000; **75**(5): 38–44.

6. McDuffie RS, Bader T. Fetal meconium peritonitis after maternal hepatitis A. *Am J Obstet Gynecol.* 1999; **180**(4): 1031–2.

7. Dandi N, Shouval D, Stein ZC, Ackerman Z. Breast milk hepatitis A virus in nursing mother with acute hepatitis A infection. *Breastfeed Med.* 2012; 7: 313–15.

8. Fawaz R, Baumann U, Ekong U et al. Guideline for the Evaluation of Cholestatic Jaundice in Infants: Joint Recommendations of the North American Society for Pediatric Gastroenterology, Hepatology, and Nutrition and the European Society for Pediatric Gastroenterology, Hepatology, and Nutrition. www.naspghan.org/files/documents/pdfs/position-papers/Guideline_for_the_Evaluation_of_Cholestatic.23.pdf.

9. Daudi N, Shouval D, Stein-Zamir C, Ackerman Z, Cara L. Breastmilk hepatitis A virus RNA in nursing mothers with acute hepatitis A virus infection. *Breastfeed Med.* 2012; 7: 313–15.

10. Fiore AE, Wasley A, Bell BP. Prevention of hepatitis A through active or passive immunization: recommendations of the Advisory Committee on Immunization Practices (ACIP0. MMWR Recomm Rep. 2006 19 May. 55(RR-7): 1–23.

11. Chaudhry SA, Koren. G. Hepatitis A infection during pregnancy. *Can Fam Physician.* 2015 Nov; **61**(11): 963–4.

12. Kao JH, Chan DS. Global control of hepatitis B virus infection. *Lancet Infect Dis.* 2002; **2**(7): 395–403.

13. Euler GL, Wooten KG, Bahghman AL, William WW. Hepatitis B surface antigen prevalence among pregnant women in urban areas: implications for testing, reporting and preventing perinatal transmission. *Paediatrics.* 2003; **111**(5 Pt 2): 1192–7.

14. World Health Organization. Hepatitis B key facts. www.who.int/news-room/fact-sheets/detail/hepatitis-b.

15. Sookoian S. Liver disease in pregnancy: acute viral hepatitis. *Ann Hepatol.* 2006; **5**: 231.

16. Jonas MM. Hepatitis B and pregnancy: an underestimated issue. *Liver Int.* 2009(suppl 1): 133.

17. World Health Organization. WHO Hepatitis B Factsheet July 2017. www.who.int/topics/hepatitis/factsheets/en/.

18. Visvanathan K, Dusheiko G, Giles M et al. Managing HBV in pregnancy. Prevention, prophylaxis, treatment and follow-up: position paper produced by Australian, UK and New Zealand key opinion leaders. *Gut.* 2016; **65**(2): 340–50.

19. Antiretroviral Pregnancy Registry. www.apregistry.com.

20. Munderi P, Wilkes H, Tumukunde D et al. Pregnancy and outcomes among women on triple-drug antiretroviral therapy (ART) in the DART trial (poster WEPEB261). Presented at the Fifth IAS Conference on HIV Pathogenesis, Treatment and Prevention, Cape Town, South Africa, 19–22 July 2009.

21. Liaw YF, Leung N, Guan R et al. Asian-Pacific consensus statement on the management of chronic hepatitis B: a 2005 update. *Liver Int.* 2005; **25**: 472.

22. Chang MS, Gavini S, Andrade PC, McNabb-Baltar J. Caesarean section to prevent transmission of hepatitis B: a meta-analysis. *Can J Gastroenterol Hepatol.* 2014; **28**: 439.

23. Yang M, Qin Q, Fang Q, Jiang LX, Nie SF. Cesarean section to prevent mother-to-child transmission of hepatitis B virus in China: a meta-analysis. *BMC Pregnancy Childbirth.* 2017; **17**: 303.

24. Maheshwari A, Ray S, Thuluvath PJ. Acute hepatitis C. *Lancet.* 2008; **372**(9635): 321–32.

25. Simmonds P. Viral heterogeneity of the hepatitis C virus. *J Hepatol.* 1999; **31**(suppl 1): 54–60.

26. Roberts EA, Yeung L. Maternal-infant transmission of hepatitis C virus infection. *Hepatology.* 2002; **36**(5 suppl 1): S106–13.

27. American College of Obstetricians and Gynecologists. Hepatitis B and Hepatitis C in Pregnancy. FAQ093, November 2013. www.acog.org/Patients/FAQs/Hepat itis-B-and-Hepatitis-C-in-Pregnancy? IsMobileSet=false.

28. Centers for Disease Control and Prevention. Testing Recommendations for Hepatitis C Virus Infection. 2014. www.cdc.gov/hepatitis/hcv/guidelinesc.htm.

29. Prasad MR, Honegger JR. Hepatitis C virus in pregnancy. *Am J Perinatol.* 2013; **30**(2): 10.1055/s–0033–1334459.

30. Royal College of Midwives, 2008. Hepatitis C, Position Statement. London: Royal College of Midwives.

31. Gupta E, Bajpai, M, Choudhary A. Hepatitis C virus: screening, diagnosis, and interpretation of laboratory assays. *Asian J Transfus Sci.* 2014; **8**(1): 19–25.

32. Centers for Disease Control and Prevention. Morbidity and Mortality Weekly Report, 2013. www.cdc.gov/ mmwr/pdf/wk/mm62e0507a2.pdf.

33. World Health Organization. Hepatitis D 23 July 2018 Key facts. www.who.int/news-room/fact-sheets/detail/ hepatitis-d.

34. Wedemeyer H, Manns MP Epidemiology, pathogenesis and management of hepatitis D: update and challenges ahead. *Nat Rev Gastroenterol Hepatol.* 2010; 7(1): 31–40.

35. World Health Organization. WHO Hepatitis D Fact Sheet July 2017. www.who.int/mediacentre/factsheets/ hepatitis-d/en/.

36. Chaudhry, SA, Verma N, Koren GNV. Hepatitis E infection during pregnancy. *Can Fam Physician.* 2015; **61**(7): 607–8.

37. WHO Hepatitis E Fact Sheet July 2017. www.who.int /mediacentre/factsheets/fs280/en/.

38. Patra S, Kumar A, Trivedi SS, Puri M, Sarin SK. Maternal and foetal outcomes in pregnant women with acute hepatitis E virus infection. *Ann Intern Med.* 2007; **147**(1): 28–33.

HIV Infection

Maimoona Ahmed

3

Introduction

The acquired immunodeficiency syndrome (AIDS) was first recognised among homosexual men in the United States in 1981. It has since then spread like wildfire, becoming one of the worst epidemics of the twentieth century, affecting all populations.

Global HIV burden is estimated at 37 million individuals, and women account for more than half of them. In the most affected countries in the world, such as in sub-Saharan Africa, 20–40 per cent of pregnant women are HIV-infected and one-third of their babies become infected.

These children are vulnerable to HIV transmission *in utero*, at birth, or through breastmilk.

Mother-to-child transmission (MTCT) accounts for 90 per cent of HIV infections among children worldwide.

The management of HIV in pregnancy has evolved over the last few decades due to an improved understanding of prevention of perinatal transmission of HIV and development of better drugs to control the infection. The successful prevention efforts can be attributed to universal testing and screening of pregnant women for HIV infection, the use of caesarean delivery (when appropriate), new and effective antiretroviral medications and avoidance of breastfeeding, when feasible. This chapter focuses on understanding the effects of HIV in pregnancy, MTCT and the intervention control strategies.

In developed countries, the introduction of antiretroviral drugs has resulted in a significant reduction in AIDS-related mortality and improved survival.

Virology

HIV is a genetic member of the *Lentivirus* genus of the *Retroviridae* family. The retrovirus genome is composed of two identical copies of single-stranded RNA molecules. The virus isolates into two types, HIV-type 1 (HIV-1) and HIV-type 2 (HIV-2).

- HIV-1 is the worldwide agent for HIV and the AIDS infections
- HIV-2 is restricted to some regions of Western and South Africa

In the majority of cases, HIV is a sexually transmitted infection and occurs by contact with or transfer of pre-ejaculate, semen and vaginal fluids. Non-sexual transmission can also occur from contaminated blood and other body fluids.

The virus cannot survive outside the bloodstream or lymphatic tissue, but transfer of non-sexual infection requires direct exposure to infected blood or secretions in the presence of skin damage, i.e. by needles (as in drug abusers) or sharp tools.[1]

A CD4 (cluster of differentiation 4) count less than 200 cells/mm^3 indicates that a person has AIDS. In general, the time from infection with HIV to the development of AIDS is approximately 10–12 years.

Seroconversion – after the initial infection, HIV continues to multiply in the lymph nodes. Lymph nodes are packed with CD4 cells, which HIV uses to reproduce. Then the nodes burst, sending the virus into the blood from three to five weeks, with an average of 22 days.

HIV levels of viral load become detectable in blood and reach very high levels (often millions of copies/mL) in three to five weeks.

A viral load test is a measurement of the amount of HIV virus in a sample of blood. This is usually reported as the number of copies per millilitre (copies/mL).

HIV and CD4

CD4 is a glycoprotein found on the surface of immune cells such as T-helper cells, monocytes, macrophages and dendritic cells. CD4 and T-helper cells are an essential part of the human immune system to fight infections and other conditions. Depletion of CD4 leaves the body vulnerable to a wide range of infections.

Normal values for CD4 cells are 500–1200 cells/mm^3.

HIV infection leads to a progressive reduction in the number of T cells expressing CD4.

CD4 tests can be used to determine efficacy of treatment.

However, viral load testing is more informative about the efficacy for therapy than CD4 counts.[2]

Clinical Presentation

The clinical picture of HIV in pregnancy is the same as that in non-pregnant women.

The World Health Organization (WHO) case definition of HIV infection includes:

- A positive result on an HIV antibody test confirmed by a positive result on a second, different HIV antibody test and/or
- A positive virologic test confirmed by a second virologic test.[3]

Stages of HIV Infection[4]

Stage 1. **Acute Primary HIV infection** (also called acute seroconversion syndrome). This generally lasts for 2–4 weeks. The infected person is usually asymptomatic but may experience flu-like symptoms. In the acute stage HIV multiples rapidly and spreads throughout the body destroying the CD4 cells. Increased level of HIV increases the risk of transmission.

Stage 2. **Chronic HIV infection.** People with chronic infection may not have any symptoms but can spread to others. Without treatment this usually advances to AIDS in approximately 10 years.

Stage 3. **AIDS**, when the immune system has been so extensively damaged that it can no longer fight off serious infections and diseases.

Symptoms of reduced immunity start to appear including: weight loss, chronic diarrhoea, night sweats, fever, persistent cough, mouth and skin problems, regular infections, serious illnesses or diseases.

Kaposi's Sarcoma and Pneumocystis Pneumonia (PCP)[5]

- Asymptomatic – persistent generalised lymphadenopathy

- Early symptomatic HIV infection (previously known as AIDS-related complex (ARC) or Class B)
- AIDS characterised by a CD4 cell count <200 cells/µl or the presence of any AIDS-defining condition
- Advanced HIV infection characterised by a CD4 cell count <50 cells/µL
- Before the introduction of antiretroviral therapy to treat HIV, about three-quarters of HIV-positive people who developed AIDS got PCP
- Antiretroviral therapy (ART) has prevented HIV-infected people from developing AIDS, and among persons who have developed AIDS, additional preventive therapy has brought this number way down. However, PCP is still the most common opportunistic infection in persons who contract AIDS.

Effects of Pregnancy on HIV

- Studies have not shown an association between pregnancy and disease progression.
- Lieve et al. investigated the effect of pregnancy on HIV disease progression and survival among HIV-infected women in rural Uganda, prior to the introduction of ART.
- HIV women who subsequently became pregnant had higher CD4 counts at enrolment and had a slower CD4 decline than those who did not become pregnant. In women who became pregnant, CD4 decline was faster after pregnancy than before ($p < 0.0001$). The survival analyses showed no significant differences between women who became pregnant and those who did not with respect to median time to CD4 count <200, AIDS or death.
- The initial comparative immunological advantage possessed by fertile women before they become pregnant is subsequently lost as a result of their pregnancy.
- Women should be informed about the potential negative effect of pregnancy on their immunological status and should be offered contraception.
- In resource-limited settings, women determined to become pregnant should be given priority for ART if eligible.[6]

Effects of HIV on Pregnancy

- Spontaneous abortion
- Stillbirth

- Low birthweight
- Prematurity
- Intrauterine growth retardation[7] [EL 1]
- Ectopic pregnancy. HIV-1 and HIV-2 infection in Africa have both been linked to a higher rate of ectopic pregnancy, which may be related to the effects of other concurrent sexually transmitted diseases
- Glucose intolerance and gestational diabetes. The development of glucose intolerance may be more common in pregnant women with HIV[8]
- Postpartum haemorrhage. HIV-positive women were more likely to have a postpartum haemorrhage

Maternal Mortality

- There were an estimated 19 000–56 000 maternal deaths attributed to HIV-related causes in 2011, contributing to some 6–20 per cent of all maternal deaths worldwide.[9] [EL 1]
- In a study by Zaba et al., HIV-infected pregnant or postpartum women had around eight times higher mortality than did their HIV-uninfected counterparts.[10]
- In Africa, it seems there is a higher mortality rate among HIV pregnant women which may be accounted for by the coexisting tuberculosis infection.
- It is important to note that many HIV-related deaths can be prevented by the implementation of high-quality obstetric care, prevention and treatment of common co-infections, and treatment of HIV with ART.

Mother-To-Child Transmission of HIV

Every mother-to-child perinatal HIV transmission indicates either a missed opportunity for prevention or, more rarely, a failure of interventions to prevent HIV infection.

Without antiretroviral preventive interventions, the risk of perinatal HIV transmission has varied between 15 and 45 per cent, depending on maternal risk factors and whether breastfeeding is practised.[11]

The most important risk factors for MTCT:

- Maternal plasma viral load
- Breastmilk viral load[12]
- Maternal immunologic status
- Clinical stage

- Low CD4 cell counts
- Anaemia
- Maternal mastitis
- Duration of membrane rupture greater than four hours

Rates of Transmission

In non-breastfeeding settings prior to the availability of antiretroviral interventions,

- 30 per cent during pregnancy
- 70 per cent during labour and delivery

In breastfeeding settings prior to the availability of antiretroviral interventions,

- 25 to 40 per cent of infant infections were estimated to occur in utero
- 50 per cent around the time of labour/ delivery or through very early breastfeeding
- 10 per cent during the reminder of breastfeeding periods

HIV RNA can be detected in colostrum and breastmilk.

Risk of transmission through breastfeeding is highest in the early months of the infant's life.

Fetal Congenital Malformations

The absence of an HIV-related dysmorphic syndrome and the lack of congenital abnormalities is a consistent finding in developed and developing countries. These findings are compatible with the view that a substantial proportion of vertical transmission occurs late in pregnancy or at the time of the delivery.

In an African study, there was no influence of HIV on congenital malformations.[13]

Diagnosis and Investigations

Early diagnosis of HIV infection in pregnancy and initiation of ART not only improves the obstetric outcomes and reduces perinatal transmission but also helps in improving the health of the mother in the long run.

Rapid Tests, Duo Test[14]

- In low-income group countries, syphilis and HIV are the major public health problem affecting the mother and their newborn baby.
- Therefore, a rapid diagnostic test for HIV and syphilis, a 'duo test' (an HIV test that looks for antibodies for HIV-1 and HIV-2 and also looks for

evidence of the p24 protein which is on the surface of the HIV particle) has been developed which can be performed with venous, arterial or capillary whole blood, or oral secretions.

- The test was 100 per cent accurate if the result is negative and 94 per cent accurate if the result is positive.[14]
- These tests are used in clinical and non-clinical settings, usually with blood from a finger prick or with oral fluid.
- The oral fluid antibody self-test provides faster results. Results are available in 20 minutes.
- For the blood test, the home collection kit involves pricking the finger to collect a blood sample, sending the sample by mail to a licensed laboratory, and then calling in for results as early as the next business day.
- These tests are available for purchase in stores and online.
- This antibody test is anonymous.
- As with other types of HIV tests, a positive result needs to be confirmed with a different test.

Antigen/Antibody

- Antigen/antibody test looks for both HIV antigens and antibodies.
- Antibodies are produced by the immune system when exposed to bacteria or viruses like HIV.
- In HIV, an antigen called p24 is produced even before antibodies develop.

Nucleic Acid Amplification Test (NAAT)

- NAAT looks for the actual virus in the blood.
- The test can give either a positive/negative result or the amount of virus present in the blood (known as an HIV viral load test).
- This test is very expensive and not routinely used for screening individuals unless they recently had a high-risk exposure and they have early symptoms of HIV infection.
- Nucleic acid testing is usually considered accurate during the early stages of infection.
- However, it is best to get an antibody or antigen/ antibody test at the same time to help the health care provider understand what a negative NAAT means.

Screening

- HIV infection does not usually cause symptoms at the early stage. Consequently people need to be screened to learn whether they are infected even if they are feeling well. They can then start treatment early and avoid giving the disease to other people.
- There is strong evidence that screening for HIV in pregnant women has many benefits. If infected pregnant women start treatment, they have a better chance for themselves and their children of staying healthy. Treatment can also reduce their chances of passing the infection to other people.
- Potential harms of screening are small. False-positive results are rare.
- All pregnant women should be screened for HIV infection as soon as possible in each pregnancy. [*CDC, RCOG & WHO recommendations*]
- Repeat testing in the third trimester is recommended for women in areas of high HIV prevalence or women known to have high risk for acquiring HIV infection. [*Grade A recommendation*]
- Pregnant women not previously tested or whose HIV status is undocumented at the time of delivery should be offered rapid screening. If the rapid HIV test in labour is reactive then ART should be started immediately while waiting for the supplemental test results.[15] [*Grade A recommendation*]

Antenatal Investigations

- A thorough history and physical examination must be performed to rule out any other health concern in the mother that would affect the fetus, such as sexually transmitted infections, tuberculosis and drug abuse.
- Newly diagnosed HIV-positive pregnant women do not require any additional baseline investigations compared with non-pregnant HIV-positive women other than those routinely performed in the general antenatal clinic. [*Grade B recommendation*]
- Accurate estimation of the gestational age should be done because early delivery may be necessary to reduce risk of perinatal transmission.
- Pregnant HIV-infected women should be screened for both hepatitis B and hepatitis C virus infections since co-infection is common in

HIV-infected patients due to shared routes of transmission (e.g. injection drug use).

- HIV-infected women without evidence of hepatitis B infection should be given HBV immunisation, since the recombinant vaccine is safe during pregnancy.[16]
- Women should also be screened for antibodies to the hepatitis C and should receive immunisation if they are hepatitis C negative.[17]
- Women should also be screened for antibodies to the hepatitis A virus (HAV). Those testing negative should receive the HAV vaccine.[18]
- Latent tuberculosis testing should be done as there is a higher risk for developing active disease.
- Screening should also be performed to rule out other sexually transmitted infections, especially maternal syphilis, to avoid another major contributing factor in adverse obstetric and neonatal outcomes.

Monitoring Disease Progression and Treatment

HIV Resistance Testing (HIVDR)

- HIV drug resistance (HIVDR) poses a potential threat to the long-term success of ART and is emerging as a threat to the elimination of AIDS as a public health problem.
- HIV resistance testing should be performed prior to initiation of treatment except for late-presenting women.[19] [*Grade C recommendation*]

CD4 Cell Count

In women who conceive on ART, there should be a minimum of one CD4 cell count at baseline and one at delivery. [*Grade D recommendation*]

Viral Load

Viral load should be performed two to four weeks after commencing ART, at least once every trimester, at 36 weeks and at delivery. [*Grade B recommendation*]

If the viral load is >1000 copies/mL near term gestation, the patient should be counselled regarding the benefits of scheduled pre-labour caesarean section (CS) at 38 weeks' gestation for the prevention of perinatal transmission.[20]

Toxicities

Toxicities associated with ART should be assessed based on the particular drug regimen. As with all HIV-infected patients, complete blood count (CBC), blood urea nitrogen (BUN) and creatinine, and liver function tests are checked prior to ART initiation and three to six months thereafter.

Urinalysis is also checked after ART initiation and every six months while on a tenofovir-containing regimen.

Liver Function Tests

In women commencing ART in pregnancy, liver function tests should be performed as per routine initiation of ART and then at each antenatal visit. [*Grade B recommendation*]

Management

The treatment is primarily aimed at benefiting the health and long-term survival of the mother and her offspring, while simultaneously reducing the risk of MTCT.

Maintaining confidentiality is essential. The care and support requires a multidisciplinary team consisting of obstetrician, paediatrician, counsellors, nutritionist and nursing staff.

ART in Pregnancy

The benefits of antiretroviral therapy during pregnancy outweigh the potential side effects or risks to both mother and baby. Hence, ART is recommended for all HIV-infected pregnant women, regardless of immune, clinical or viral status.

Women Already on ART

It is recommended that women conceiving on an effective ART regimen should continue this even if it contains efavirenz (EFV) or does not contain zidovudine (AZT). [*Grade B recommendation*]

Exceptions are:

- Protease inhibitor (PI) monotherapy should be intensified to include (depending on tolerability, resistance and prior antiretroviral history) one or more agents that cross the placenta.
- The combination of stavudine and didanosine should not be prescribed in pregnancy.

Women Not Already on ART

All women should have commenced ART by week 24 of pregnancy. Any woman presenting after 28 weeks should start ART without delay.[21] [*Grade B recommendation*]

First-Line Therapy[22]

Polytherapy

- A once-daily fixed-dose combination of tenofovir + lamivudine + EFV is recommended as first-line ART in pregnant and breastfeeding women, including the first trimester of pregnancy. [*Grade A recommendation*]
- This first-line regimen for pregnant and breastfeeding women with HIV has low cost, is available as a fixed-dose combination, is safe for both pregnant and breastfeeding women and their infants, is well tolerated, has low monitoring requirements and a low drug-resistance profile, and is compatible with other drugs used in clinical care.
- The PROMISE (Promoting Maternal–Infant Survival Everywhere) Study was started in 2012 with the aim of determining how best to safely reduce the risk of HIV transmission from mother to baby during pregnancy and after delivery and assure benefits of ART for the health of the mother. Their findings supported the WHO recommendations for ART in pregnancy as the best-suited regimen.
- The British HIV Association recently changed its recommendation to allow EFV to be used in the first trimester.
- If the viral load is unknown or >100 000 HIV RNA copies/mL, a three- or four-drug regimen that includes raltegravir is suggested.
- An untreated woman presenting in labour at term should be given a stat dose of nevirapine (NVP) and commence fixed-dose zidovudine with lamivudine. [*Grade B recommendation*]

Monotherapy

Zidovudine monotherapy can be used in women planning a caesarean section who have a baseline viral load of <10 000 HIV RNA copies/mL and a CD4 of >350 cells/μL. [*Grade A recommendation*]

Elite Controllers

- Elite controllers are a small subset of people living with HIV who are able to maintain suppressed viral loads for years without ART; still HIV continues to replicate even in elite controllers.
- Initiating ART in HIV elite controllers remains controversial, as current evidence does not definitively demonstrate that the benefits of ART outweigh risk in this group of the HIV population.
- In developed countries, where first-line ART regimens have minimal toxicities, treatment of elite controllers should be strongly considered. Treatment has the potential to minimise the size of the HIV reservoir, dampens immune activation and diminishes risk of transmission.[23,24]

Long-Term Nonprogressors (LTNP)

- Long-term nonprogressors (LTNP) are a small group of people with HIV who do not take ART and still maintain CD4 counts in the normal range indefinitely.
- The CD4 count is the strongest predictor of HIV progression.
- However, in a 2017 study, Sophie Grabar and colleagues followed 171 LTNP patients for five years and found that one-third of LTNP patients lost their status (with lower baseline CD4 cell counts and CD4/CD8 ratio). Their data suggest that all LTNP patients should begin combination ART without delay.[25]
- The above study is in line with the results of the INSIGHT-START trial, which showed a clear clinical benefit of immediate vs deferred ART in asymptomatic adults with CD4 cell counts above 500/mm^3, especially in those with high plasma HIV RNA and a CD4/CD8 ratio below 0.5.[26]

ART Medications and Adverse Effects[27]

Zidovudine, Lamivudine, Stavudine, Didanosine, Emtricitabine

Maternal side effects include mitochondrial toxicity: myopathy, peripheral neuropathy, hepatic steatosis and lactic acidosis.

There is no evidence of teratogenicity, no increased risk of spontaneous abortions, stillbirths, preterm births and low birthweight.

In newborns it may cause mitochondrial toxicity where mitochondria become damaged or decline significantly in number.

Abacavir, Tenofovir Disoproxil Fumarate

Maternal toxicity includes hypersensitivity reactions, renal toxicity, bone density loss.

There is no evidence of teratogenicity, no increased risk of spontaneous abortions, stillbirths, preterm births and low birthweight.

In newborns it may cause mitochondrial toxicity: anaemia, neutropenia.

Efavirenz, Nevirapine

Maternal side effects include central nervous system toxicity, rash, hyperlipidaemia, elevated hepatic transaminases, serious maternal skin and liver toxicity.

There are no fetal risks.

Protease Inhibitors: Lopinavir/Ritonavir, Darunavir, Atazanavir

Maternal risks include insulin resistance, hyperglycaemia, diabetes, hyperlipidaemia, lipodystrophy and hepatotoxicity.

There is an increased incidence of preterm birth.

Prevention of MTCT[28,29]

Without interventions the risk of mother-to-child transmission of HIV during pregnancy, delivery and postpartum via breastfeeding is 20–45 per cent.

- Identification of HIV-infected pregnant women by routine antenatal screening
- Combination antiretroviral regimens antepartum, intrapartum
- Postnatal infant prophylaxis together with scheduled caesarean section in certain situations
- Prevention of breastfeeding reduces the transmission rates to 2 per cent

However, in 2009 and based on the World Health Organization (WHO) Breastfeeding Antiretroviral and Nutrition Study held in Malawi, the risk of HIV transmission is reduced to just 1.8 per cent for infants given the antiretroviral drug nevirapine daily while breastfeeding for six months. This led to a WHO recommendation that HIV-positive mothers or their infants take antiretroviral drugs throughout the period of breastfeeding and until the infant is 12 months old. This means that the child can benefit from breastfeeding with very little risk of becoming infected with HIV.[30]

Mode of Delivery

Women should continue taking their ART regimen during labour and delivery or scheduled caesarean delivery.

The British HIV Association (BHIVA) guidelines stipulate that mode of delivery should be decided on the basis of viral load (VL) at 36 weeks' gestation. [*Grade B recommendation*]

- VL <50 copies/mL: vaginal delivery (including cases for planned vaginal birth after previous CS)
- VL 50–399 copies/mL: CS at around 38–39 weeks is recommended
- VL >499 copies/mL: CS at around 38–39 weeks

Labour Considerations[31]

The following should be avoided unless there are clear obstetric indications. [*Good practice point*]

- Artificial rupture of membranes
- Routine use of fetal scalp electrodes for fetal monitoring
- Fetal blood sampling
- Operative delivery with forceps or vacuum extractor

Management of Spontaneous Rupture of Membranes (ROM)

- Term ROM:
  - o If viral load is <50 copies, induction of labour should be started.
  - o If viral load is 50–999 HIV RNA copies/mL, CS should be the mode of delivery.
- PROM at 34–37 weeks
  - o If viral load is <50 copies, induction of labour should be started.
  - o If viral load is 50–999 HIV RNA copies/mL, CS should be the mode of delivery. However, group B *Streptococcus* prophylaxis in line with national guidelines should be offered.
- P-PROM < 34 weeks
  - o Offer steroids for lung maturity.
  - o Require a multidisciplinary team approach to decide the mode of delivery.

Intrapartum Intravenous Infusion of Zidovudine

- For women with a viral load of >1000 HIV RNA copies/mL plasma who present in labour, or with ruptured membranes or who are admitted for planned CS[32] [*Grade B recommendation*]

- For untreated women presenting in labour or with ruptured membranes in whom the current viral load is not known[32] [*Grade B recommendation*]

Special Obstetric Considerations

Invasive prenatal diagnostic testing:

- Should not be performed until after the HIV viral load is known
- Should be deferred until viral load has been adequately suppressed to below the level of detection
- If the test cannot be delayed, highly active antiretroviral therapy (HAART) including raltegravir should be started and single-dose nevirapine should be given two to four hours prior to the procedure

Vaginal Birth after Caesarean Section (VBAC)

Vaginal birth after caesarean section (VBAC) should be offered to women with a viral load <50 HIV RNA copies/Ml. [*Grade B recommendation*]

The decision should be based on a woman's choice, indication for previous caesarean and current obstetric factors.

Intrapartum Epidural Use

Studies suggest that epidural anaesthesia can be used safely regardless of the ART regimen.

Postpartum Haemorrhage and Methergine Use

Oral or parenteral methergine are often used as first-line management for postpartum haemorrhage due to uterine atony. In women on potent CYP 3A4 inhibitors including protease inhibitors, use of ergotamines has been associated with an exaggerated vasoconstrictive response. Other alternatives like PG F2-alpha, misoprostol or oxytocin are to be used.

Human Immunodeficiency Virus Discordant Couples[33]

HIV-uninfected pregnant women with HIV-infected partners may present for consultation. Recommendations are:

- To review and encourage safe sexual practices, including consistent use of barrier contraception.
- The HIV-infected partner should be on an ARV regimen with maximal or complete suppression of viral load. In the partner study, which looked at the risk of HIV transmission when viral load is undetectable on HIV treatment (ART), there were no HIV transmissions after nearly 900 couples had sex without condoms more than 58 000 times. It is still safer to use barrier contraception.
- Pre-exposure prophylaxis (PrEP):
  - Periconception pre-exposure prophylaxis (PrEP) may minimise HIV transmission risk within discordant couples.
  - PrEP is the use of daily oral tenofovir disoproxil fumarate (TDF) or co-formulated TDF/emtricitabine (TDF/FTC) by HIV-uninfected individuals to maintain blood and genital drug levels sufficient to prevent HIV acquisition. Pregnancy is not a contraindication to PrEP.
  - When taken consistently, PrEP has been shown to reduce the risk of HIV infection in people who are at high risk by up to 92 per cent. PrEP is much less effective if it is not taken consistently.
  - PrEP is an effective HIV prevention policy and can be combined with condoms and other prevention methods to provide greater protection than when used alone. To be effective, the drug must be taken every day. A health care provider should see patients for follow-up every three months.
- A plan for HIV screening during pregnancy: as a high-risk patient, first-, second- and third-trimester screening is appropriate. If women present to labour and delivery without documented negative serology at 36 weeks, rapid intrapartum testing should be performed.
- Donor sperm: in discordant couples with an HIV-infected man, the safest reproductive option is using donor sperm from an HIV-uninfected man.
- Sperm preparation techniques (if donor sperm is not an acceptable option) coupled with intrauterine insemination (with or without ovulation induction), in vitro fertilisation, or intracytoplasmic sperm injection have been reported to be effective in avoiding seroconversion in uninfected women and offspring.

Management of Newborn[34]

Infant prophylaxis:

- All infants born to HIV-infected mothers should receive antiretroviral post-exposure prophylaxis as soon as possible, ideally within the first 6–12 hours after delivery to decrease the risk of HIV acquisition. [*Grade A recommendation*]

The precise prophylactic regimen depends on the mother's use of antepartum antiretroviral agents and her viral load near delivery.

• Infants Born to Mothers on ART with Viral Load <100 copies/mL

Should receive daily NVP/AZT for six weeks. This provides added early postpartum protection, especially for those who were not compliant, started late therapy and did not achieve full viral suppression.

• Infants Born to Mothers who are at High Risk

○ Mothers who received no ART or less than six weeks' ART during pregnancy

○ Mothers who received only intrapartum ART

○ Mothers who received antepartum ART but viral load >100 copies/mL

In the above situations, infants should receive dual therapy for six weeks (AZT twice daily and NVP once daily for six weeks) and if breastfeeding should continue for 12 weeks in total.[35]

Pneumocystis Pneumonia (PCP) Prophylaxis

Pneumocystis pneumonia (PCP) is a serious fungal infection caused by the fungus *Pneumocystis jirovecii*.

It is more common in immunocompromised individuals (e.g. HIV-infected people). Symptoms include fever, cough, difficulty breathing, chest pain, chills, fatigue (tiredness).

PCP prophylaxis, with co-trimoxazole, should be initiated from the age of four weeks.[36] [EL 1]

HIV Testing in the Newborn

• In exclusively non-breastfed infants, molecular diagnostics for HIV infection should be performed on the following occasions.[37] [*Grade B recommendation*]

○ During the first 48 hours and prior to hospital discharge

○ Two weeks post-cessation of infant prophylaxis (six weeks of age)

○ Two months post-cessation of infant prophylaxis (12 weeks of age)

○ On other occasions if additional risk

○ HIV antibody testing for seroconversion should be performed at age 18 months

• In breastfed infants additional monthly testing of both mother and infant is recommended.

Breastfeeding[38]

The choices that can be offered for breastfeeding differ depending on whether it is a resource-rich setting or resource-poor setting.

• In a resource-rich setting, due to the high risk of transmission during breastfeeding, it is advised that all mothers known to be HIV-positive, regardless of antiretroviral therapy and infant PEP, should be advised to exclusively formula feed from birth. [*Grade A recommendation*]

• In a resource-poor setting, however, the answer is not so simple. The WHO proposes exclusive breastfeeding for the first six months of life unless replacement feeding is 'Acceptable, Feasible, Affordable, Sustainable and Safe' referred to as AFASS criteria. [*Grade A recommendation*]

• Exclusive breastfeeding confers nutritional and immunological benefits on the infant.

The infant feeding options should be discussed with the mother in the antenatal period and she should be supported in her choice of feeding regimen.

Postpartum Care

• ART should be continued postpartum regardless of immune, clinical or viral status. This will reduce the risk of disease progression, prevent HIV sexual transmission and reduce the risk of MTCT in subsequent pregnancies.[20]

• In women opting for replacement feeds, lactation suppressants should be given along with advice about emptying the breast, cold compress and cabbage leaves to relieve symptoms of engorgement.

• **Contraception advice** is of utmost importance to avoid unplanned pregnancies.

• Some methods, such as combined oral hormonal pills, progesterone-only pills and implants, may interact with antiviral medications, especially protease inhibitors.

• Long-acting progesterone has been recommended as a reliable form of contraception.

• Barrier contraception should be used as it provides dual protection against unplanned pregnancy and sexually transmitted infections (STIs).[39]

• Antiretroviral therapy can be initiated in all pregnant and breastfeeding women regardless of gestational age or WHO clinical stage and at any CD4 count and be continued lifelong.

Conclusion

In the current circumstances, with proper medications and care, women living with HIV can expect a normal pregnancy and birth.

Through early antenatal screening, timely initiation of ART, careful monitoring under a multidisciplinary team, optimal management in labour, compliance with advice regarding breastfeeding and infant ART prophylaxis, mother-to-child transmission of HIV can be kept to a minimum.

In HIV in pregnancy, we are not just treating the mother medically, but also offering a more holistic management that caters for the emotional, economical and societal aspects of this disease.

References

1. Cunningham AL. Virology of HIV. *Pathology – Journal of the RCPA*. 2009; **41**: 39.

2. US Department of Veterans Affairs. HIV/AIDS. CD4 count (or T-cell count). www.hiv.va.gov/patient/diagnosis/labs-CD4-count.asp.

3. World Health Organization. AIDS and HIV Case Definitions. www.who.int/hiv/strategic/surveillance/definitions/en/.

4. US Department of Health and Human Services. Aids Info, The Stages of HIV Infection. 27 July 2018. aidsinfo.nih.gov/understanding-hiv-aids/fact-sheets/19/46/the-stages-of-hiv-infection.

5. Huang L, Cattamanchi A, Davis JL, et al. HIV-associated pneumocystis pneumonia. *Proc Am Thorac Soc*. 2011; **8**(3): 294–300.

6. Lieve VD, Shafer LA, Mayanja BN, Whitworth JA, Grosskurth H. Effect of pregnancy on HIV disease progression and survival among women in rural Uganda. *Trop Med Int Health*. 2007; **12**(8): 920–8.

7. Ezechi OC, Gab-Okafor CV, Oladele DA et al. Pregnancy, obstetric and neonatal outcomes in HIV positive Nigerian women. *Afr J Reprod Health*. 2013; **17**(3): 160–8.

8. Hitti J, Anderson J, McComsey G et al. Effect of protease inhibitor-based antiretroviral therapy on glucose tolerance in pregnancy. Abstract. 13th Conference on Retroviruses and Opportunistic Infections. February 2006.

9. Calvert C, Ronsmans C. The contribution of HIV to pregnancy-related mortality: a systematic review and meta-analysis. *AIDS*. 2013; **27**(10): 1631–9.

10. Zaba B, Calvert C, Marston M, Isingo R, Nakiyingi-Miiro J, Lutalo T. Effect of HIV infection on pregnancy-related mortality in sub-Saharan Africa: secondary analyses of pooled community-based data from the network for Analysing Longitudinal Population-based HIV/AIDS data on Africa (ALPHA). *Lancet*. 2013; **381**(9879): 1763–71.

11. De Cock KM, Fowler MG, Mercier E et al. Prevention of mother-to-child HIV transmission in resource-poor countries: translating research into policy and practice. *JAMA*. 2000; **283**: 1175.

12. Nduati R, Mbori-Ngacha D, John G, Richardson B, Kreiss J. Breastfeeding in women with HIV. *JAMA*. 2000; **284**: 956.

13. European Collaborative Study. Perinatal findings in children born to HIV-infected mothers. *Br J Obstet Gynecol*. 1994; **101**: 136–41.

14. Centers for Disease Control and Prevention. HIV/AIDS HIV Basics. Testing. Screening for Human Immunodeficiency Virus (HIV). www.cdc.gov/hiv/basics/testing.html.

15. US Preventive Services Task Force. Screening for Human Immunodeficiency Virus (HIV). file:///C:/Users/pc/Downloads/hivfact.pdf.

16. Taylor GP, Dhar J, Kennedy MJ, Shea SO. British HIV Association guidelines for the management of HIV infection in pregnant women 2012 (2014 interim review). 2014; 15: 1–77.

17. Polis CB, Shah SN, Johnson KE, Gupta A. Impact of maternal HIV coinfection on the vertical transmission of hepatitis C virus: a meta-analysis. *Clin Infect Dis*. 2007; **44**: 1123.

18. Centers for Disease Control and Prevention. Guidelines for vaccinating pregnant women, Hepatitis A. 2013. www.cdc.gov/vaccines/pubs/preg-guide.htm#hepa.

19. Clutter DS, Jordan MR, Bertagnolio S, Shafer RW. HIV-1 drug resistance and resistance testing. *Infection, Genetics and Evolution*. 2016; **46**: 292–307.

20. World Health Organization. Consolidated guidelines on the use of antiretroviral drugs for treating and preventing HIV infection, second edition. June 2016. www.who.int/hiv/pub/arv/arv-2016/en/.

21. Therapy HIVA, Data C. Antiretroviral Therapy (ART) in pregnant women with HIV infection: overview of HIV Antiretroviral Therapy (ART) in pregnancy. 2018; 3–8.

22. Abrams EJ. 2017. Safety and dosing of antiretroviral medications in pregnancy. In: Mofenson LM, ed. UpToDate. Retrieved August 2017 from John GC, Kreiss J. Mother-to-child transmission of human immunodeficiency virus type 1. *Epidemiol Rev*. **1996**; **18**: 149. www.uptodate.com/contents/.

23. US Department of Health and Human Services. Aids Info. HIV/AIDS Glossary. Elite Controllers. https://aidsinfo.nih.gov/understanding-hiv-aids/glossary/3127/elite-controllers.

24. Promer J, Karris MY. Current treatment options for HIV elite controllers: a review. *Infectious Diseases*. 2018. doi:10.1007/s40506-018-0158-8.

25. Grabar S, Selinger-Leneman H, Abgrall S, Pialoux G, Weiss L, Costagliola D. Loss of long-term non-progressor and HIV controller status over time in the French Hospital Database on HIV. *PLoS/ONE*. 2017; **12**(10). https://journals.plos.org/plosone/article?id=10.1371/journal.pone.0184441.

26. Insight Start Study Group, Lundgren JD, Babiker AG et al. Initiation of antiretroviral therapy in early asymptomatic HIV infection. *N Engl J Med*. 2015; **373** (9): 795–807. pmid:26192873.

27. Abrams EJ. 2017. Safety and dosing of antiretroviral medications in pregnancy. In: Mofenson LM, ed. UpToDate. Retrieved August 2017 from John GC, Kreiss J. Mother-to-child transmission of human immunodeficiency virus type 1. *Epidemiol Rev*. 1996; **18**: 149. www.uptodate.com/contents/.

28. Townsend CL, Cortina-Borja M, Peckham CS et al. Low rates of mother-to-child transmission of HIV following effective pregnancy interventions in the United Kingdom and Ireland, 2000–2006. *AIDS*. 2008; **22**: 973.

29. Mandelbrot L, Tubiana R, Le Chenadec J et al. No perinatal HIV-1 transmission from women with effective antiretroviral therapy starting before conception. *Clin Infect Dis*. 2015; **61**: 1715.

30. World Health Organization. Breast is always best, even for HIV-positive mothers. 2009. www.who.int/bulletin/volumes/88/1/10-030110/en/.

31. Myani CN, Nicolaou E, Bera E et al. Guideline on invasive obstetric procedures in the HIV-infected pregnant woman. *South Afr J Obstet Gynecol*. 2012; **18**(1): 3–5.

32. Recommendations for the use of Antiretroviral Drugs in pregnant women with HIV infection and interventions to reduce Perinatal transmission in the United States. https://aidsinfo.nih.gov/guidelines.

33. World Health Organization. WHO issues new guidance for discordant couples. https://sciencespeaksblog.org/2012/04/18/breaking-who-issues-new-guidance-for-discordant-couples/.

34. Krist AH, Crawford-Faucher A. Management of newborns exposed to maternal HIV infection. *Am Fam Physician*. 2002; **65**(10): 2049–205.

35. Alidina Z, Wormsbecker AE, Urquia, M, MacGillivray J, Taerk E, Yudin MH, Campbell DM. HIV prophylaxis in high risk newborns: an examination of sociodemographic factors in an inner city context. *Can J Infect Dis Med Microbiol*. 2016; 2782786.

36. Centers for Disease Control and Prevention. Guidelines for Prophylaxis against Pneumocystis carinii Pneumonia for Persons Infected with Human Immunodeficiency Virus. www.cdc.gov/mmwr/preview/mmwrhtml/00001409.htm.

37. Nielsen-Saines K, Watts DH, Veloso VG et al. Three postpartum antiretroviral regimens to prevent intrapartum HIV infection. N Engl J Med. 2012; **366** (25): 2368–79.

38. World Health Organization. Infant feeding for the prevention of mother-to-child transmission of HIV. 10 December 2018. www.who.int/elena/titles/hiv_infant_feeding/en/.

39. Fakoya A, Lamba H, Mackie N et al. British HIV Association, BASHH and FSRH guidelines for the management of the sexual and reproductive health of people living with HIV infection 2008. 2008; **9**(9): 681–720.

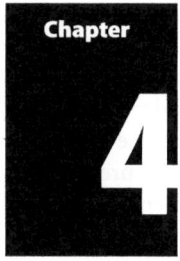

Herpes Infections and Measles

Rashda Imran

In humans, eight different types of herpes viruses have been reported so far, which belong to three subgroups. These subgroups are based on the site of latency (defined as the persistence of viral genomes in cells that do not produce infectious virus) and most frequently infected cell types.

- α-group viruses

    This group includes herpes simplex virus types 1, 2 (HSV1, HSV2) and herpes zoster virus (VZV), which infect epithelial cells and produce latent infection in neurons.

- Lymphotrophic β-group viruses

    This group includes *Cytomegalovirus* (CMV), human herpes virus-6 (*Roseolovirus* more commonly known as the sixth disease or *Roseola Infantum*, and human herpes virus-7 (not yet classified).

- γ-group viruses

    These viruses produce latent infection mainly in lymphoid cells and include Ebstein B virus (EBV) and Kaposi's sarcoma-associated herpes virus KSHV/HHV-8, which causes Kaposi sarcoma.[1]

Herpes Simplex Virus Infection

Herpes simplex is a very common infectious disease globally, affects both women and men and is caused by both known types of viruses, herpes simplex virus 1 (HSV1) and herpes simplex virus 2 (HSV2).

- HSV1 is mainly transmitted by oral to oral contact and may cause cold sore, gingiva-stomatitis or rare life-threatening disseminated visceral infections and encephalitis. It is usually acquired in childhood.
- HSV2 is sexually transmitted, causes genital herpes and is usually acquired later in life. Genital herpes simplex virus (HSV) is a recurrent disease that can occur throughout life and has no known cure.[2] Genital herpes negatively affects the quality of life and work productivity of patients.[2]

Virology and Pathogenesis

HSV1 and 2 are double-stranded DNA viruses, distinguished by their surface glycoprotein that exhibit only 50 per cent of genetic homology with one another, so infection with one type does not prevent infection from the other.

Pathogenesis and Transmission

The incubation period after contact transmission is four to six days.

Acute infection starts as HSV (1 or 2) enters the body through the skin or mucosa by direct sexual contact with secretions or mucosal surfaces of an infected person and replicates at the site of entry. It produces infectious virions and causes vesicular lesions of the epidermis. The viruses then spread to sensory neurons that innervate the primary site of replication.

Primary HSV infection resolves in a few weeks in an immune-competent host, but the virus remains latent in cells. From the sensory ganglia it reactivates and travels down the axon to the skin on the mucosal surface, resulting in symptomatic shedding or clinically apparent disease. Asymptomatic shedding is the most common mechanism of sexual HSV transmission.[3]

Risk of transmission appears to be greatest when active vesicular lesions are present and during the prodromal phase (early sign or symptom which often indicates the onset of a disease before more diagnostically specific signs and symptoms develop).

The patients should be advised to abstain from sexual contact during this time.

Transmission can occur in the absence of lesion recurrence as a result of subclinical viral shedding.

The efficacy of condoms to prevent sexual transmission has not been formally assessed. However, in a multivariable analysis, condom use during more than 25 per cent of sex acts was associated with protection against HSV2 acquisition for women but not for men.[4] [EL 2, *B recommendation*]

Genital Herpes

Signs and Symptoms (Primary and Latent Stages and Recurrent Episodes)

Primary Herpes

The first infection with either herpes simplex virus type 1 (HSV1) or type 2 (HSV2) is the primary infection. The first herpes outbreak is the most severe, particularly in women. Symptoms tend to resolve within two to three weeks.

The signs of a primary episode of genital herpes in women:

- **Multiple blisters** in the genital area (vagina, vulva, buttocks, anus and thighs). Blisters on the outer labia may crust over and heal.
- **Painful ulcers.** The blisters then turn into painful ulcers. New lesions may develop between five and seven days after the first group appears.
- **Lymph node involvement.** The infection may affect the groin lymph nodes which may be tender and swollen.
- **Systemically,** there may be flu-like symptoms, joint pains, fever and headache.

The Latent Stage

This is an asymptomatic stage. After the initial outbreak, the virus travels to the bundle of nerves at the base of the spine, where it remains dormant for or a period of time.

Recurrent Infection (Episodes)

Recurrence occurs frequently in many patients, especially in those with HSV type 2.

Recurrent episodes of genital herpes occur when the virus travels through nerves to the skin's surface, causing an outbreak of ulcers. The recurrent episodes are usually milder than the initial outbreak.

In the recurrent episodes, the ulcers may develop in the same area as those of the first outbreak, or may appear in other areas.

Around 50 per cent of infected people with a recurrent outbreak experience mild symptoms (itching, tingling, or pain in the buttocks, legs or hips).

Recurrences tend to become less frequent and less severe after the first year.

The clinical features of primary or recurrent herpes do not differ in pregnancy and non-pregnant women except for the fact that recurrence appears to increase in frequency over the course of pregnancy.

The incidence of reactivation of latent genital HSV virus infection and asymptomatic virus shedding on any day in pregnancy is 1 per cent.[5]

Complications of Genital Herpes

The most serious rare clinical complication is disseminated herpes, which may present with pneumonia, encephalitis, hepatitis, disseminated skin lesions or a combination of these conditions.

It is more commonly reported in pregnancy, particularly in immunocompromised women.

The maternal mortality associated with disseminated disease (involvement of the central nervous system (CNS), liver and adrenal dysfunction, shock and coagulopathy) is as high as 50 per cent.[6]

Psychological complications of genital herpes are sometimes very distressing and may affect sexual life and future relations, particularly with the knowledge it is not a curable disease.

Laboratory Diagnosis[7]

Direct Virus Isolation

Swabs taken from the base of the lesion (vesicles should be unroofed with a needle or scalpel blade) and placed in viral transport medium are the most accurate method as they directly demonstrate the virus HSV DNA detection and allow for virus typing.[7] [EL 1, *A recommendation*]

Virus typing of HSV1 and HSV2 is recommended in all patients with first-episode genital herpes to guide further counselling and management.

However, culture sensitivity is low, especially for recurrent lesions, and declines as lesions heal.

Polymerase Chain Reaction (PCR)

PCR is a technique to amplify any trace amounts of DNA (and in some instances, RNA) located in or on almost any liquid or surface where DNA strands may be deposited. Viruses contain DNA (or RNA) genetic material such as sequences unique to their species, and to the individual member of that species.

If a sample contains segments of DNA or RNA, PCR amplifies these unique sequences.

These amplified unique consequences can then be used to determine with a very high degree of accuracy the identity of the source pathogenic organism.

Nucleic Acid Amplification Test

The same technique as for the PCR is utilised for a nucleic acid amplification test.

Women with suspected genital herpes should be referred to a genitourinary medicine physician to confirm or exclude the diagnosis by viral PCR, advise on management of genital herpes and arrange a screen for other sexually transmitted infections (STIs).

Serological Testing

Serological testing for immunoglobulin G (IgG) has high false-negative results at low index values (1.1–3.5).

Screening

Routine screening for HSV in pregnancy is not recommended.

Fetal Vertical Transmission and Fetal Implications

Rarely, congenital herpes may occur as a result of transplacental intrauterine infection.

Case reports suggest that the skin, eyes and CNS may be affected and there may be fetal growth restriction or fetal death.[8] [EL 2]

Herpes infection can be passed from mother to child during pregnancy or childbirth.

Factors associated with transmission to the fetus *in utero* include:[9]

- The type of maternal infection (primary or recurrent)
- The presence of transplacental maternal neutralising antibodies
- The duration of rupture of membranes before delivery
- The use of fetal scalp electrodes and the mode of delivery
- The risks are greatest when a woman acquires a new infection (primary genital herpes) in the third trimester, particularly within six weeks of delivery, as viral shedding may persist, and the baby is likely to be born before the development of protective maternal antibodies. Development of antibodies to HSV usually requires four to six weeks. These antibodies cross the placenta and reduce the transmission risk from 50 per cent in case of primary infection to 0–4 per cent in case of recurrent disease.

Fetal implications may include:

- Primary infection occurring in the first or second trimester is associated with an increase in spontaneous abortion and/or prematurity and fetal growth restriction.
- Transplacental transmission causes severe *in utero* congenital infection. The fetal manifestations include microcephaly, hepatosplenomegaly, intrauterine growth restriction (IUGR) and intrauterine fetal death (IUFD).

Neonatal Herpes[10]

- Neonatal herpes is very rare but is a serious viral infection with a high morbidity and mortality. This virus could affect skin, eyes, CNS etc.
- Neonatal infection occurs as the result of an infection at the time of birth.
- Neonatal herpes may be caused by HSV1 or HSV2.
- Most cases of neonatal herpes occur as a result of direct contact with infected maternal secretions. In 25 per cent of cases, a close relative is the possible source of postnatal infection.
- Postnatal infection may occur as a result of exposure to oro-labial herpes infection.

Neonatal herpes is divided into three groups:

1. Disease localised to skin, eye and/or mouth[10]
   These comprise approximately 30 per cent of cases and have the best prognosis. With appropriate antiviral treatment, the ocular and neurological morbidity is less than 2 per cent.
2. Local CNS disease (encephalitis alone)[9]
   Infants with local CNS disease often present late (generally between 10 days and four weeks of age). With timely antiviral treatment, mortality from local CNS disease is around 6 per cent and neurological morbidity (which may be lifelong) is 70 per cent.
3. Disseminated infection with multiple organ involvement[9]
   Disseminated infection carries the worst prognosis; with appropriate antiviral treatment, mortality is around 30 per cent, and 17 per cent have long-term neurological sequelae.

Management of the Neonate

Babies born by Caesarean Section in Mothers with Primary HSV Infection in the Third Trimester

These babies are at low risk.

- No active treatment is required for the baby.
- Normal postnatal care of the baby with a neonatal examination at 24 hours of age, after which the baby can be discharged from the hospital if well and feeding is established.
- Parents should be educated regarding good hand hygiene and due care to reduce risk of postnatal infection.
- Parents should ask for medical help if they have concerns and should look for skin, eye and mucous membrane lesions, lethargy/irritability and poor feeding.

Babies Born by Spontaneous Vaginal Delivery in Mothers with a Primary HSV Infection within the Previous Six Weeks

These babies are at high risk of disease and transmitted infection.

- If the baby is well:
  - Swabs of the skin, conjunctiva, oropharynx and rectum should be sent for diagnosis of infection (herpes simplex PCR).
  - Empirical treatment with intravenous (IV) aciclovir (20 mg/kg every eight hours) should be initiated until evidence of active infection is ruled out.
  - Breastfeeding should continue unless the mother has herpetic lesions around the nipples.
  - Warning signs of early infection (poor feeding, lethargy, fever or any suspicious lesions) should prompt patients to seek medical help.
- If the baby is unwell:
  - Swabs of the skin, lesions, conjunctiva, oropharynx and rectum should be taken to confirm infection.
  - A lumbar puncture should be performed even if CNS features are not present.
  - Intravenous aciclovir (20 mg/kg every eight hours) should be initiated until there is no evidence of active infection.

Babies Born to Mothers with Recurrent HSV Infection in Pregnancy with or without Active Lesions at Delivery

These babies have a low risk of infection because maternal IgG will be protective.

- Normal postnatal care of the baby with a neonatal examination at 24 hours of age, after which the baby can be discharged from hospital if well and feeding is established.
- Parents should be educated regarding good hand hygiene and due care and are advised to seek medical help if they have concerns.
- If there are any concerns, intravenous aciclovir (20 mg/kg every eight hours) should be given while awaiting cultures.

Treatment of the Mother[11]

Primary Infection

First or Second Trimester Acquisition until 27+6 Weeks of Gestation

- Pregnant women with suspected genital herpes should be referred to a genitourinary medicine physician to confirm the diagnosis by viral PCR, arrange proper management and arrange a screen for other STIs.
- Aciclovir in standard doses (400 mg three times daily, usually for five days) is not licensed in pregnancy but is safe to use. Its use is associated with a reduction in the duration and severity of symptoms and a decrease in the duration of viral shedding.
- Paracetamol and topical lidocaine 2 per cent gel can be offered for symptomatic relief. Neither is harmful in pregnancy in standard doses.
- Because of less experience with the valaciclovir and famciclovir in pregnancy, they are not recommended as first-line treatment in pregnancy.
- Daily suppressive aciclovir 400 mg three times daily from 36 weeks of gestation reduces HSV lesions at term and hence the need for delivery by caesarean section.
- Providing that delivery does not ensue within the next six weeks, the pregnancy should be managed expectantly, and vaginal delivery anticipated.

Third Trimester Acquisition (from 28 Weeks of Gestation) of Primary Genital Herpes[11]

- Treatment should not be delayed. It will usually involve the use of oral (or intravenous for disseminated HSV) aciclovir in standard doses (400 mg three times daily, usually daily until delivery).
- Caesarean section should be recommended to all women presenting with primary episode genital herpes lesions within six weeks of the expected date of delivery or at the time of delivery, in order to reduce exposure of the fetus to HSV which may be present in maternal genital secretions.

Recurrent and Secondary Infection

It is sometimes difficult to differentiate between primary and secondary infection.

- If available, the presence of antibodies of the same type as the HSV isolated from genital swabs at the time of primary infection would confirm this episode to be a recurrence rather than a primary infection and elective caesarean section would not be indicated to prevent neonatal transmission.
- In women who choose to deliver vaginally, particularly in the presence of primary genital herpes lesions, invasive procedures (application of fetal scalp electrodes, fetal blood sampling, and artificial rupture of membranes and/or instrumental deliveries) should be avoided.[12]
- With recurrent genital herpes, the risk of neonatal herpes is low (0–3 per cent for vaginal delivery) even if lesions are present at the time of delivery.
- Daily suppressive aciclovir 400 mg three times daily should be considered from 36 weeks of gestation.
- Prior to 36 weeks treatment is not recommended.

There is no increased risk of preterm labour, preterm prelabour rupture of membranes or fetal growth restriction associated with women seropositive for HSV.

Primary Herpes Infection and Preterm Rupture of Membranes

- If immediate delivery is indicated, then caesarean section is the best option.
- If conservative management is decided based upon obstetric and other reasons, then the mother should be offered IV aciclovir 5 mg/kg every eight hours.

- Prophylactic corticosteroids should be considered for lung maturity.

Recurrent Herpes Infection and Preterm Rupture of Membranes (PPROM)

- In the case of PPROM before 34 weeks, expectant management is appropriate, including oral aciclovir 400 mg three times daily for the mother, with antenatal steroids for the baby.
- After 34 weeks, it may be best to deliver by caesarean section.

Postpartum

Maternal oro-labial or ano-genital lesions require proper hand washing and contact prevention to avoid exposure of the infant.

Those with oral herpetic lesions (cold sores) should not kiss the neonate.

Aciclovir use in breastfeeding could be considered if needed.

Breastfeeding is not recommended if there are active lesions on the breast.

Management of HIV-Positive Women with HSV Infection[12]

HIV-positive women with primary genital HSV infection in the last trimester of pregnancy should be managed according to the recommendations for all women with primary genital HSV infection.

There is some evidence that HIV antibody positive women with genital HSV ulceration in pregnancy are more likely to transmit HIV infection independent of other factors. However, this is not a consistent finding across all studies.

Women who are HIV antibody positive and have a history of genital herpes should be offered daily suppressive aciclovir 400 mg three times daily from 32 weeks of gestation to reduce the risk of transmission of HIV infection, especially in women where a vaginal delivery is planned. Starting therapy at this earlier gestation than usual should be considered in view of the increased possibility of preterm labour in HIV-positive women.

The mode of delivery should be according to obstetric factors and HIV parameters such as HIV viral load.

Herpes Zoster

Herpes simplex viruses 1 and 2 cause oral and genital herpes infection; herpes zoster virus causes chickenpox and shingles.

Virology and Epidemiology of Herpes Zoster Virus

Herpes zoster virus (HZV), a DNA virus, belongs to the α-group of herpes family. It causes chickenpox (varicella zoster infection) and shingles (herpes zoster).

- Chickenpox or 'varicella' infection is the primary herpes zoster varicella virus infection. It is a common childhood infection.

  - The virus is spread by direct contact with infected vesicles or airborne droplets followed by mucosal invasion of the upper respiratory tract and conjunctiva.
  - The virus is also directly shed from vesicles and may be transferred by heavily contaminated clothing or bedding until all the vesicles have crusted over.
  - Chickenpox is characterised by the presence of a generalised, pruritic rash that develops into vesicles, then pustules and finally crusts.[13]
  - The rash is mostly on the head and trunk but can occur in any area of the skin and conjunctiva.
  - Varicella can develop between 1 and 16 days of life in infants born to mothers with active varicella around the time of delivery.
  - Asymptomatic infection is unusual; mild cases may go unrecognised.
  - Children are contagious from one to two days before the onset of the rash until all lesions have crusted over and dried, usually after five to six days.
  - The incubation period is 10–21 days, but most children usually become ill 14–16 days after contact.
  - In the UK, 90 per cent of adults over the age of 18 years are seropositive for VZV. Chickenpox is common, so most pregnant women exposed to the virus are immune and only three in 1000 pregnancies are complicated by primary infection.

In the USA, more than 90 per cent of the antenatal population is immune to chickenpox due to the presence of VZV IgG antibodies because of previous exposure.

Table 4.1 Differences between chickenpox and shingles

Chickenpox	Shingles
Affects children	Usually in adults
Symptoms: fever, flu-like symptoms and swollen glands	Itching, fever, muscle pain
Rash: tiny blisters which dry to form scabs	The rash (typically on the torso or face) grows into pus-filled blisters which turn into crusts
Infectivity: highly contagious	Not in itself contagious, but virus can spread and cause chickenpox

Shingles (**herpes zoster**) is a painful skin rash.

Shingles is caused by reactivation of the varicella zoster virus, the same virus that causes chickenpox. The symptoms and signs are:

- One-sided stabbing pain, tingling, itching, burning, or stinging sensation, which appears before the appearance of the rash by a few days.
- The rash usually follows a dermatome distribution. It is a fluid-filled blistering red rash, typically on the torso or face.
- Systemic symptoms may include headache, fever and chills, nausea, body aches.

Shingles can be treated with antiviral medication and pain medication.

The prognosis for shingles is generally favourable.

Complications

- Post-herpetic neuralgia, which is persistent nerve pain after the rash disappears
- Bacterial infections of the skin and soft tissues in children, including group A streptococcal infections
- Infection of the lungs (pneumonia)
- Infection or inflammation of the brain (encephalitis, cerebellar ataxia)
- Bleeding problems (haemorrhagic complications)
- Bloodstream infections (sepsis)

Laboratory Diagnosis

Immunoglobulin M (IgM) serologic testing: considerably less sensitive than PCR testing of skin lesions.

It can provide evidence for a recent active VZV infection, but cannot discriminate between a primary infection and reinfection or reactivation from latency.

Direct fluorescent antibody assay (DFA) and viral culture: these techniques are generally not recommended because they are less sensitive than PCR and will take longer to generate results.

Polymerase chain reaction (PCR): To detect VZV in skin lesions (vesicles, scabs, maculopapular lesions), vesicular lesions or scabs, if present, are the best for sampling.

Differential Diagnoses

Chickenpox is usually distinctive, but other causes of vesicular rash might be considered, including herpes simplex (not usually disseminated), herpes zoster (usually dermatomal), hand, foot and mouth disease (coxsackievirus), enterovirus, impetigo and syphilis.

Chickenpox in Pregnancy[14]

Pregnant women who develop chickenpox during pregnancy are exposed to increased morbidity:

- Pneumonia, with a 10–14 per cent incidence[21,22]
- Hepatitis
- Encephalitis

Rarely, it may result in death.

Fetal Implications

- The risk of spontaneous miscarriage does not increase if chickenpox occurs in the first trimester. [EL 2]
- Fetal effects of varicella can manifest as congenital fetal varicella syndrome (FVS).[15]

FVS is a recognised complication of infection in the first half of pregnancy, affecting approximately 0.4 per cent of infants born to mothers infected up to 12 weeks, and 2 per cent of those infected between 13 and 20 weeks of gestation.

Some of the manifestations include chorioreinitis, cerebral cortical atrophy, hydronephrosis and cutaneous and bony leg defects.

These manifestations do not appear at the time of infection. They occur subsequent to herpes zoster reactivation *in utero*. [EL 2]

There have been rare cases of FVS reported in infants exposed between 20 and 28 weeks' gestation.

Neonatal Varicella[16]

- Varicella infection of the newborn refers to early infection in early neonatal life (usually up to 10 days postpartum). It occurs because of maternal infection near the time of delivery, or immediately postpartum, or from contact with a person other than the mother with chickenpox or shingles in the immediate postpartum period.
- Neonates are at the highest risk if maternal infection occurs between one and four weeks before delivery. Up to 50 per cent of babies are infected and approximately 23 per cent develop clinical varicella, due to the lack of transfer of protective maternal antibodies and the relative immaturity of the neonatal immune system. Mortality is thought to be up to 30 per cent without active treatment.
- Women should be referred to a fetal medicine specialist for advice after resolution of acute disease. A detailed ultrasound examination or amniocentesis to detect varicella DNA by PCR may be offered.
- Shingles (herpes zoster) in the mother does not present a risk to the infant.

Management of Chickenpox in Pregnancy[17]

If a woman develops varicella infection/chickenpox during pregnancy, she should be informed of potential adverse maternal and fetal sequel, the risk of transmission to fetus and the options available for prenatal diagnosis. [EL 1]

The incidence of pneumonia complicating varicella in pregnancy has been quoted at 10–14 per cent but this is based on small case series.

Pregnant Women Who Have Been in Contact with Chickenpox or Shingles

- A careful history should be taken to ascertain immunity through previous infection, and the significance of exposure.
- Pregnant women who are uncertain about their immunity history should be checked for immunity through an IgG immunity measurement.
- If the pregnant woman who had a significant exposure is not immune to VZV, she should be

offered varicella zoster immunoglobulin (VZIG) as soon as possible. VZIG is effective when given up to 10 days after contact. A second dose of VZIG may be required if a further exposure is reported and three weeks have elapsed since the last dose.

Pregnant Women Who Develop Chickenpox

- Oral aciclovir (800 mg five times/day for 7 days) should be prescribed for pregnant women with chickenpox if they present within 24 hours of the onset of the rash. Aciclovir is not licensed for use during pregnancy, but is safe. Women should be informed if an unlicensed medication is offered. VZIG has no therapeutic role once chickenpox has developed.
- Oral aciclovir is prescribed if they are 20+0 weeks of gestation or beyond.
- Use of aciclovir before 20+0 weeks should also be considered.
- Intravenous aciclovir (10–15 mg/kg (or 500 mg/ m^2) intravenously every eight hours for ≥7 d) should be given to all pregnant women with severe chickenpox.
- Women who develop symptoms or signs of severe chickenpox, develop any respiratory symptoms or whose condition deteriorates should be referred immediately to hospital. If admitted they should be isolated from other women, babies and susceptible staff.
- A neonatologist should be informed of the birth of all babies born to women who have developed chickenpox at any gestation during pregnancy.
- Time and route of delivery should be individualised.
- Women are allowed to breastfeed even if they are vaccinated.
- Seronegative women should be offered postpartum vaccination.

Timing and Mode of Delivery

The timing and mode of delivery is individualised. Delivery during viraemia period, while chickenpox vesicles are active, may be extremely hazardous. It may precipitate maternal haemorrhage or coagulopathy due to thrombocytopenia or hepatitis.

In rare cases delivery may be required to help in assisted ventilation if severe varicella pneumonia develops.

Neonatal Management

- There is significant risk of neonatal varicella infection if the woman acquires infection in the last four weeks of pregnancy. It requires at least seven days for maternal antibodies to transfer to fetus to provide passive immunity.
- The neonatologist should be informed of maternal chickenpox infection regardless of gestation at time of infection.
- VZIG is recommended for all infants whose mothers develop chickenpox seven days before to seven days after delivery. Intravenous aciclovir should be given to these infants if they develop chickenpox, whether or not they received VZIG. Shingles in the first two years of life is thought to be a reactivation of chickenpox acquired *in utero*.

Prevention of Varicella during Pregnancy

- At booking, immunity history as a result of previous exposure or vaccination should be ascertained.
- If she has had a history of infection, she needs to be reassured of immune status.
- If she has never had infection in the past or is known to be seronegative for chickenpox, she is advised to avoid contact with chickenpox or shingles during pregnancy.
- Women should inform the midwife or general practitioner if they are exposed to chickenpox in pregnancy.
- Pregnant women with uncertain or no previous history of chickenpox should be tested for immunity.

Primary Prevention of Chickenpox

There are two varicella vaccines currently licensed in the UK:

Varilrix (GSK)

Varivax (SPMSD)

Both are live attenuated vaccines (contraindicated during pregnancy) and are administered in two separate doses four to eight weeks apart. Women who receive varicella vaccine postpartum can safely breastfeed.

Herpes Virus-6 during Pregnancy

Human herpes virus (HHV)-6 and HHV-7 are β-lymphotropic viruses. They cause universal infection during infancy or early childhood.[18]

Primary infection with HHV-6 causes an undifferentiated febrile illness, with a subset of children developing roseola infantum (occurs in 9- to 12-month-old infants with an abrupt onset of high fever (40°C), which lasts for three days with non-specific complaints; a febrile seizure occurs in 15 per cent of patients followed by a mild, pink, morbilliform exanthem).

HHV-6 reactivation seems common during pregnancy, and transfer of HHV-6 to the fetus may occur in ~1 per cent of pregnancies. However, in a study in 107 mother–infant pairs, there was no indication that the congenital HHV-6 infection causes fetal harm, as all the children were apparently healthy.

Epstein–Barr Virus (EBV) Infection

In a nested control study in Norway, there was no association between EBV antibody status and fetal death. Women with significant EBV reactivation had a significantly shorter duration of pregnancy, and associated smaller babies, compared with women without significant reactivation. In this study, it was suggested that only a limited number (2–6 per cent) of women have significant EBV reactivation in pregnancy.[19]

Other than treating symptoms, there is no specific treatment for EBV disorders or associated diseases.

Currently, there are no antiviral drugs or vaccines available.

Measles

Measles is a highly contagious airborne infectious disease that is contracted through contact with an infected person. Most adults would have been vaccinated against the virus during their childhood.

If left untreated during pregnancy in women who are not vaccinated, it can cause miscarriage, stillbirths or preterm labour.

Virology

Measles is caused by the measles virus, a single-stranded, negative-sense, enveloped RNA virus of the genus *Morbillivirus* within the family *Paramyxoviridae*.

It is a highly contagious virus, to the extent that 90 per cent of nearby non-immune people will also become infected if they are in close contact with an infected person. The virus spreads by coughing and sneezing via close personal contact or direct contact with secretions. Humans are the only natural hosts of the virus, and no other animal reservoirs are known to exist.[20]

Prevalence

Worldwide, global measles deaths have decreased by 84 per cent worldwide in recent years – from 550 100 deaths in 2000 to 89 780 in 2016. However, measles is still common in many developing countries, particularly in parts of Africa and Asia. The World Health Organization estimates that 7 million people were affected by measles in 2016. The overwhelming majority (more than 95 per cent) of measles deaths occur in countries with low per capita incomes and weak health infrastructures.[21]

Even in some countries where vaccination has been introduced, rates may remain high. Measles is a leading cause of vaccine-preventable childhood mortality.

In the USA, measles was declared eliminated since 2000. However, the annual number of cases has ranged from a low of 37 in 2004 to a high of 667 in 2014.

In Europe in 2013–14, there were almost 10 000 cases in 30 European countries. Most cases occurred in unvaccinated individuals, and over 90 per cent of cases occurred in five European nations: Germany, Italy, Netherlands, Romania and the United Kingdom. Between October 2014 and March 2015, a measles outbreak in the German capital Berlin resulted in at least 782 cases. In 2017, numbers continued to increase in Europe to 21 315 cases, with 35 deaths.[22]

Signs and Symptoms

- A four- to seven-day fever (can be as high as 40°C (104°F)
- Cough
- Coryza (head cold, fever, sneezing)
- Conjunctivitis
- Rashes: a generalised red maculopapular rash. It begins several days after the fever starts. It starts on the back of the ears and, after a few hours, spreads to the head and neck before spreading to cover most of the body, often causing itching. Overall,

the disease from infection with the measles virus usually resolves after about three weeks.[23]

Complications

- Otitis media
- Bronchopneumonia
- Laryngotracheobronchitis
- Acute encephalitis in one of every 1000 infected cases. It may result in permanent brain damage
- Sub-acute sclerosing panencephalitis (SSPE) is a rare, but fatal, degenerative disease of the CNS characterised by behavioural and intellectual deterioration and seizures that generally develop 7–10 years after measles infection
- Death due to neurologic and respiratory complications may occur, in one or two in every 1000 children

The above complications are more common in pregnant women than in non-pregnant women.

Laboratory Diagnosis of Measles

Antibody Testing

- IgM
  - IgM antibodies are usually detected in serum after four days post-onset of rash with a 90–100 per cent sensitivity, and can be detected for up to two to three months.
  - IgM may support a clinical diagnosis of recent/acute phase infection with the virus.

- IgG
  - The presence of detectable IgG-class antibodies, in the absence of IgM-class antibodies, indicates prior exposure to the measles virus through infection or immunisation. These individuals are considered immune to measles infection.
  - The absence of detectable IgG-class antibodies suggests the lack of a specific immune response to immunisation or no prior exposure to the measles virus. These individuals are considered non-immune to measles virus infection.

- IgG avidity
  - IgG avidity enzyme immunoassays differentiate early primary infection from distant secondary infection.
  - A low IgG avidity index of 30 indicates a recent infection, while a high IgG index of 70 indicates old infection.
  - IgG avidity is also used to detect success or failure of immunity after vaccination.

Polymerase Chain Reaction (PCR)

RNA detection by the reverse transcriptase–polymerase chain reaction (RT-PCR), using serum, urine or pharyngeal exudate specimens, provides more sensitive markers. [EL 2]

Isolation of Measles Virus

Measles virus can be isolated from clinical specimens, including throat swab, conjunctival swabs, nasopharyngeal aspirates or urine.

Maternal Implications

In a retrospective survey in France, of women who had measles and required hospital admission while being pregnant between January and December 2011, pneumonia occurred in 4 women (30.8 per cent), while other maternal complications included fever (11 women; 84.6 per cent) and elevated liver enzymes (2/6 women; 33.3 per cent).[24]

Fetal Implications

In unvaccinated pregnant women:

- Miscarriage
- Stillbirths
- Preterm labour
- There is no strong evidence to associate measles infection with congenital anomalies

Mother-to-Child Transmission (Congenital Measles)

- Congenital measles is the presence of the rash at birth or within the first 10 days of life, in a newborn whose mother was infected with measles within 10 days of delivery.
- Provision of pooled human immune globulin after delivery can decrease the risk of congenital measles.

Immunity for Measles Infections

A person is considered immune:

- If there is a definite positive history of measles disease
- If there is documented evidence of having received two doses of a measles-containing vaccine (MMR) administered at least four weeks apart and with both doses administered ≥ 12 months of age
- If a positive measles antibody test confirms immunity

Management of Women Who Are Not Immune and Are Exposed to Measles Infection

- Because of their increased risk for measles-related morbidity and mortality, pregnant women without evidence of measles immunity who are exposed to measles should receive IV immunoglobulin at a dose of 400 mg/kg within six days of exposure. Intravenous administration is recommended so that doses are high enough to reach levels of measles antibodies expected to be protective. A rapid IgG antibody test can be used to document measles immunity, provided that immunoglobulin administration is not delayed.[25]
- In a hospital environment, any contact not known to be immune, and who is admitted or within the hospital during the potentially contagious period of measles (10–14 days after exposure), should be cared for in single-room isolation.
- NHIG may not always prevent measles but decreases the severity of the disease, and increases the incubation period to 21 days. Therefore contacts given NHIG should be isolated from day 10 to day 21 if still within the hospital.[26]

Management of Women with Suspected or Known Measles during Pregnancy

- Measles should be suspected in patients presenting with fever, rash, cough, coryza and conjunctivitis. Measles infection should then be confirmed by detection of measles-specific IgM antibody and measles RNA real-time polymerase chain reaction.
- Patients should be asked about recent international travel, and history of measles illness in their communities.

- Patients with suspected measles should be isolated promptly in an airborne infection isolation room, with a facemask.
- All health care personnel caring for the patient should have evidence of measles immunity.
- Appropriate personal protective equipment should be used by all health care providers caring for the patient, even those with documented immunity.
- There is no available specific treatment. Pregnant women diagnosed with measles should receive supportive and symptomatic care.
- Hospitalisation may be indicated for treatment of complications (bacterial superinfection, pneumonia or dehydration). Antibiotics may be administered to combat infection.
- Febrile patients may become dehydrated, IV rehydration is required.
- Fever management with standard antipyretics is appropriate.

- **Antiviral Therapy**

There are no controlled trials for antiviral therapy for measles. There is no approved US Food and Drug Administration (FDA) antiviral treatment for measles.

Management of the Neonates of Measles-Infected Mothers

- There is an increased risk of severe disease in neonates born to mothers who have measles within 10 days of delivery. The paediatrician caring for the neonate should be made aware of potential for congenital measles.
- Infants younger than 12 months of age with exposure to measles should receive measles immunoglobulin intramuscularly at a dose of 0.5 mL/kg of body weight (max = 15 mL).
- There are limited data on whether well neonates born to mothers with measles need to be separated from their mothers. The specific situation should be discussed with infection control and public health experts to weigh the benefits against the risks of isolating the neonate from the mother until she is no longer infectious (four days after onset of her rash).

Breastfeeding

- In several maternal viral diseases, such as hepatitis, herpes, measles, mumps and rubella, among others, the virus may be excreted into human milk. However, except for infections caused by retroviruses, human immunodeficiency virus (HIV-1), human T-lymphotropic virus type I (HTLV I) and human T-lymphotropic virus type II (HTLV II), transmission via human milk has little epidemiological relevance. Therefore, in general, there is no formal contraindication for breastfeeding in most cases of viral diseases, except for diseases caused by retroviruses.
- In immune mothers, breastfeeding protects against measles infection.
- In a measles-infected nursing mother, the infant should receive immunoglobulin, and the mother should be isolated for 72 hours after the appearance of the rash.
- However, expressed breastmilk can be given to the infant because secretory IgA begins to be secreted 48 hours after the appearance of the rash in the mother.[27]

Prevention

- The mainstay of prevention is vaccination before pregnancy.
- Women who are trying to become pregnant and who do not have a definite history of a previous exposure or a proper vaccination of two doses should either check for their immunity or consider getting the measles vaccine again.
- Pregnant women who are not immune, or are uncertain of their immunity or immunisation status, should avoid exposure to large crowds, especially in areas where there may international visitors, e.g. tourists. They should also avoid contact with children who have not been immunised.
- Families are advised to vaccinate their children against measles and other vaccine-preventable illnesses.
- Non-immune pregnant women should have vaccination after delivery as the vaccine is contraindicated during pregnancy.
- Non-immune pregnant women who had a measles exposure should report to their carers to receive immunoglobulin.

Conclusion

Measles viral infection is rare. However, outbreaks still happen. Measles infection has deleterious maternal and fetal implications. Women who are trying to get pregnant should check their immunity and if not immune should follow the above prevention precautions.

References

1. Carter J, Saunders V. *Virology, Principles and Applications*, 2nd ed. New York: John Wiley & Sons; 2016.

2. Beauman JG. Genital herpes: a review. *Am Fam Physician.* 2005; **72**(8): 1527–34.

3. Kodle DM, Cory L. Recent progress in HSV immunology and vaccine research. *Clin Microbiol Rev.* 2003; **16**(1): 96–113.

4. Wald A, Langenberg AG, Krantz E et al. The relationship between condom use and herpes simplex virus acquisition. *Ann Intern Med.* 2005; **143**(10): 707–13.

5. Johnston C, Corey L. Current Concepts for Genital Herpes Simplex Virus Infection: Diagnostics and Pathogenesis of Genital Tract Shedding. American Society of Microbiology, Clinical Microbiology Reviews. https://cmr.asm.org/.

6. Hussain, NY, Uriel A, Mammen C, Bonington A. Disseminated herpes simplex infection during pregnancy, rare but important to recognise. *Qatar Med J.* 2014(1): 61–4.

7. Sauerbrei A. Herpes genitalis: diagnosis, treatment and prevention. *Geburtshilfe Frauenheilkd.* 2016; **76**(12): 1310–17.

8. Foley E, Clarke E, Beckett VA et al. Management of Genital Herpes in Pregnancy. October 2014. BASHH and the Royal College of Obstetricians and Gynaecologists. www.bashhguidelines.org/media/1060/management-genital-herpes.pdf.

9. Brown Z. Preventing herpes simplex virus transmission to the neonate. *Herpes.* 2004; **11**(suppl 3): 175A–86A.

10. British Paediatric Surveillance Unit. BPSU 21st Annual Report 2006–2007. London: British Paediatric Surveillance Unit/Royal College of Paediatrics and Child Health; 2007.

11. Clinical Effectiveness Group (British Association for Sexual Health and HIV). *National Guideline for the Management of Genital Herpes.* Macclesfield: BASHH; 2007.

12. Heng MC, Heng SY, Allen SG. Co-infection and synergy of human immunodeficiency virus-1 and herpes simplex virus-1. *Lancet.* 1994; **343**(8892): 255–8.

13. Centers for Disease Control and Prevention. Chickenpox (Varicella). About chickenpox. www.cdc.gov/chickenpox/about/index.html.

14. Lamont RF, Sobel JD, Carrington D et al. Varicella-zoster virus (chickenpox) infection in pregnancy. *BJOG.* 2011; **118**: 1155–62.

15. Birthistle K, Carrington D. Fetal Varicella Syndrome – a reappraisal of the literature. *J Infection.* 1998; **36**(suppl 1): 25–9.

16. Sauerbrei A, Wutzler P. Neonatal varicella. *J Perinatol.* 2001; **21**(8): 545–9.

17. Royal College of Obstetricians and Gynaecologists. Chickenpox in Pregnancy. RCOG Green-top Guideline No. 13.

18. Dahl H, Fjaertoft G, Norsted T et al. Reactivation of human herpesvirus 6 during pregnancy. *J Infectious Dis.* 1999;**180**(6): 2035–8.

19. Eskild A, Bruu A-L, Stray-Pedersen, B, Jenumd P. Epstein–Barr virus infection during pregnancy and the risk of adverse pregnancy outcome. *BJOG.* 2005, **112**: 1620–4.

20. Centers for Disease Control and Prevention. Measles. www.cdc.gov/measles/hcp/index.html.

21. World Health Organization. Measles. www.who.int/immunization/diseases/measles/en/.

22. World Health Organization. Europe observes a 4-fold increase in measles cases in 2017 compared to previous year. February 2018. www.euro.who.int/en/media-centre/sections/press-releases/2018/europe-observes-a-4-fold-increase-in-measles-cases-in-2017-compared-to-previous-year.

23. Measles. Merck Manuals Professional Edition. January 2018.

24. Casalegno S, Huissoud C. Rudigoz R, Massardier J, Gaucherand P, Mekkia Y. Measles in pregnancy in Lyon France, 2011. *Int J Gynaecol Obstet.* 2014; **126**(3): 248–51.

25. Department for Health and Wellbeing, Government of South Australia. South Australian Perinatal Practice Guideline. Measles and measles contacts in pregnancy. www.sahealth.sa.gov./Measles+and+measles+contacts+in+pregnancy_PPG_v4_1.pdf?MOD=AJPERES&CACHEID=ROOTWORKSPACE-b9f4a8004ee4fe8e97779fd150ce4f37-mg-yJEQ.

26. Rasmussen SA, Jamieson DJ. What obstetric health care providers need to know about measles and pregnancy. *Obstet Gynecol.* 2015; **126**(1): 163–70.

27. Lamounier JA, Moulin ZS, Xavier CC. Recommendations for breastfeeding during maternal infections. *Jornal de Pediatria.* (Porto Alegre) 2004; **80**(5) suppl.

Zika Virus

Youssef Abo Elwan

History

Zika virus was discovered for the first time in April 1947 in Uganda at Zika forest near Victoria Lake, when a veterinarian and his monkey had the same symptoms (fever, malaise, conjunctivitis and drowsiness). In 1952 infection was proven by a rise in Zika virus-specific antibodies in a Nigerian female.[1]

The first outbreak occurred in April 2007 in Africa and Asia. The second outbreak occurred in May 2015 in South America and Mexico.

In July 2015 some cases were reported in Malaysia, India, Thailand and upper Egypt. The third outbreak occurred at the end of 2016 at the Olympic Games in Brazil.

Virology, Pathogenesis

Zika virus is an arthropod-borne virus, a member of the virus family *Flaviviridae*, genus *Flavivirus* and transmitted by *Aedes aegypti* mosquito. The virus is transmitted through mosquito bites, blood transfusion, sexual contact (from male to female) and from mother to fetus.[2]

The incubation period is three to seven days.

- It is a neurotropic virus which particularly targets neural progenitor cells.
- Studies suggest the hypothesis that maternal infection leads to placental infection and injury, followed by transmission of the virus to the fetal brain, hence killing neuronal progenitor cells and disrupting neuronal proliferation, migration and differentiation, slowing brain growth and reducing viability of neural cells.[3,4]
- In the placenta, the virus infects and then replicates in placental macrophages (Hofbauer cells), and to a lesser extent in cytotrophoblasts.[5]

- In a series from Brazil and in other case series, there was immune-histochemical and molecular evidence of virus persistence in the brain of newborns with microcephaly and severe arthrogryposis who died shortly after birth.[6,7] [EL 2]

Clinical Manifestations

Clinical manifestations of Zika virus infection occur in 20 per cent of patients:

- Acute onset low grade fever
- Maculopapular pruritic rash
- Arthralgia (mostly in small joints of hands and feet)
- Non-purulent conjunctivitis[8]

Diagnosis

- **Clinical manifestation of infection,** history of exposure in epidemiologic areas or those who travel to Zika virus infection prone area, or had unprotected sexual contact with a person who meets these criteria.
- **Antigen antibody testing:** antibody response to all related flavivirus infections (dengue viruses, West Nile virus and/or in women vaccinated against yellow fever virus) has been known to be cross-reactive.

  In populations previously exposed to any of the above-mentioned conditions antibody detection of ZIKV is not specific.
- **Real-time reverse transcriptase–polymerase chain reaction (rRT-PCR) for Zika virus RNA** (in serum, urine or whole blood). PCR tests should be carried out within two weeks of first suspicion of infection.
- **Nucleic acid assays** in the whole blood.

Differential Diagnosis

- Dengue fever
- Parvovirus
- Rubella
- Measles
- Leptospirosis
- Malaria
- Rickettsial infection.

Congenital Infection

- The risk for vertical transmission can occur throughout pregnancy and affect the fetus of both symptomatic and asymptomatic mothers.
- If a woman is infected during pregnancy, the overall risk of birth defect or abnormality ranges from 6 to 42 per cent.[9] [EL 2 & 3]
- In endemic areas, or on clinical suspicion of Zika viral infection (maculopapular pruritic rash, arthralgia, conjunctivitis or fever), pregnant women should be offered screening to exclude or confirm Zika virus infection.

Fetal Implications and Features of Congenital Zika Virus Syndrome

- **Microcephaly** (head circumference > 2 standard deviations below the mean of the standard growth charts for sex, age and gestational age).

In some cases, congenitally infected offspring of women during the first or second trimester have a normal head circumference at birth but may subsequently develop microcephaly in the first year of life.[10]

Estimates of the risk of microcephaly exposure range from 1 to 4 per cent.

- **Central nervous system abnormalities** (ventriculomegaly, intracranial calcifications).[11]
- **Positional abnormalities** (club foot and arthrogryposis) may be of neurogenic origin.
- Miscarriage.
- Stillbirth.
- IUGR.
- Hydrops fetalis.

Placental insufficiency is the mechanism postulated for fetal loss later in pregnancy.

Management and Prevention

There is no specific treatment for Zika virus infection. Rest and supportive therapy such as proper hydration and administration of acetaminophen to relieve fever and pain.

The World Health Organization (WHO) has issued initial guidance on psychosocial support for patients and families affected by Zika virus infection and associated complications.

Diagnosis of Fetal Infection

- **Ultrasound examination** every three to four weeks to look for signs of congenital infection and monitor fetal growth with laboratory evidence of recent Zika virus infection in women.[12]
- **Magnetic resonance imaging** (MRI) is more sensitive for diagnosis of fetal brain abnormalities.[13]
- **Amniocentesis** should be considered and tailored to individual clinical circumstances, if ultrasound examination is abnormal.[14]

  o The sensitivity and specificity of Zika virus RT-PCR testing of amniotic fluid are not known and likely depend on the timing of amniocentesis after onset of maternal infection.
  o A positive RT-PCR result on amniotic fluid should be considered suggestive of fetal infection.
  o If the fetus is abnormal and RT-PCR is negative, evaluation for other causes of the fetal abnormalities should be considered.
  o As the duration of amniotic fluid PCR positivity is unknown, a negative RT-PCR does not definitively exclude fetal Zika virus infection.

Delivery

Delivery timing, route and place of delivery are according to obstetric practices and standards.

Breastfeeding

According to the WHO:[15]

- 'There are currently no documented reports of Zika virus being transmitted to infants through breastfeeding.'
- 'In countries with ongoing transmission, no adverse neurological outcomes have been reported

to date in infants with postnatally acquired Zika virus.'

- 'Based on the available evidence, suggests that the benefits of breastfeeding for the infant and mother outweigh any potential risk of transmission through breast milk.'

Consequently the WHO issued the following recommendation: 'Infants born to mothers with suspected, probable or confirmed infection, or who reside in or have travelled within 2 weeks to areas of ongoing Zika virus transmission, should start breastfeeding within 1 h of birth. They should exclusively breastfeed for 6 months and have timely introduction of adequate, safe and properly fed complementary foods, while continuing breastfeeding up to 2 years of age or beyond.'

Prevention

- Unless absolutely necessary, avoid travel to areas with known mosquito transmission of Zika virus.
- Observe mosquito protective measures. (Using mosquito repellents, wearing long-sleeved shirts and long trousers, sleeping or resting in screened or air-conditioned rooms and using mosquito nets.) Avoid unprotected sexual intercourse, ideally for six months for both men and women who have travelled to endemic area.
- There is no vaccine for prevention of Zika virus infection.

Conclusion

Zika virus is a mosquito-borne virus transmitted by *Aedes* mosquitoes and is known to circulate in Africa, the Americas, Asia and the Pacific.

Its main complication is fetal microcephaly, CNS abnormality, miscarriage, stillbirth, IUGR and hydrops fetalis.

There is no specific treatment or any immunisation.

References

1. World Health Organization. The history of Zika virus. www.who.int/emergencies/zika-virus/timeline/en/.

2. Armstrong N, Hou, WH, Tang QY. Biological and historical overview of Zika virus. *World J Virol.* 2017; 6(1): 1–8.

3. Costello A, Dua T, Duran P et al. Defining the syndrome associated with congenital Zika virus infection. *Bull World Health Organ.* 2016; 94(6): 406–6A.

4. Garcez PP, Loiola EC, Madeiro da Costa R et al. Zika virus impairs growth in human neurospheres and brain organoids. *Science.* 2016; 352(6287): 816–18.

5. Quicke KM, Bowen JR, Johnson EL et al. Zika virus infects human placental macrophages. *Cell Host Microbe.* 2016; 20(1): 83–90.

6. Martines RB, Bhatnagar J, de Oliveira Ramos AM et al. Pathology of congenital Zika syndrome in Brazil: a case series. *Lancet.* 2016; 388(10047): 898–904.

7. Hazin AN, Poretti A, Turchi Martelli CM, Huisman TA, Microcephaly Epidemic Research Group et al. Computed tomographic findings in microcephaly associated with Zika virus. 2016; *N Engl J Med.* 374(22): 2193–5.

8. Petersen EE, Staples JE, Meaney-Delman D et al. Interim guidelines for pregnant women during a Zika virus outbreak, United States, 2016. *MMWR Morb Mortal Wkly Rep.* 2016; 65(2): 30–3.

9. Honein MA, Dawson AL, Petersen EE et al. Birth defects among fetuses and infants of US women with evidence of possible Zika virus infection during pregnancy. *JAMA.* 2017; 317(1): 59–68.

10. van der Linden V, Pessoa A, Dobyns W et al. Description of 13 infants born during October 2015–January 2016 with congenital Zika virus infection without microcephaly at birth – Brazil. *MMWR.* 2016; 65(47): 1343–8.

11. Rasmussen SA, Jamieson DJ, Honein MA et al. Zika virus and birth defects – reviewing the evidence for causality. *N Engl J Med.* 2016; 374(20): 1981–7.

12. Carvalho FH, Cordeiro KM, Peixoto AB et al. Associated ultrasonographic findings in fetuses with microcephaly because of suspected Zika virus (ZIKV) infection during pregnancy. *Prenat Diagn.* 2016; 36(9): 882–7.

13. Griffiths PD, Bradburn M, Campbell MJ et al. Use of MRI in the diagnosis of fetal brain abnormalities in utero (MERIDIAN): a multicentre, prospective cohort study. *Lancet.* 2016; 389(10068): 538–46.

14. Maykin M, Pereira JP Jr, Moreira M, Nielsen-Saines K, Gaw S. Role of amniocentesis in the diagnosis of congenital Zika syndrome. *Am J Obstet Gynaecol.* 2018; 219(6): 652.

15. World Health Organization. Infant feeding in areas of Zika virus transmission. Last updated 11 April 2017. www.who.int/elena/titles/zika_breastfeeding/en/.

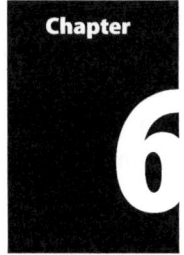
Parvovirus

Mohammed Hamed

Many viral infections can result in significant adverse maternal and fetal effects if acquired during pregnancy. Some of these adverse outcomes are easily preventable.

Introduction

Parvovirus B19 is a single-stranded DNA virus of the family *Parvoviridae* and genus *Erythrovirus*; it is responsible for erythema infectiosum. It is also known as fifth disease because it was the fifth of six classic exanthematous diseases of childhood.[1]

Epidemiology

- Parvovirus B19 infection is extremely common. Seropositivity rates are 5–10 per cent among children aged two to five years, increasing to 50 per cent by age 15 years and 60 per cent by age 30 years. A small percentage of adults every year acquire the infection, resulting in a cumulative incidence of approximately 90 per cent in adults older than 60 years.
- The annual conversion rate among pregnant women is 15 per cent.[2]
- Nursery school teachers have a three-fold higher risk of acute infection than other pregnant women, and other school teachers have a 1.6-fold increased risk. The population-attributable risk of infection in susceptible pregnant women is about 55 per cent from their own children and 6 per cent for occupational exposure.

People at Increased Risk

- Mothers of preschool children
- School age children
- Workers at daycare centres
- School teachers

Assessment of immunity at the beginning of the pregnancy can be considered in these populations.

Signs and Symptoms

Infection is often asymptomatic, and up to 50 per cent of non-pregnant women, and up to 70 per cent of infected pregnant women are asymptomatic.[3]

1 Prodromal Illness

- fever (15–30 per cent)
- malaise
- headache
- myalgia
- nausea
- rhinorrhea

Symptoms typically begin five to seven days after initial infection and are caused by the initial viraemia which dissipates within two to three days.

2 A Diffuse Maculopapular Rash

- The rash appears approximately one week later.
- It is a bright red macular exanthem which appears on the cheeks and is often associated with circumoral pallor.
- It may later fade to a lacy erythematous rash.
- The rash may be pruritic.
- It may spread gradually towards the distal extremities.
- The classic 'slapped cheek' rash is much more common in young children.
- The rash corresponds to the appearance of immunoglobulin M (IgM) in the serum and signals the clearance of viraemia.[4]

3 'Gloves-and-Socks' Syndrome (PPGSS)

- Erythematous exanthem of the hands and feet with a distinct margin at the wrist and ankle joints.
- It is mainly seen in young adults.
- It initially presents with painful erythema and induration of the hands.
- The skin changes may progress to petechia, purpura and bulla with skin sloughing. PPGSS usually resolves in one to three weeks without scarring.

4 Transient Small Joint Arthropathy

- May be the main clinical presentation in adults.
- Most have some joint pain.
- A few may progress to frank arthritis.
- Arthritis usually improves in one to three weeks but may persist for months.

5 Transient Aplastic Crisis (TAC)

- Parvovirus infection rarely causes transient aplastic crisis as it has an affinity for hematopoietic system cells.
- The anaemia, however, may be significant in those with underlying haematologic disorders including sickle cell disease, hereditary spherocytosis, pyruvate kinase deficiency, thalassemia and autoimmune haemolytic anaemia.

Pathogenesis

Mode of transmission is through respiratory secretions and hand-to-mouth contact.[5]

Other modes of transmission are blood product infusion and transplacental transfer which occurs in up to 33 per cent of cases. Infected patients are contagious for 5–10 days after exposure, only during the week before the onset of the rash. Approximately 50 per cent of women are at risk if exposed to an infected household member.

Outbreaks usually occur yearly, with larger epidemics every four to five years, and may last up to six months.

Without known exposure, about 1–3 per cent of susceptible pregnant women will develop serologic evidence of infection in pregnancy, rising to over 10 per cent in epidemic periods.[6]

Diagnosis of Maternal Infection

Parvovirus serology (enzyme-linked immunoassay (ELISA), radioimmunoassay, or immunofluorescence)

- For detection of anti-parvovirus B19 immunoglobulin M (IgM) and immunoglobulin G (IgG) antibodies

Polymerase chain reaction (PCR) testing for parvovirus B19

- To detect viral DNA present in the blood or other tissues/fluids
- The differentiation between acute and chronic infection requires standard DNA hybridisation or quantitative (real-time) PCR in combination with serologic assays for B19-specific IgG, IgM, or both[7]
- Monitoring the quantitative PCR viral load in neonates with congenital parvovirus infection helps direct follow-up and the need for transfusions[7]
- PCR may be performed on fetal serum or amniotic fluid to detect virus[7]

Management of Maternal Infection

- Maternal parvovirus B19 infection is managed with symptomatic therapy.
- There is no specific antiviral treatment.
- High-dose intravenous immunoglobulin is occasionally used for treating persistent aplastic anaemia associated with parvovirus B 19 infection.
- Maternal complications are uncommon. Parvovirus infection is usually a self-limited viral infection.

Pregnancy and Parvovirus

Over 50 per cent of pregnant women in the USA are immune to parvovirus.

Pregnancy does not appear to affect the course of the infection, but infection may expose the fetus to the risks of miscarrying, hydrops fetalis and fetal loss.

The transmission rate of maternal parvovirus infection to the fetus is 17–33 per cent.

Fetal Implications

- Spontaneous abortion

Spontaneous abortion or fetal death occurs in less than 10 per cent of infected pregnancies. Most usually occur between 10 and 20 weeks' gestation, and the spontaneous abortions 4–6 weeks after infection.

The spontaneous loss rate of fetuses affected with parvovirus B19 before 20 weeks' gestation is 13.0 per cent, and after 20 weeks' gestation is 0.5 per cent.[8]

- Congenital anomalies

Currently, there does not appear to be any evidence that parvovirus infection increases the risk of congenital anomalies in humans, though there have been case reports of central nervous system, craniofacial, musculoskeletal and eye anomalies.[9]

- Fetal loss

If infection is acquired before 19–20 weeks' gestation (14.8 per cent), the fetal loss rate is higher than if the infection is acquired after 20 weeks (2.3 per cent).[10]

- Hydrops fetalis

Ultrasound picture of hydrops fetalis includes: [11,12]

  ○ Ascites
  ○ Skin oedema
  ○ Pleural and pericardial effusions
  ○ Placental oedema
  ○ Possible mechanisms for hydrops include fetal anaemia due to transplacental infection, combined with the shorter half-life of fetal red blood cells (especially during the hepatic stage of hematopoiesis)
  ○ Other possible causes include fetal viral myocarditis leading to cardiac failure, and impaired hepatic function caused by direct damage to hepatocytes and indirect damage due to haemosiderin deposits
  ○ Parvovirus infection accounts for 8–10 per cent of non-immune hydrops, although some studies found molecular evidence in 18–27 per cent of cases of non-immune hydrops

Long-Term Neonatal Outcome

Most infants do not have long-term adverse sequelae. Further research is needed. However, case reports showed hepatic insufficiency, myocarditis, transfusion-dependent anaemia and central nervous system abnormalities.

Parvovirus itself, in the absence of hydrops or significant fetal anaemia, does not seem to cause long-term neurological morbidity.

Table 6.1 Interpretation of maternal blood results after suspected infection

IgM	IgG	
Negative	Negative	SUSCEPTIBLE – test should be repeated in 3 weeks if symptoms/history to determine if antibodies appear
Positive	Negative	ACUTE INFECTION – infection occurred at least 3, but less than 7, days ago; fetus is at risk and requires monitoring
Positive	Positive	SUB-ACUTE INFECTION –infection occurred more than 7, but less than 120, days ago; fetus is at risk and requires careful evaluation (recent infection, check stored blood for recent seroconversion). If IgG is rising, then this indicates recent infection; if it remains static, then older infection

However, severe anaemia and fetal hydrops may be an independent risk factor for long-term neurological sequelae. Moreover, myocarditis can lead to severe dilated cardiomyopathy and may even require heart transplantation.

If a pregnant woman is exposed or develops signs and symptoms suggestive of parvovirus infection:

IgM and IgG Serology Testing for Immunity

- IgM indicates acute infection and usually appears within two to three days of acute infection and may persist up to six months.
- The presence of IgG and no IgM indicates immunity and there is no risk to the fetus.
- If both IgM and IgG are negative, the woman is not immune and the fetus is exposed to the risk of infection.
- The presence of both IgM and IgG may suggest recent infection in the last 7–120 days. Comparing to the stored blood if available may confirm seroconversion, indicating recent infection.

Middle Cerebral Artery Peak Systolic Velocity to Diagnose Fetal Anaemia

- In an anaemic fetus, changes in cardiac output and blood-flow velocities are reflected by an increase in peak systolic velocity in the middle cerebral artery.

- Middle cerebral artery peak systolic velocity (MCA PSV) is a reliable non-invasive method to diagnose fetal anaemia.

  It reduces the number of invasive procedures in the management of fetuses at risk of fetal anaemia due to parvovirus infection.[13]

  It should be utilised both before the first cordocentesis for fetal blood transfusion and to help decide if there is a need for repeat fetal blood transfusion.

  MCA has a sensitivity of 83–100 per cent, and a specificity of 78.6–93 to 100 per cent for diagnosis of anaemia.

  The reference test for the diagnosis of fetal anaemia is peak systolic velocity of the MCA more than 1.5 multiple of median (MOM).

Diagnosis of Fetal Infection

- Polymerase chain reaction (PCR) for detection of viral DNA in the amniotic fluid.
- Cordocentesis and examination of the fetal blood for viral DNA by PCR. The presence of parvovirus B19 IgM in fetal blood cannot be relied upon to make the diagnosis of fetal infection. The fetus does not begin to make its own IgM until 22 weeks' gestation.

Management of Fetal Hydrops

- **Women should be referred to a maternal–fetal medicine specialist** for serial ultrasounds to detect evidence of hydrops for 8–12 weeks after infection, as the development of hydrops may be delayed.
- **Ultrasound follow-up**There are no randomised trials of the frequency of ultrasounds required; however, most specialists perform ultrasonographic assessment weekly or every two weeks.

  Ultrasound assessment of the fetus should include Doppler measurement of the MCA peak systolic velocity to assess for fetal anaemia.
- **Expectant management**
  - Expectant management is indicated if hydrops fetalis is estimated to be mild either because of ultrasound findings, middle cerebral artery peak velocity or cordocentesis result for fetal anaemia and reticulocyte count. Expectant management requires a very careful balance.
  - Expectant management is a reasonable option if the haemoglobin levels are above 9.3 g/dL.

  - Expectant management is also reasonable with a MCA-PSV below 1.5 MOM.
- **Delivery**

  Delivery after a course of steroids for lung maturity is indicated if hydrops occurs after a reasonable degree of maturity in the third trimester as extrauterine blood transfusion is safer than cordocentesis and intrauterine transfusion.
- **Cordocentesis and intrauterine blood transfusion**[15]
  - This is indicated if there is severe hydrops and guided by the MCA-PSV.
  - Cordocentesis is then carried out to indicate the degree of anaemia.
  - If the haemoglobin level is below 9.3 g/dL packed red cells are transfused into the umbilical vein, or intra-cardiac and/or intraperitoneal transfusion.
  - The upper limit of gestational age for transfusion is case- and centre-dependent. Two to three transfusions may be required before resolution of the fetal hydrops or anaemia, which usually occurs three to six weeks after the first transfusion.

Complications of Invasive Management

- Complications are due to the periumbilical blood sampling procedure itself.
- The overall fetal loss rate of 1–5 per cent depends on operator experience, with most centres reporting loss rates of 1–2 per cent.
- Cordocentesis is associated with:
  - Infection
  - Bleeding
  - Fetal bradycardia
  - Premature rupture of the membranes and pregnancy loss[16]

  A summary of 14 studies involving a total of 1436 cases of fetal parvovirus infection found a survival rate of 82 per cent with transfusion compared with 55 per cent in those who were not transfused.[17] [EL 1]

Conclusion

- Parvovirus infection should be suspected in cases of fetal hydrops or intrauterine fetal death. [EL 2]

- Routine screening for parvovirus immunity in low-risk pregnancies is not recommended. [EL 2]
- Pregnant women who are exposed to, or who develop symptoms should be assessed to see whether they are susceptible to infection (non-immune) or have a current infection by testing for IgG and IgM status. [EL 2]
- If IgG is present and IgM is negative, the woman is immune and should be reassured that she will not develop infection and that pregnancy will not be affected. [EL 2]
- If a recent infection has been diagnosed, referral to an obstetrician or a maternal–fetal medicine specialist should be considered. [EL 3]
- Women should be counselled regarding risks of fetal transmission, fetal loss and hydrops, and serial ultrasounds should be performed every 1–2 weeks, up to 12 weeks after infection.
- Doppler measurement of the middle cerebral artery peak systolic velocity should be done to detect hydrops/anaemia and fetal blood sampling and intravascular transfusion performed if present.[18] [EL 2]

References

1. American Academy of Pediatrics Committee on Infectious Diseases. Parvovirus B19. In: Kimberlin DW, Brady M, Jackson SA, Long SS, eds. *2015 Red Book: Report of the Committee on Infectious Diseases*, 30th ed. Elk Grove Village, IL: American Academy of Pediatrics; 2015: 593–6.

2. Lamont RF, Sobel JD, Vaisbuch E et al. Parvovirus B19 infection in human pregnancy. *BJOG.* 2011; **118**: 175–86.

3. Brown KE. Parvovirus B19. In: Bennett JE, Dolin R, Blaser M, eds. *Mandell, Douglas and Bennett's Principles and Practice of Infectious Diseases*, 8th ed. Philadelphia: Churchill Livingstone Elsevier; 2015. Vol. 2: 1840–7.

4. Dijkmans AC, de Jong EP, Dijkmans BA et al. Parvovirus B19 in pregnancy: prenatal diagnosis and management of fetal complications. *Curr Opin Obstet Gynecol.* 2012; **24**: 95–101.

5. de Jong EP, Walther FJ, Kroes AC, Oepkes D. Parvovirus B19 infection in pregnancy: new insights and management. *Prenat Diagn.* 2011; **31**: 419–25.

6. Landry ML. Parvovirus B19. *Microbiol Spectr.* 2016; **4**(3): 1–13.

7. Healthline Editorial Team. Diagnosis of Parvovirus in Pregnancy. How is Parvovirus B19 Diagnosed in the Mother? Health line newsletter. www.healthline.com/health/pregnancy/infections-parvovirus-b19#1.

8. Giorgio E, De Oronzo MA, Iozza I et al. Parvovirus B19 during pregnancy: a review. *J Prenat Med.* 2010; **4**(4): 63–6.

9. Desilets V, Audibert F, SOGC Genetics Committee. Investigation and management of non-immune fetal hydrops. SOCG Clinical Practice Guidelines, No. 297, October 2013. *J Obstet Gynaecol Can.* 2013; **35**: 923–38.

10. Dijkmans AC, de Jong EP, Dijkmans BA et al. Parvovirus B19 in pregnancy: prenatal diagnosis and management of fetal complications. *Curr Opin Obstet Gynecol.* 2012; **24**: 95–101.

11. Norton, ME, Chauhan SP, Dashe JS. Society for Maternal-Fetal Medicine (SMFM) Clinical Guideline #7: nonimmune hydrops fetalis. *Am J Obstet Gynecol.* 2015; **212**(2): 127–39.

12. von Kaisenberg CS, Jonat W. Fetal parvovirus B19 infection. *Ultrasound Obstet Gynecol.* 2001; **18**: 280–8.

13. Borna S, Mirzaie F, Hanthoush-Zadeh S, Khazardoost S, Rahimi-Sharbaf F. Middle cerebral artery peak systolic velocity and ductus venosus velocity in the investigation of nonimmune hydrops. *J Clin Ultrasound.* 2009; **37**: 385–8.

14. Argoti PS. Bebbington M, Adler, M, Johnson A, Moise KJ. Serial intrauterine transfusions for a hydropic fetus with severe anemia and thrombocytopenia caused by parvovirus: lessons learned. *AJP Rep.* 2013; **3**(2): 75–8.

Influenza

Adel Elkady, Prabha Sinha and Soad Ali Zaki Hassan

Introduction

Influenza is a contagious viral respiratory illness caused by influenza viruses that infects the nose, throat and sometimes the lungs. It can cause mild to severe illness, and at times can lead to significant morbidity and mortality.

- There are four types of seasonal influenza viruses, types A, B, C and D.
- Influenza A and B viruses circulate and cause seasonal epidemics of disease.
- Influenza A virus subtypes include: subtype A (H1N1) and A (H3N2). The A (H1N1) caused the pandemic in 2009. Only influenza type A viruses are known to have caused pandemics.
- Influenza B viruses are not classified into subtypes.
- Influenza C virus is detected less frequently and usually causes mild infections; it does not present public health importance.
- Influenza D viruses primarily affect cattle and are not known to infect or cause illness in humans.[1]

Prevalence

Worldwide, annual epidemics are estimated to result in about 3 to 5 million cases of severe illness, and about 290 000 to 650 000 deaths.

In the USA, flu-related hospitalisations since 2010 ranged from 140 000 to 710 000, while flu-related deaths are estimated to have ranged from 12 000 to 56 000.[2]

The effects of seasonal influenza epidemics in developing countries are not fully known. Research estimates that 99 per cent of deaths in children under five years of age with influenza-related lower respiratory tract infections are found in developing countries.

Signs and Symptoms

There is usually a sudden onset of fever, dry cough, headache, muscle and joint pain, severe malaise, sore throat and a runny nose.

Influenza illnesses range from mild to severe and even death.

Transmission and Infectivity

- Infection is transmitted when an infected person coughs or sneezes.
- Infection droplets containing viruses are dispersed into the air and can spread up to 1 metre. Persons breathing in the proximity will inhale the infected droplets and become infected.
- The virus can also be spread by hands contaminated with influenza viruses.

The incubation period is from one to four days.

Diagnosis of Influenza

There are a number of diagnostic influenza tests available. They detect the virus in the respiratory system.

Rapid Influenza Diagnostic Tests (RIDTs)

RIDTs work by detecting the antigens of the virus. These tests can provide results within approximately 10–15 minutes, but are not as accurate as other flu tests.

Rapid Molecular Assays

This test detects genetic material of the virus. They are more accurate than RIDTs.

In addition, specialised laboratories in hospitals or state public health laboratories have more accurate and sensitive tests performed on nasal swabs or the back of the throat.

Direct Antigen Detection/Reverse Transcriptase–Polymerase Chain Reaction (RT-PCR)[3]

This means virus isolation or detection of influenza-specific RNA, from throat, nasal and nasopharyngeal secretions or tracheal aspirate or washings.

Differential Diagnosis

Other Respiratory Viruses

Rhinovirus, respiratory syncytial virus, parainfluenza and adenovirus may also present as influenza-like illness (ILI), making it difficult to differentiate on clinical signs and symptoms.

Common Cold

- Influenza and the common cold are both respiratory illnesses.
- They are caused by different viruses. Because of the similarity of signs and symptoms, it can be difficult to tell the difference between them.
- In general, in influenza the symptoms are worse and more intense.
- Colds generally do not result in serious health problems, such as pneumonia, bacterial infections, or hospitalisations.

Maternal Implications

- Influenza (flu) is more likely to cause severe illness in pregnant women than in women who are not pregnant.
- Changes in the immune system, heart and lungs during pregnancy make pregnant women (and women up to two weeks postpartum) more prone to severe illness from flu, including illness resulting in hospitalisation.
- Evidence suggests that pregnant women are even more vulnerable during pandemics.
- Pregnant women with influenza were five times more likely to be hospitalised than non-pregnant women, and the risks increase with advancing gestations.[4] [EL 2]
- The risks of influenza in pregnant women have been observed in pandemic and non-pandemic seasons.
- Influenza in pregnant women may be complicated by acute severe cardiopulmonary complications. [EL 1]
  - During the H1N1 influenza pandemic of 2009–10, pregnant women were more likely to be hospitalised or admitted to intensive care units (ICUs), and were at higher risk of death than non-pregnant adults.[5]
  - In one study of the 1918, H1N1 influenza pandemic, half of the pregnant women had

pneumonia and there was a 27 per cent case fatality rate.
  - In the H2N2 influenza pandemic in 1957–58, one-half of women of reproductive age who died from pandemic influenza were pregnant.[6,7]
  - In a systematic review of 120 studies reporting on 3110 pregnant women from 29 countries with H1N1 influenza, pregnant women accounted for approximately 6 per cent of individuals who were hospitalised, were admitted to an ICU and died as a result of H1N1 2009 pandemic influenza A (H1N1).[8] [EL 1]

Fetal Implications

Early Pregnancy Loss

In a case series from the 1918 H1N1 pandemic, one-quarter of women with uncomplicated influenza and more than half of those with pneumonia had a pregnancy loss.[6]

Small for Gestational Age

A Canadian population-based cohort study found that infants born to women who were hospitalised for a respiratory illness during influenza season over 13 years had a significantly increased risk of being born small for their gestational age and a lower mean birthweight.[9] [EL 2]

Preterm Birth

In a UK series of 256 women with 2009 H1N1 influenza, there was a four-fold increased likelihood of preterm birth.

Perinatal Mortality

In this same UK study, there was an increased perinatal mortality rate (39 per 1000 births compared to 7 per 1000 in women without influenza).[10]

Management of Flu during Pregnancy

Early treatment is important for pregnant women.

There are antiviral drugs that can treat flu illness and prevent serious flu complications.

The US Centers for Disease Control and Prevention (CDC) recommend prompt treatment for people who have influenza infection or suspected influenza infection and who are at high risk of serious flu complications, such as pregnant women.

- Treatment should begin as soon as possible because antiviral drugs work best when started early (within 48 hours after symptoms start).
- Antiviral drugs can make flu illness milder and make patients feel better faster. They may also prevent serious health problems that can result from flu illness.
- Antipyretics if there is fever.

When to Seek Emergency Medical Care[11]

- Difficulty breathing or shortness of breath
- Pain or pressure in the chest or abdomen
- Sudden dizziness
- Confusion
- Severe or persistent vomiting
- High fever that is not responding to treatment
- Decreased or absent fetal movements

Antiviral Medications for Influenza

During pregnancy, the antiviral medications most widely used are:

- The neuraminidase inhibitors oseltamivir (at a therapeutic dose of 75 mg twice daily and a prophylactic dose of 76 mg once daily)
- Zanamivir (at a therapeutic dose of 10 mg two inhalations twice daily and a prophylactic dose of 5 mg two inhalations once daily)

Both medications are effective against influenza A and B.

Zanamivir is an inhaled drug and has little systemic absorption.

Oseltamivir (Tamiflu) is an oral medication that is absorbed systemically.

- Treatment is most effective if taken early within 12 hours, and should ideally be started within 24–48 hours of the onset of symptoms.
- These antiviral medications are considered both safe and effective.
- In controlled trials and a meta-analysis, antiviral medications reduced the duration, severity and risk of complications in higher-risk populations including pregnant women.[12] [EL 1]
- Both medications are US Food and Drug Administration (FDA)-approved for treatment of influenza.

- Both medications are category C; however, these medications should still be used to treat influenza during pregnancy as the benefits have proven to far exceed the risks.
- The FDA believes that the benefits of antiviral therapy outweigh the potential for risks from the drugs.[13]
- Studies from different countries, before the recent H1N1 pandemic, and many since, have confirmed there is no increased risk for congenital anomalies, or preterm birth or adverse birth outcomes (low birthweight, low APGAR scores, neonatal seizures, stillbirth or neonatal death) among children exposed to antiviral medications while *in utero*.[14]

Breastfeeding

Breastmilk concentrations for both oseltamivir and zanamivir are lower than doses used in children.[14]

Prevention and Protection

The combined use of vaccination and antiviral medications when appropriate can decrease the risks of influenza in pregnancy by reducing the likelihood of acquiring infection and ameliorating its effects.

Vaccination

- Getting a flu shot is the first and most important step in protecting against flu.
- Studies in young healthy adults show that getting a flu shot reduces the risk of illness by 40–60 per cent during seasons when the flu vaccine is well matched to circulating viruses.
- There are also studies that show that a baby whose mother was vaccinated during her pregnancy is protected from flu infection for several months after they are born, until the baby is old enough to be vaccinated.
- For pregnant women, the inactivated influenza vaccine (IIV) or the recombinant influenza vaccine (RIV) can be given.
- The nasal spray flu vaccine (live attenuated influenza vaccine or LAIV) should not be used.
- The CDC and US Advisory Committee on Immunization Practices (ACIP) recommend that pregnant women be vaccinated during any trimester of their pregnancy.

- The efficacy and safety of flu vaccination for pregnant women have been proven over many years and after use with millions of women.
- Immunogenicity and efficacy data from the 2009–10 influenza A (H1N1) pandemic were very similar among pregnant women when compared to seasonal influenza vaccination.

Good Health Habits

To prevent transmission, people are advised to:

- Cover their mouth and nose when coughing/sneezing
- Wash their hands regularly
- Avoid close contact with people who are sick

People who are sick are advised to:

- Keep their distance from others
- Stay at home
- Avoid touching other people's eyes, nose or mouth[15]

Avian Influenza Transmission

- Infected birds shed avian influenza virus in their saliva, mucus and faeces.
- Avian influenza A viruses usually do not infect people, but rare cases of human infection with these viruses have been reported.
- The spread of avian (bird) influenza from one ill person to another is very rare.

Preventing Human Infection with Avian Influenza A Viruses

- Avoid close contact with sources of exposure (infected poultry).
- Those with close contact with infected birds may be given influenza antiviral drugs, which are 70–90 per cent effective.[16]

Conclusion

Influenza is an important cause of morbidity and mortality for pregnant women. Vaccination and early antiviral therapy are the cornerstones for prevention and management.

References

1. World Health Organization. Influenza (Seasonal). Fact sheet. Reviewed January 2018. www.who.int/mediacentre/factsheets/fs211/en/.

2. Centers for Disease Control and Prevention. Key Facts about Seasonal Flu Vaccine. www.cdc.gov/flu/protect/keyfacts.htm.

3. Centers for Disease Control and Prevention. Diagnosing Flu. www.cdc.gov/flu/about/qa/testing.htm.

4. Influenza info for Health Professionals. The University of Auckland Advisory Center. www.influenza.org.nz/impact-influenza-infection-during-pregnancy.

5. Yudin MH. Risk management of seasonal influenza during pregnancy: current perspectives. *Int J Women's Health.* 2014; **6**: 681–9.

6. Harris JW. Influenza occurring in pregnant women: a statistical study of thirteen hundred and fifty cases. *JAMA.* 1919; **72**: 978–80.

7. Freeman DW, Barno A. Deaths from Asian influenza associated with pregnancy. *Am J Obstet Gynecol.* 1959; **78**: 1172–5.

8. Mosby LG, Rasmussen SA, Jamieson DJ. 2009 pandemic influenza A (H1N1) in pregnancy: a systematic review of the literature. *Am J Obstet Gynecol.* 2011; **205**(1): 10–18.

9. McNeil SA, Dodds LA, Fell et al. Effect of respiratory hospitalization during pregnancy on infant outcomes. *Am J Obstet Gynecol.* 2011; **204**(6 suppl 1): S54–7.

10. Pierce M, Kurinczuk JJ, Spark P, Brocklehurst P, Knight M. Perinatal outcomes after maternal 2009/H1N1 infection: national cohort study, UKOSS. *BMJ.* 2011; **342**: d3214.

11. Centers for Disease Control and Prevention. Pregnant Women & Influenza (Flu). www.cdc.gov/flu/protect/vaccine/pregnant.htm.

12. Aoki FY, Allen UD, Stiver HG, Evans GA. The use of antiviral drugs for influenza: guidance for practitioners 2012/2013. *Can J Infect Dis Med Microbiol.* 2012; **23**(4): e79–92.

13. US Food and Drug Administration. Treatment of Influenza During Pregnancy. www.fda.gov/drugs/drugsafety/informationbydrugclass/ucm184917.htm.

14. Xie HY, Yasseen AS, Xie RH et al. Infant outcomes among pregnant women who used oseltamivir for treatment of influenza during the H1N1 epidemic. *Am J Obstet Gynecol.* 2013; **208**(4): 293.e1–7.

15. Centers for Disease Control and Prevention. Preventing the Flu: Good Health Habits Can Help Stop Germs. www.cdc.gov/flu/protect/habits.htm.

16. Centers for Disease Control and Prevention. Avian Influenza A Virus Infections in Humans. www.cdc.gov/flu/avianflu/avian-in-humans.htm.

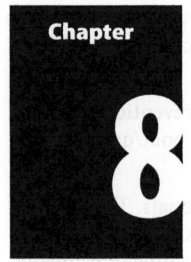

Cytomegalovirus

Tarek El Shamy

Introduction

Cytomegalovirus (CMV) is a double-stranded DNA virus and is a member of the *Herpesviridae* family.[1]

For women of reproductive age, the greatest risk for exposure is through contact with the urine or saliva of young children.[1]

Routes of Transmission of Maternal Infection

CMV-infected individuals shed the virus in body fluids, such as urine, saliva, blood, tears, semen and breastmilk. CMV is spread from an infected person in the following ways:

- From direct contact with urine or saliva, especially from babies and young children
- Through sexual contact
- From breastmilk
- Through transplanted organs and blood transfusions[1]

Prevalence

In developed countries:

- Up to 70 per cent of the population are infected.
- In the United States, over 50 per cent of adults by age 40 have been infected with CMV.
- The prevalence of congenital CMV infection has been reported to vary from approximately 0.2 per cent to 2 per cent.[2]

In developing countries:

- Over 90 per cent of people are ultimately infected.
- The congenital CMV birth rates ranged from 0.6 per cent to 6.1 per cent (systematic review of 11 population-based studies).[3] [EL 1]

Signs and Symptoms of Maternal Cytomegalovirus

Most people are asymptomatic. But if symptoms occur:

- Fever
- Night sweats
- Tiredness and uneasiness
- Sore throat
- Swollen glands
- Joint and muscle pain
- Low appetite and weight loss

Above symptoms will generally disappear after two weeks.

Complications of Maternal Cytomegalovirus Infection

- Pneumonia with hypoxemia, or low blood oxygen
- Mouth ulcers that can be large
- Problems with vision, including floaters, blind spots and blurred vision
- Hepatitis
- Encephalitis
- CMV is the leading cause for non-hereditary sensorineural hearing loss (SNHL)

Types of Maternal Infection during Pregnancy

- A new first-time infection during the pregnancy
- A reinfection with a different CMV strain
- A reactivation of a previous infection

Primary Maternal Infection

Primary maternal CMV infection during pregnancy usually occurs following contact with infected bodily fluids such as urine or saliva, especially from young children.[2] Infection can be also acquired through sexual contact, transfusion of blood and blood products, whereas airborne infection is unlikely.

After a primary CMV infection, the virus remains dormant but reactivation and viral shedding is common. Reinfection with a different strain of the virus has also been reported.[3]

Primary maternal infection is responsible for 25 per cent of congenital CMV infections in the United States.[2]

Clinical Picture of Primary Maternal Infection

Ninety per cent of women with primary CMV infection are asymptomatic.

Symptomatic group may present with non-specific symptoms (fever, headache, pharyngitis, myalgia, arthralgia and fatigue).

Reactivation or reinfection with a different strain passes without clinical manifestations.

Diagnosis of Maternal Cytomegalovirus Infection

History

The majority of primary HCMV infections in immunocompetent individuals are clinically asymptomatic.

Fewer than 5 per cent of pregnant women with primary infection are reported to have symptoms.

However, careful clinical history may be extremely useful for detecting minor clinical symptoms and dating the onset of infection.

In a survey involving 244 pregnant women with primary HCMV infection, clinical symptoms were present in 166 (68.1%), with fever (60.2%), fatigue (48.8%) and headache (26.5%) being the most frequent symptoms.[4] [EL 2]

Immune Responses

- *Immunoglobin M (IgM)*
  - o CMV-specific IgM antibodies are produced during the primary infection and persist for three or four months.
  - o However, immunocompromised individuals may fail to produce IgM with primary infection. The presence of CMV IgM cannot be used by itself to time the infection or diagnose primary

CMV infection because IgM can also be present during secondary CMV infection, which includes reinfection with a different strain or reactivation of latent CMV acquired in the past.
  - o IgM-positive results in combination with low immunoglobin G (IgG) avidity results are considered reliable evidence for primary infection.

- *Immunoglobulin G (IgG)*
  - o Measurement of CMV IgG in paired samples taken one to three months apart can be used to diagnose primary infection.
  - o Seroconversion (first sample IgG negative, second sample IgG positive) is clear evidence for recent primary infection.[4]
  - o Specific IgG of low avidity is an excellent single serum indicating recent primary infection within the last three months.[5]

Viral Isolation, Detection of Virus and Viral Products in Maternal Blood

- CMV can be recovered from multiple body fluids such as saliva, urine and vaginal secretions for a variable period.
- The isolation of the virus from these sites confirms infection, but will not differentiate between a new primary or recurrent infection.
- However, virus detection in blood has been reported to be diagnostic of primary CMV infection in immunocompetent individuals.

Diagnosis of Recurrent Maternal CMV Infection

Recurrent infection occurs when the initial CMV infection reactivates during pregnancy or due to a different CMV strain.[4]

IgG avidity describes the proportion of IgG bound to the antigen following treatment with denaturing agents.

A high IgG avidity index of 70 CMV at 6–18 weeks' gestation can identify all women who would have an infected fetus/newborn (100 per cent sensitivity).[5]

Congenital CMV Infection

In about 30 per cent of cases, congenital infection passes from mother to baby when a previous latent CMV reactivates during pregnancy.

Only about 1–7 per cent of women are infected for the first time with CMV (primary CMV) during pregnancy; 30–40 per cent of those with primary infection will pass it on to the baby.[6]

About 10–15 per cent of babies with congenital infection will have symptoms at birth; up to 60 per cent of these will have serious complications later in life.

Fetal Implications of Congenital CMV

- Miscarriage
- Growth restriction
- Intrauterine death
- Microcephaly
- Hepatosplenomegaly[6]

Mother-to-Child Transmission

During pregnancy, mother-to-child transmission occurs predominantly via transplacental transfer. The virus is then transmitted to the fetus, where the virus is replicated in multiple tissues.

Ascending infection from the maternal genital tract is thought to be rare but possible antepartum.

Perinatal transmission can also occur through ingestion or aspiration of cervico-vaginal secretions at delivery or ingestion of breastmilk post-delivery.

Term infants (with no underlying immunodeficiency) who acquire CMV infection from breastmilk do not develop clinical sequelae from the infection.

Third trimester primary infection seems to be associated with a high fetal transmission rate, but the outcomes are favourable for the infant.[7,8] [EL 1–]

The transmission rates vary from 14.2 to 52.4 per cent and are significantly related to gestational age at the time of maternal infection (34.8, 42 and 58.6 per cent at first, second and third trimester infection, respectively).[9]

Most congenital CMV infections (75–90 per cent) are asymptomatic at birth.

About 10–25 per cent of these infants will develop neurological sequelae such as sensorineural hearing loss, delayed psychomotor development and visual impairment.

Approximately 5–20 per cent of infants born to mothers with primary CMV are overtly symptomatic, with intrauterine growth restriction, microcephaly, hepatosplenomegaly, petechia, jaundice, chorioretinitis,

thrombocytopenia, seizures or anaemia. Thirty per cent of these infants may die.

Diagnosis of Fetal Congenital Infection

Imaging

Ultrasound, and magnetic resonance imaging (MRI) can be used for the diagnosis of fetal CMV infection sequel.

The spectrum of imaging findings varies widely. Findings include:

- Intrauterine growth retardation
- Hydrops or ascites
- Fetal intracranial calcification: mainly periventricular calcification (hyperechogenic foci)
- Fetal hydrocephalus
- Heterogeneous appearing parenchyma
- Microcephaly
- Intraventricular adhesions
- Intra-hepatic calcification
- Hepatomegaly
- Echogenic bowel

These findings may indicate CMV infection and are also an indication for invasive testing after proper counselling of the parents.[10]

Invasive Testing

- Fetal blood (cordocentesis) can be used for both determination of CMV-specific IgM antibody and quantification of viral load.[11]
- Diagnosis of fetal infection by testing for fetal IgM via cordocentesis is not currently recommended because of the associated risks. CMV-infected fetuses do not develop specific IgM until late in pregnancy, resulting in poor sensitivity.
- Amniotic fluid can be tested for isolation of the virus (polymerase chain reaction (PCR) technique for CMV DNA detection).
- In a study of 242 women by Enders et al., a sensitivity of 100 per cent was achieved by combining detection of CMV-DNA and CMV-specific IgM in fetal blood or by combined testing of AF and fetal blood for CMV-DNA or IgM antibodies.[11] [EL 2]

Prenatal Therapy

There is currently no proven effective therapy for congenital CMV. Thus parents are faced with the difficult choice of whether to terminate the pregnancy once congenital fetal CMV infection is confirmed.

Antiviral Drugs

Ganciclovir, valganciclovir, cidofovir, foscarnet and valaciclovir antiviral agents are of moderate effectiveness in treating CMV infection in the adult, particularly the immunocompromised patient, and have no proven value in preventing or treating congenital CMV infection.

With the exception of valaciclovir, their teratogenic and toxic effects preclude their use in pregnancy.[12]

Recently published results of a phase II, multicentre, open-label study that evaluated the efficacy of high-dose oral valaciclovir (8 g daily) in pregnant women carrying a moderately CMV-infected fetus showed encouraging results. However, with the limitation in the study (the sample size and the study design), this therapeutic option should be further investigated before antiviral therapy may be considered in pregnant women.[13,14]

Hyperimmuno Globulin (HIG)

Given the conflicting results of different studies, HIG is not currently routinely recommended for the treatment of women with primary CMV infection in pregnancy, and should be reserved for use in the research setting.

In case of primary infection, HIG may help if

- The infection occurred up to 14 weeks
- It is a very recent primary infection
- Treatment starts as soon as possible

Vaccination

There are no available vaccines yet.

Treatment of the Newborn

Congenital CMV should be confirmed at birth (e.g. urine or oral swab for CMV PCR within three weeks of birth).

Treatment of congenital CMV infection is indicated when there is evidence of central nervous system (CNS) involvement, or if there is serious end-organ disease (hepatitis, pneumonia and thrombocytopenia).

Ganciclovir is the cornerstone of antiviral therapy in newborn babies with congenital CMV infection.

Ganciclovir is well tolerated in the newborn and has proven its safety and efficacy.[15] [EL 1] It is useful in the management of severe, focal, end-organ disease in infants.

In a randomised control trial, ganciclovir showed long-term neurodevelopmental benefit for some infants with congenital CMV infection.[16] [EL 1]

However, it is important to note that once therapy is completed, infants resume excretion of CMV in urine and saliva.

Treatment should be started in the first month of life.

Six weeks of intravenous ganciclovir therapy is recommended. Infants need to be closely observed for toxicity, especially neutropenia.

Use of antivirals for treating babies with congenital CMV infection who have no signs at birth is not currently recommended.

Delivery and Breastfeeding

CMV infection is not a contraindication for vaginal delivery, and caesarean section should be reserved for obstetric indication.

Although CMV infection can be acquired by consumption of breastmilk of the infected mother, there have been no reports of long-term sequelae. Following delivery, the newborn should have thorough assessment and the developmental milestones should be monitored, especially hearing.[17]

Screening for Congenital Cytomegalovirus (CMV)

Routine CMV screening does not meet several of the criteria for an effective screening test. Specifically, until now there has been no effective treatment during pregnancy.

Consequently, routine prenatal screening is not recommended outside the research setting.

The UK National Screening Committee (UK NSC), the American College of Obstetricians and Gynecologists (ACOG) and the Centers for Disease Control and Prevention (CDC) do not recommend routine maternal screening for CMV.

However, serological testing for CMV is offered to women who:

- Have developed influenza-like symptoms, or symptoms of glandular fever (with negative test results for Epstein–Barr virus) or of hepatitis (with negative test results for hepatitis A, B and C) during pregnancy
- Or in whom routine ultrasound detects fetal abnormalities suggestive of possible CMV infection, such as ventriculomegaly, microcephaly, calcifications, intraventricular synechiae, intracranial haemorrhage, periventricular cysts, cerebellar hypoplasia, cortical abnormalities, echogenic bowel, small for gestational age, pericardial effusion, ascites and fetal hydrops[18]

Preventive Measures

As there is no licensed vaccine yet, the only available prevention is simple hygiene-based measures:

- Hand washing after contact with urine or saliva
- Avoiding sharing utensils, drinks or food with young children
- Pregnant women working with young children (e.g. in daycare units) should be educated regarding increased risk of CMV infection and its effects on the unborn child
- Pregnant women requiring blood transfusion should be transfused with blood from CMV seronegative donors

Conclusion

CMV is the most common viral infection that leads to serious neonatal and long-term sequelae including congenital sensorineural deafness, neurodevelopmental delay and first trimester infection. Prenatal sonographic findings are associated with increased risk of long-term disability.

New primary maternal infection presents the greatest risk of transmission and severity.

Major advances in the availability of the IgG avidity test facilitate the diagnosis of primary infection. Fetal infection may be confirmed with amniocentesis or cordocentesis.

Ganciclovir is the cornerstone of antiviral therapy in newborn babies with congenital CMV infection.

Based on current evidence, neither the Royal College of Obstetricians and Gynaecologists (UK) nor the National Collaborative Centre for Women's and Children Health (UK) recommends routine CMV screening for pregnant women.

Prevention of infection still remains the cornerstone to avoid the sequelsae of congenital CMV infection.

References

1. virology-online.com/viruses/CMV.htm.

2. Kenneson A, Cannon MJ. Review and meta-analysis of the epidemiology of congenital cytomegalovirus (CMV) infection. *Rev Med Virol.* 2007; **17**(4): 253–76.

3. Lanzieri TM, Dollard SC, Bialek SR, Grosse SD. Systematic review of the birth prevalence of congenital cytomegalovirus infection in developing countries. Int *J Infect Dis.* 2014; **22**: 44–8.

4. Revello MG, Gerna G. Diagnosis and management of human cytomegalovirus infection in the mother, fetus, and newborn infant. *Clin Microbiol Rev.* 2002; **15**(4): 680–715.

5. Lazzarotto T, Varani S, Spezzacatena P et al. Maternal IgG avidity and IgM detected by blot as diagnostic tools to identify pregnant women at risk of transmitting cytomegalovirus. *Viral Immunology.* 2009, **13**(1): 137–41.

6. Stagno S, Pass RF, Cloud G et al. Primary cytomegalovirus infection in pregnancy: incidence, transmission to fetus, and clinical outcome. *JAMA.* 1986; **256**: 1904–8.

7. Schleiss MR. Role of breast milk in acquisition of cytomegalovirus infection: recent advances. *Curr Opin Pediatr.* 2006; **18**: 48–52.

8. Feldman B, Yinon Y, Tepperberg M, Yoeli R, Schiff E, Lipitz S. Pregestational, periconceptional, and gestational primary maternal cytomegalovirus infection: prenatal diagnosis in 508 pregnancies. *Am J Obstet Gynecol.* 2011; **205**: e1–6.

9. Enders G, Daiminger A, Bäder U, Exler S, Enders M. Intrauterine transmission and clinical outcome of 248 pregnancies with primary cytomegalovirus infection in relation to gestational age. *J Clin Virol.* 2011; **52**: 244–6.

10. Di Muzio B. Congenital cytomegalovirus infection results from intra-uterine fetal infection by cytomegalovirus (CMV). Radiopaedia. https://radiopaedia.org/articles/congenital-cytomegalovirus-infection.

11. Enders G, Bäder U, Lindemann L, Schalasta S, Daiminger A. Prenatal diagnosis of congenital cytomegalovirus infection in 189 pregnancies with known outcome. *Prenatal Diagnosis.* 2001; **21**(7): 605.

12. Duff P. Diagnosis and management of CMV infection in pregnancy. *Perinatology.* 2010; **1**: 1–6.

13. Marsico C, Kimberlin DW. Congenital cytomegalovirus infection: advances and challenges in diagnosis, prevention and treatment. *Ital J Pediatr.* 2017; **43**: 38.

14. RCOG Scientific Impact Paper No. 56. Congenital Cytomegalovirus Infection: Update on Treatment. First published 15 November 2017.

15. Kimberlin DW, Lin CY, Sánchez PJ et al. Effect of ganciclovir therapy on hearing in symptomatic congenital cytomegalovirus disease involving the central nervous system: a randomized, controlled trial. *J Pediatr.* 2003; **143**(1): 16–25.

16. Swanson E, Schleiss MR. Congenital cytomegalovirus infection: new prospects for prevention and therapy. *Pediatr Clin North Am.* 2013; **60**(2): 335–49.

17. Navti O, Hughes BL Tang JW, Konje J. Comprehensive review and update of cytomegalovirus infection in pregnancy. *The Obstetrician & Gynaecologist.* http://onlinetog.org. 2016.

18. Centers for Disease Control and Prevention. Babies Born with Congenital CMV Infection. www.cdc.gov/cmv/congenital-infection.html.

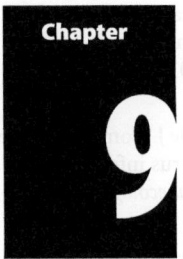

Chapter

9

Dengue Fever

Adel Elkady, Prabha Sinha and Soad Ali Zaki Hassan

Dengue fever is a mosquito-transmitted viral infection. It is common in most tropical and subtropical countries.

Approximately 390 million dengue virus infections occur each year, of which 500 000 require hospitalisation.[1]

The *Aedes aegypti* mosquito is the primary host of dengue.

The virus is transmitted to humans through the bites of infected female mosquitoes of the species *Aedes aegypti*. This vector can also transmit other infections (chikungunya, yellow fever and Zika infection).[1]

The virus has an incubation period of 4–10 days.

An infected mosquito can transmit the virus for the rest of its life.

Severe dengue (also known as dengue haemorrhagic fever) was first recognised in the 1950s during dengue epidemics in the Philippines and Thailand.

Today, severe dengue is one of the leading causes of hospitalisation and death among children and adults in these regions.

There are four distinct, closely related, serotypes of the virus that cause dengue (DEN-1, DEN-2, DEN-3 and DEN-4). Recovery from infection by one provides lifelong immunity against that particular serotype. Cross-immunity to the other serotypes after recovery is only partial and temporary.

Further infections by other serotypes increase the risk of developing severe dengue.[2]

Transmission

Infected symptomatic or asymptomatic humans are the main carriers as the virus multiplies, serving as a source of the virus for uninfected mosquitoes.

Patients who are already infected with the dengue virus can transmit the infection (for 4–5 days; maximum 12) via *Aedes* mosquitoes after their first symptoms appear.

Signs and Symptoms

Symptomatic patients show:

- High fever (40°C)
- Severe headache
- Pain behind the eyes
- Muscle and joint pains
- Nausea and vomiting
- Swollen glands
- Rash

Complications

Severe dengue is potentially deadly due to:

- Plasma leaking
- Fluid accumulation
- Respiratory distress
- Severe bleeding because of thrombocytopenia
- Organ impairment

Warning Signs of Death

- Decrease in temperature (below 38°C/100°F)
- Severe abdominal pain
- Persistent vomiting, with blood in the vomitus
- Rapid breathing
- Bleeding gums, fatigue
- Restlessness

Death follows quickly in the next 24–48 hours unless proper medical care is immediately offered.

Prompt medical care should be offered as soon as possible to avoid death.

Maternal Implications

- Pre-eclampsia
- Thrombocytopenia
- Increased caesarean section rate

In a retrospective analysis of 2738 deliveries, 14 cases were diagnosed with dengue fever. The commonest complication was haemorrhagic fever and thrombocytopenia (21 per cent). The same review suggested conservative management, but platelet transfusion was indicated in cases of severe thrombocytopenia (<20 000), if there were haemorrhagic complications or there was an operative delivery.[3] [EL 1−]

A systemic review of 30 published studies (19 case reports, 9 case series and 2 comparison studies), among women with dengue infection during pregnancy, showed high rates of caesarean deliveries (44.0 per cent) and pre-eclampsia (12.0 per cent).[4] [EL 1−]

The rate of vertical transmission varies between 18.5 and 22.7 per cent depending on the calculation method used and the stage of pregnancy, as it is more frequent when maternal dengue occurs late during pregnancy. [EL 1]

Fetal Implications

Fetal implications are preterm birth and low birthweight.

A retrospective study by Friedman et al. published in 2014, including 86 exposed infants whose mothers had a laboratory-confirmed case of symptomatic dengue fever, detected increased risks for low birthweight (odds ratio 2.06–2.23) as well as preterm birth (odds ratio 1.9–3.34).

The infants who had low birthweight were also likely to be preterm, suggesting that these infants were low birthweight because of shorter duration of gestation, rather than impaired fetal growth *in utero*.[5] [EL 2]

Maternal Treatment

There is no specific treatment for dengue fever.

Maintenance of the patient's body fluid volume is critical to severe dengue care.

Medical care by physicians and nurses with experience of the effects and progression of the disease can save lives, decreasing mortality rates from more than 20 per cent to less than 1 per cent.

Fetal Therapy

There is no known *in utero* treatment; however, the disease does not seem to cause any congenital abnormalities, and supernova care (a team for dedicated, personalised, professional and patient-centred health care) seems to prevent preterm birth.

Immunisation

In late 2015 and early 2016, the first dengue vaccine, Dengvaxia (CYD-TDV) by Sanofi Pasteur, was registered in several countries for use in individuals 9–45 years of age living in endemic areas.

The World Health Organization recommends that countries should consider introduction of the dengue vaccine CYD-TDV only in geographic settings where epidemiological data indicate a high burden of disease.

Prevention and Control

Currently, the main prevention is to combat vector mosquitoes through:

- Preventing mosquitoes from accessing egg-laying habitats
- Disposing of solid waste properly
- Applying appropriate insecticides to water storage outdoor containers
- Using personal household protection such as window screens, long-sleeved clothes, insecticide-treated materials, coils and vaporisers
- Spraying of insecticides during outbreaks as one of the emergency vector-control measures
- Clinical detection and management of dengue patients to reduce mortality rates from severe dengue[6]

Conclusion

Dengue fever is a viral infection. The main complication is thrombocytopenia.

In pregnant women it causes pre-eclampsia, increased caesarean section rates, prematurity and low birthweight.

With prompt treatment of severe cases, mortality can be reduced to 1 per cent.

References

1. Bhatt S, Gething PW, Brady OJ et al. The global distribution and burden of dengue. *Nature*. 2013; **496**: 504–7.

2. World Health Organization. Dengue and severe dengue. 2 February 2018. www.who.int/en/news-room/fact-sheets/detail/dengue-and-severe-dengue.

3. Chitra TV, Panicker S. Maternal and fetal outcome of dengue fever in pregnancy. *J Vector Borne Dis.* 2011; **48**: 210–13.

4. Pouliot SH, Xiong X, Harville E et al. Maternal dengue and pregnancy outcomes: a systematic review. *Obstet Gynecol Surv.* 2010; **65**(2): 107–18.

5. Friedman EE, Dallah F, Harville EW et al. Symptomatic dengue infection during pregnancy and infant outcomes: a retrospective cohort study. *PLoS Negl Trop Dis.* 2014; **8**(10): e3226.

6. Centers for Disease Control and Prevention. Dengue fever. Prevention. www.cdc.gov/dengue/prevention/index.html.

Rubella

Rania Hassan Mostafa Ahmed

Introduction

Rubella is an acute viral illness with characteristic maculopapular rash and low-grade fever.

Up to 50 per cent of cases may pass unnoticed without any symptoms. The disease occurs more commonly in young children.

The most devastating consequence occurs when rubella infects a pregnant female early during the period of embryogenesis, with serious multiple birth defects, known as congenital rubella syndrome (CRS).

Microbiology and Transmission/ Epidemiology

Rubella virus is an enveloped positive-stranded RNA virus, belonging to the *Togaviridae* family.[1]

The virus is directly transmitted by direct or droplet contact from nasopharyngeal secretions.[2]

The virus replicates in the respiratory mucosa and cervical lymph nodes, before reaching the target organs via systemic circulation.

The average incubation period is 17 days (range: 12–23 days).

Rubella is most infectious when the rash is erupting; however, the infectious period extends from seven days before to seven days after rash onset.

Maternal viraemia may occur five to seven days after exposure, when the virus spreads throughout the body, with transplacental transfer and infection of the fetus also occurring.

Before the availability of rubella vaccines, rubella was a common disease occurring primarily among young children.

Incidence was highest during the spring, with epidemics every six to nine years.

Clinical Picture[3]

- Low-grade fever
- Mild, maculopapular rash

The rash occurs in 50–80 per cent of cases, characteristically starting on the face, then becoming generalised within 24 hours, and lasting for about three days.

- Lymphadenopathy

  Lymphadenopathy may precede rash, and often involves posterior auricular or suboccipital lymph nodes, but can be generalised, and lasts from five to eight days.

- Arthritis/arthralgia

  Adults, more commonly women, may develop arthritis/arthralgia that usually lasts 3–10 days.[4]

- Thrombocytopenia is a rare sign
- Neurological disorders are also a rare occurrence
- About 25–50 per cent of infections are asymptomatic

The following case definition for rubella was approved by the Council of State and Territorial Epidemiologists (CSTE) in 2012:

Suspected: Any generalized rash illness of acute onset that does not meet the criteria for probable or confirmed rubella or any other illness.

Probable: In the absence of a more likely diagnosis, an illness characterized by all of the following:

- acute onset of generalized maculopapular rash; and
- temperature greater than 99.0°F or 37.2°C, if measured; and
- arthralgia, arthritis, lymphadenopathy, or conjunctivitis; and
- lack of epidemiologic linkage to a laboratory-confirmed case of rubella; and
- Non-contributory or no serologic or virologic testing.

Confirmed: A case with or without symptoms who has laboratory evidence of rubella infection confirmed by one or more of the following:

- isolation of rubella virus; or
- detection of rubella-virus specific nucleic acid by reverse transcriptase–polymerase chain reaction (RT-PCR); or
- significant rise between acute- and convalescent-phase titres in serum rubella IgG antibody level by any standard serologic assay; or
- positive serologic test for rubella IgM antibody (not explained by MMR vaccination during the previous 6–45 days, and not otherwise ruled out by more specific testing in a public health laboratory)

OR

An illness characterized by all of the following:

- Acute onset of generalized maculopapular rash; and
- Temperature greater than 99.0°F or 37.2°C; and
- Arthralgia, arthritis, lymphadenopathy, or conjunctivitis; and
- Epidemiologic linkage to a laboratory-confirmed case of rubella.'

Diagnosis of Maternal Infection[5]

ELISA Serologic Testing

Enzyme-linked immunoassay (ELISA) serologic testing for IgM/IgG antibodies is the mainstay of laboratory diagnosis.

It is best carried out within 7–10 days after the onset of the rash or a history of exposure and should be repeated two to three weeks later.

IgM

- Rubella virus immunoglobulin M (RV-IgM) appears within three days after the rash and generally disappear in 4–12 weeks.

IgG

- Rubella virus immunoglobulin G (RV-IgG) detected by ELISA appear slightly later (five to eight days after the onset of the rash) and persists throughout life.
- RV-IgG reaches a steady state at any time from a few days to a few weeks.
- The maximal and residual RV-IgG rates are extremely variable, depending on the patient tested and the assay used.
- A high RV-IgG titre is not necessarily a marker of a recent primary infection.

The Presence of a Rubella Infection is Confirmed By:

- A positive serologic test for rubella-specific IgM, which indicates recent infection
- A four-fold rise in rubella IgG antibody titre between acute and convalescent serum specimens, which also indicates recent infection
- High IgG titres (10 IU/mL or greater) indicate old infection and probable immunity
- A high IgG avidity index indicates old infection and possible immunity.

Isolation of rubella virus in nasopharyngeal secretions by RT-PCR.

This relies on a positive culture of the rubella virus in a clinical specimen from the patient (nasopharyngeal secretions).

Complications

- Arthralgia or arthritis may complicate up to 70 per cent of adult women with rubella
- Thrombocytopenic purpura
- Encephalitis
- Guillain–Barré syndrome (a disorder in which the body's immune system attacks part of the peripheral nervous system). Symptoms include varying degrees of weakness or tingling sensations in the legs. Symmetrical weakness and abnormal sensations spreading to the arms and upper body may occur in rare cases

Fetal Implications[6]

Rubella easily crosses the placenta of infected pregnant women.

Rubella infection during pregnancy carries substantial risks to the fetus, especially during the first trimester:

- Miscarriages
- Fetal deaths/stillbirths
- Severe birth defects; what is known as congenital rubella syndrome (CRS)

Congenital Rubella Syndrome (CRS)[7]

The risk of fetal infection and/or fetal damage is mainly related to the timing of maternal infection.

Infection During the First 8–10 Weeks

Maternal infection occurring in the first 8–10 weeks of pregnancy causes fetal damage in up to 90 per cent of affected pregnancies, usually with multiple defects.

Infection during the 11th to 16th Weeks

The risk of damage reduces to 10–20 per cent.

Infection Occuring During 16–20 Weeks

The risk has on rare occasions been reported after 20 weeks, with sensorineural deafness being the prominent abnormality in the second trimester.

- Maternal rubella infection early during the period of embryogenesis leads to congenital rubella syndrome associated with:
  - Ophthalmic abnormalities (microphthalmia, cataracts and retinopathy)
  - Cardiac abnormalities (patent ductus arteriosus and pulmonary artery hypoplasia)
  - Auditory impairment (sensorineural deafness)
  - Central nervous system manifestations (mental or psychomotor retardation and language delay)
  - Thrombocytopenic purpura
  - Hemolytic anaemia
  - Hepatosplenomegaly
  - Meningoencephalitis

Prenatal Diagnosis of Fetal Infection [8,9]

A prenatal diagnosis of congenital infection is recommended when a maternal infection is diagnosed or suspected.

Prenatal diagnosis is based on the detection of RV-IgM in fetal blood or on the detection of the viral genome in amniotic fluid (AF), fetal blood or chorionic villus biopsies.

Postnatal Diagnosis of Congenital Infection

Congenital infection is diagnosed postnatally by the detection of a specific RV-IgM by immunocapture ELISA, with sensitivity and specificity that approach 100 per cent.

If the RV-IgM test is positive, a congenital infection might be confirmed by isolating the rubella virus or by detecting the viral genome in nasopharyngeal swabs, urine and oral fluid using RT-PCR.

Confirming postnatal diagnosis of a congenital infection is important, to provide a specific follow-up plan if an infection is discovered (including neurological and hearing monitoring).

Prevention/Vaccination

Prevention of congenital infection from rubella is the major goal of rubella vaccination.

The rubella virus was isolated in 1961, and vaccines were developed in 1969 – the shortest time period from virus identification to vaccine ever.

The World Health Organization (WHO) recommends all countries that have not yet introduced rubella vaccine to consider doing so, making use of existing, well-established measles immunisation programmes.

In 2015, the WHO Region of the Americas became the first in the world to be declared free of endemic transmission of rubella.

The vaccine is a live attenuated strain, giving long-lasting immunity similar to that induced by natural infection.[5] It is primarily administered as the combined measles, mumps, rubella (MMR) vaccine.

Because it is a live attenuated vaccine, and to avoid any teratogenic risk, it is not recommended during pregnancy. Accordingly, also pregnancy should be avoided for 28 days following vaccination.

However, this risk is not yet clinically proven, and several studies have reported absence of CRS after inadvertent vaccination during pregnancy.[10]

Vaccination side effects (febrile seizures, anaphylaxis, thrombocytopenic purpura or encephalitis) are very rare.

Screening

- *Non-pregnant women* of childbearing age should be routinely assessed for evidence of immunity, and if none is found they should be immunised.
- *Pregnant women* who lack evidence of immunity should receive the first dose of MMR immediately postpartum before discharge from the health care facility, with the second dose four weeks after that.

Fetal Ultrasound Findings[11]

The most common ultrasound abnormalities:

- Cardiac (septal defects)
- Ocular (cataracts and microphthalmia) defects
- Microcephaly
- Hepatomegaly, splenomegaly

- Intrauterine growth retardation

No studies have been done that have determined the frequency of occurrence of these abnormalities.

A preliminary study that analysed the role of ultrasonography (USG) for the prenatal diagnosis of congenital infection defined the specificity of USG at 100 per cent and the sensitivity at 11 per cent. However, this was a small series.

Management

Management of rubella infection in pregnancy depends mainly on the gestational age at time of infection.

- Infection before18 weeks: high probability of fetal damage and major defects, hence termination of pregnancy could be offered in accordance with local rules and regulations.
- Infection after 18 weeks has no great risk of congenital rubella syndrome and no intervention is required.

Infant management: (adopted from South Australian Perinatal Practice Guidelines). [EL 2 & 3]

- All personnel caring for the newborn should have received rubella vaccination.
- The newborn must be assessed by the paediatrician at delivery including: physical examination for evidence of congenital rubella syndrome (growth restricted, eye/cardiac abnormalities, rash, haematological abnormalities, pneumonitis, osteitis).
- Neonatal investigations (cord blood IgM serology; maternal blood for IgG, IgM serology; rubella PCR and culture from urine, pharyngeal and conjunctival tears) should be carried out if the woman had or was exposed to rubella infection during pregnancy.
- Breastfeeding is *not* contraindicated.

Conclusion

Rubella virus infection of a pregnant mother in the first 1–18 weeks of pregnancy leads to serious fetal and congenital health sequelae.

There has been significant progress in preventing CRS since the discovery of the teratogenic potential of the rubella virus in 1941, and the introduction of vaccination in 1996.

The significance of IgM in the diagnosis of acute infection has been partially established in the diagnosis of maternal infection.

The measurement of RV-IgG avidity helps to differentiate recent from old infection.

Prenatal diagnoses of fetal infection performed by RT-PCR on AF are very reliable.

In developing countries, increased rates of vaccination are necessary.

References

1. Weinberg J, Brownlee J. Rubella Virus. Infectious Disease Advisor. www.infectiousdiseaseadvisor.com/infectious-diseases/rubella-virus/article/609681/.

2. Centers for Disease Control and Prevention. Rubella (German Measles, Three-Day Measles). www.cdc.gov/rubella/lab/serology.html.

3. South Australian Maternal & Neonatal Clinical Network. South Australian Perinatal Practice Guidelines – Rubella infection in pregnancy. Last revised: September 2015. www.sahealth.sa.gov.au/wps/wcm/connect/d81813804eedb835b2b8b36a7ac0d6e4/.

4. WHO – Rubella fact sheet. http://origin.who.int/mediacentre/factsheets/fs367/en/.

5. Bouthry E, Picone O, Hamdi G, Grangeot-Keros L, Ayoubi J-M, Vauloup-Fellous C. Rubella and pregnancy: diagnosis, management and outcomes. *Prenatal Diagnosis.* 2014; **34**(13): 1246–53.

6. SOGC Clinical Practice Guidelines. Rubella in Pregnancy. No. 203, February 2008. https://sogc.org/wp-content/uploads/2013/01/guiJOGC203CPG0802.pdf.

7. Toizumi M, Vo HM, Dang DA, Moriuchi H, Yoshida LM. Clinical manifestations of congenital rubella syndrome. *Vaccine.* 2019; **37**(1): 202–9.

8. Best JM, Enders G. Laboratory diagnosis of rubella and congenital rubella. *Perspect Med Virol.* 2006; **15**: 39–77.

9. Revello MG, Baldanti F, Sarasini A, Zavattoni M, Torsellini M, Gerna G. Prenatal diagnosis of rubella virus infection by direct detection and semiquantitation of viral RNA in clinical samples by reverse transcription-PCR. *J Clin Microbiol.* 1997; **35**(3): 708–13.

10. Demicheli V, Rivetti A, Debalini MG et al. Vaccines for measles, mumps and rubella in children. *Cochrane Database Syst Rev.* 2012; **2**: CD004407.

11. Migliucci A, Di Fraja D, Sarno L, Acampora E, Mazzarelli LL, Quaglia F. Prenatal diagnosis of congenital rubella infection and ultrasonography: a preliminary study. *Minerva Ginecol.* 2011; **63**: 485–9.

Molluscum Contagiosum

Adel Elkady, Prabha Sinha and Soad Ali Zaki Hassan

Molluscum contagiosum (MC) is a benign, skin infection.

It presents as pearly dome-shaped papules, with a central dell or depression. It is caused by the molluscum contagiosum virus (MCV) which is the most common poxvirus to infect humans.

Poxviruses are brick-shaped (240 nm by 300 nm) and have a complex internal structure including a double-stranded DNA genome (130–260 kb) and associated enzymes.

Poxvirus infections are characterised by the production of skin lesions. Smallpox, a poxvirus with serious consequences, has been eradicated since 1980.

Varicella or chickenpox is not the same group as the smallpox and other poxviruses. The virus has three genotypes, but the MCV genotype 1 is responsible for 98 per cent of cases of MC in the United States. The genotype MCV 2 is responsible for sexually transmitted MC, and consequently is not detected in children prior to sexual debut. Genotype 3 is also associated with congenital infection.

The genotype MCV 2 has been detected in vaginal lesion specimens.[1]

Spread of Virus and Transmission[2]

- Direct skin-to-skin contact with an infected person, maybe during play or in a swimming pool.
- Shared items, e.g. towels, shaving utensils.
- One part of a person's body to another part.
- Through sexual contact. Sexually acquired molluscum is rare in younger children, but becomes quite common during adolescence and young adulthood, after sexual debut.

Clinical Picture

- Small, skin dome-shaped bumps with dimpling in centre.
- Itching and tenderness.

- Translucent, pearly or flesh-coloured bumps that may turn grey and drain white or waxy substance.
  - Multiple lesions may occur in clusters.
  - Symptoms may last from several weeks to several years.
  - Molluscum contagiosum usually affects the face, trunk, arms and legs of children.
  - In adults, the genitals, abdomen and inner thighs are the common sites.

Congenital Molluscum Contagiosum

MC genotype MCV 2 has been detected in vaginal lesion specimens. Mother-to-child transmission is thought to occur during vaginal delivery. There have so far been few cases of congenital MC reported in the literature. In those reported cases, lesions appeared at different postnatal periods ranging from one week to three months. However, in all cases mother's MC was confirmed, indicating the possibility of congenital MC. Infants with congenital MC show the same cutaneous lesions as in the adult MC.[2]

Treatment

- Cryotherapy
- Curettage
- Laser surgery
- Topical therapy – destruction of the lesion with a variety of chemicals (e.g. liquid nitrogen, 0.7 per cent cantharidin)[3]
  - In immunocompetent people, molluscum contagiosum lesions usually go away without treatment within six months to two years.
  - In immunocompromised people, the lesions usually persist and spread indefinitely, hence treatment may be specifically indicated.

Conclusion

Molluscum contagiosum is a self-limiting skin disease caused by the molluscum contagiosum virus which is a poxvirus group. Although rare, cases of congenital molluscum contagiosum appear between 1 and 12 weeks postpartum.

It is important not to confuse this disease with chickenpox. Chickenpox is an acute viral infection affecting the skin and nerves. It is caused by the herpes zoster varicella virus, which belongs to the herpes viruses group, while the poxvirus group is a different virus strain.

References

1. Scholz J, Rosen-Wolff A, Bugert J et al. Epidemiology of Molluscum contagiosum using genetic analysis of the viral DNA. *J Med Virol*. 1989; 27: 87–90.

2. O' Connell C, Oranje A, Van Gysel D, Silverberg NB. Congenital molluscum contagiosum: report of four cases and review of the literature. *Paed Dermatol*. 2008; 25(5): 553–6.

3. Centers for Disease Control and Prevention. Molluscum contagiosum, treatment options. www.cdc.gov/pox virus/molluscum-contagiosum/treatment.html.

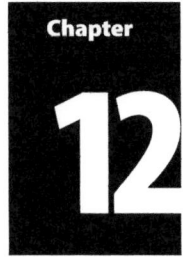

Chapter

12

Ebola

Adel Elkady, Prabha Sinha and Soad Ali Zaki Hassan

Ebola virus disease (EVD) was first recognised in 1976, when there was an outbreak of viral haemorrhagic fever near the Ebola River in Zaire (now the Democratic Republic of the Congo (DRC)) with multiple subsequent outbreaks confined to sub-Saharan Africa and spread to Europe and the USA by human transportation.[1]

Ebola disease is rare but causes severe viral haemorrhagic disease.

EVD is a filovirus infection, thought to be transmitted to humans from an unknown animal reservoir. Bats or non-human primates are suggested to be the most likely species involved in the occurrence of sporadic human outbreaks.

There are five identified species of EVD. Zaire ebolavirus is the most lethal strain.

Animal-to-human transmission is thought to be through the wild animal meat consumption. Human-to-human transmission is through mucosal contact with infected body fluids.

Incubation period is up to 21 days (median five to nine days).

EVD and Pregnancy

Maternity services have been particularly vulnerable to nosocomial Ebola infection, therefore it is important to devise a plan for management of pregnant women during an Ebola outbreak.[2,3]

Unfortunately, limited evidence does suggest that pregnant women are likely to be at increased risk of severe illness and death when infected with Ebola virus.

Pregnant women with EVD also appear to be at increased risk of fetal loss and pregnancy-associated haemorrhage. Reports of Ebola outbreaks suggest that the incidence of spontaneous miscarriage, prematurity and neonatal death is very high. Neonates do not survive for more than a few days to weeks.[4,5]

In a study by Mupapa et al., mortality among pregnant women with Ebola haemorrhagic fever was slightly but not significantly higher than the overall mortality observed during the Ebola epidemic in Kikwit, DRC (77 per cent; 245/316 infected persons). [EL 2]

Effect of Ebola Virus on Pregnancy

- Ebola viral disease's interaction with pregnancy is poorly understood and remains a challenge for health care providers.
- It is not well established whether pregnant women are at higher risk than the general population.
- However, a small series of case reports does suggest that pregnant women are at risk of severe morbidity and death, perhaps due to decreased immunity during pregnancy itself. There has been no fetal survival in these women; however, the cause of death remains unknown.
- It is established that Ebola virus does infect the placenta, therefore it is likely that the fetus has placental transmission of the virus. These viruses are detected in the amniotic fluid, meconium, umbilical cord, buccal swab and vaginal secretion.
- Ebola virus persists in amniotic fluid even after maternal blood is negative for reverse transcription–polymerase chain reaction (RT-PCR) tests. Therefore it is important for health care personnel to take necessary precautions in delivery and avoid contact with body fluid from pregnant women who had been infected and are currently in the convalescent period.[7]
- Women with active disease and who survive without pregnancy loss may transmit the virus during delivery and pose a potential risk of transmitting infection.
- Women who become pregnant after they recover from an Ebola infection pose little risk to the unborn fetus during the new pregnancy, especially if infection occurs at least 20 weeks after negative

blood result for RT-PCR tests for Ebola virus in maternal blood.[8]

- There is no evidence to show that women who survive EVD and subsequently become pregnant pose a risk for Ebola virus transmission.

Signs and Symptoms during Pregnancy

Health care providers should be aware of the signs and symptoms of Ebola virus, as early signs and symptoms are non-specific and may be confused with malaria, typhoid or influenza.

A history of fever, recent travel to the epidemic zone or any contact with an infected person should raise suspicion of Ebola infection.

Symptoms of EVD include:

- Fever
- Severe headache
- Muscle pain
- Weakness
- Fatigue
- Diarrhoea
- Vomiting
- Abdominal (stomach) pain
- Unexplained haemorrhage (bleeding or bruising)

Symptoms usually appear within 8–10 days of contact and can be confused with influenza (flu) or malaria.

Transmission

- Initial spread occurs through an Ebola virus-infected animal (bat or non-human primate). After that, the virus spreads from person to person, involving a large number of people (epidemic).
- The spread is through direct contact and through broken skin or mucous membranes in the eyes, nose or mouth, or direct contact with blood or body fluids (urine, saliva, sweat, faeces, vomit, breastmilk and semen).
- Proper cleaning and disposal of instruments including needles and syringes are important. Preferably, disposable instruments should be used.[10]
  - Ebola virus is not usually transmitted by food. However, it may spread through the handling and consumption of meat from wild animals.
  - There is also no evidence that mosquitoes or other insects can transmit Ebola virus.

Fetal Implications of Ebola Virus Infection

- Miscarriage
- Intrauterine fetal death
- Neonatal death

Diagnosis

Clinical

This may be difficult as symptoms are very similar to other diseases (typhoid, malaria, flu). Therefore these symptoms should be combined with history of recent travel to an epidemic country and contact history.

Once suspected the person should be isolated.

Blood test should be carried out to confirm the diagnosis.

Nucleic acid amplification testing (NAAT) is currently the gold standard diagnostic test and is performed in category 4 biosafety facilities. [EL 2]

The low sensitivity of NAAT during the first 72 hours of symptoms may require repeat testing.

As it is a communicable disease, public health should be informed and contact tracing is required.

Treatment of Women

The general care or medical treatment remains the same as for non-pregnant adults.

- Replacement of fluid and electrolytes.
- Maintenance of blood pressure.
- Oxygen therapy is important.
- Symptomatic treatment, e.g. pain relief and temperature-lowering medications.
- Any pregnant woman suspected of having Ebola should be isolated and handled in the same way as any other suspect/confirmed patient until proven not to have Ebola. Begin the same standard treatment as for any other patient admitted to the Ebola treatment centre (ETC).
- Currently, there is no antiviral treatment for Ebola.

Obstetric Management

- Obstetric management should be focused on early treatment of haemorrhagic complications. These patients have increased incidence of coagulation failure and very high fetal loss in the form of spontaneous miscarriage and antepartum haemorrhage.

- Blood transfusion and re-transfusing filtered blood should be considered.
- Active management of the third stage is recommended with the use of 600 µg of misoprostol and continue with oral tablets after delivery.
- There are no data available to suggest which mode of delivery, caesarean section versus vaginal delivery, is superior or has more benefits in relation to maternal and neonatal outcomes.
- However, vaginal delivery seems to be the safer option, according to the guidelines from the Royal College of Gynaecologists (RCOG) based on Médecins Sans Frontières (MSF).
- There is very high neonatal mortality, and hardly any neonatal survivals were noted. It is hard to establish whether these neonates had transplacental transmission or if they were infected during delivery through vaginal route or any other cause.
- It is not known whether early intervention or delivery improves the maternal outcome.

Treatment of the Newborn

Infants can be treated with monoclonal antibodies (ZMapp), a buffy coat transfusion from an Ebola survivor, and the antiviral GS-5734. However, there is no consensus over the treatment of the newborn, as not many fetuses survive after the infection.

Breastfeeding and Ebola Virus[13,14]

There are very limited data for breastfeeding and its effect on neonates as not many pregnancies end in live birth. However, it is recommended that breastfeeding should be discouraged in these women as evidence suggests the presence of Ebola virus in the breastmilk.

Breastfeeding is safe and should be encouraged in a recurrent pregnancy if there is no Ebola virus genetic material detected in the breastmilk.

Prevention of Infection for Health Care Workers and Relatives

Personal Protective Equipment (PPE)

Anyone in direct contact with the woman during labour or in the hospitalisation period should take proper precautions and have PPE protection and be properly instructed how to put it on and take it off.

Proper training should be given to all involved on how to use PPE.

PPE includes some of the following items:
- Hearing-protective devices, earmuffs and earplugs
- Respiratory protective equipment
- Eye and face protection, such as safety glasses and face shields
- Safety helmets
- Skin protection, such as gloves, gauntlets and sunscreen

Limited Direct Contact

- Number of health care providers for the patient should be limited, and they and visitors, spouse or relatives should have limited contact.
- Direct contact should be emphatically discouraged wherever possible.
- Visitors have the same risk as the patient and should be informed regarding the risk. If they have come across the patient they should be screened.
- Pregnant health care worker should be discouraged from providing care to the infected woman because of increased risk for mother and her baby.

Summary

- Ebola is a rare but severe and often deadly disease.
- Survival depends on good supportive clinical care and the patient's immunity to the infection.
- Ebola virus antibodies can be detected in the blood up to 10 years after recovery.
- Maternal mortality remains high (approximately 95 per cent).
- Perinatal mortality virtually reaches 100 per cent for infected pregnant women.

Guidelines from RCOG Based on Médecins Sans Frontières (MSF)[13] [EL 2 & 3]

- Maternal mortality remains high (approximately 95%)

- Perinatal mortality virtually 100% for infected pregnant women.
- Ebola virus remains positive in breast milk and amniotic fluid even after woman become sero-negative, therefore remains infective.
- Guidelines suggest assessment of health care work and advice to have minimal number and minimal contact with the patient.
- Body fluid exposure should be avoided, consequently any invasive procedure should be avoided including caesarean section.
- Spontaneous vaginal delivery should be contemplated.
- Fetal monitoring, repeated vaginal examination and artificial rupture of membrane, episiotomy and suturing should be avoided as increases the risk to health care worker.
- Suspected cases of Ebola virus should be isolated for 21 days from the exposure.
- Delivery should only take place within a designated high-risk area with easy access to decontamination for healthcare staff. Patient should not be moved to a delivery room, and the labour ward should be isolated in a side room.
- In case of intrauterine death, spontaneous labour should be awaited and placenta and baby should be disposed of carefully as per protocol.
- Medical treatment should be considered for induction, termination of pregnancy, management of Post-partum hemorrhage.
- In case of live birth baby he/she should be treated as Ebola virus positive, can be breast fed and mother should be informed that baby is likely to die soon.
- Medical milk suppression should be carried out in case of still birth and expressed milk should be properly disposed.

References

1. Centers for Disease Control and Prevention. Ebola Virus Disease. www.cdc.gov/vhf/ebola/pdf/ebola-factsheet.pdf. 2015.

2. Hayden EC. Ebola's lasting legacy. *Nature.* 2015; **519**: 24–6.

3. Maganga DG, Kapetshi J, Berthet N et al. Ebola virus disease in the Democratic Republic of Congo. *N Engl J Med.* 2014; **371**: 2083–91.

4. Mupapa K, Mukundu W, Bwaka MA et al. Ebola hemorrhagic fever and pregnancy. *J Infect Dis.* 1999; **179**(suppl 1): S11–12.

5. Jamieson DJ, Uyeki TM, Callaghan WM, Meaney-Delman D, Rasmussen SA. What obstetrician-gynecologists should know about Ebola: a perspective from the Centers for Disease Control and Prevention. *Obstet Gynecol.* 2014; **124**(5): 1005–10.

6. Wamala JF, Lukwago L, Malimbo M et al. Ebola hemorrhagic fever associated with novel virus strain, Uganda, 2007–2008. *Emerg Infect Dis.* 2010; **16**(7): 1087–92.

7. Caluwaerts S, Fautsch T, Lagrou D et al. Dilemmas in managing pregnant women with Ebola: 2 case reports. *Clin Infect Dis.* 2016; **62**: 903–5.

8. Kamali A, Jamieson DJ, Kpaduwa J et al. Pregnancy, labor, and delivery after Ebola virus disease and implications for infection control in obstetric services, United States. *Emerg Infect Dis.* 2016; **22**(7): 1156–61.

9. World Health Organization (WHO). Laboratory guidance for the diagnosis of Ebola virus disease: interim recommendations. www.who.int/. 2014.

10. Sterk E. *Filovirus Haemorrhagic Fever Guideline.* Barcelona: Médecins Sans Frontières; 2008.

11. Kaner J, Schaak S. Understanding Ebola: the 2014 epidemic. *Globalization and Health.* 2016; **12**: 53.

12. Centers for Disease Control and Prevention. Ebola (Ebola Virus Disease). Diagnosis. www.cdc.gov/vhf/ebola/diagnosis/index.html.

13. Médecins Sans Frontières (MSF) International. Guidance paper Ebola Treatment Centre (ETC): Pregnant & lactating women. 2014.

14. CDC's Ebola (Ebola virus disease). Recommendations for breastfeeding/infant feeding in the context of Ebola.

Chikungunya

Shabnum Sibtain

Introduction

Chikungunya is a vector-borne infection which is caused by the chikungunya virus.

It is transmitted to humans by infected female mosquitoes (*Aedes aegypti* and *Aedes albopictus* also called tiger mosquito) which breed in stagnant water and are also responsible for dengue fever.[1]

These mosquitoes bite only during the daytime, and the peak activity is in the early morning and late afternoon.

The first chikungunya outbreak occurred in southern Tanzania in 1952. The disease is caused by a ribonucleic acid (RNA) virus that belongs to the *Alphavirus* genus of the family *Togaviridae*. The virus's name comes from the Makonde language of Tanzania and means to bend up. It describes the stooped appearance of sufferers with joint pain.

Chikungunya has clinical features similar to those of dengue and Zika and can be misdiagnosed in areas where they are common.

Prevalence

Chikungunya is prevalent mostly in Africa, Asia and the Indian subcontinent. The virus has led to major epidemics in Asia and Africa since 2004. In 2013 it appeared as an emerging infection in America. An outbreak in 2015 affected several countries around America.[2]

Symptoms

- High-grade fever
- Joint pain which is often debilitating and can last for variable duration from a few days to weeks, several months or even years
- Gastrointestinal symptoms, abdominal pain, may also occur

Most of these symptoms are very general, therefore the clinician should be vigilant, especially if symptoms persist for more than a few days.[3]

Signs and Symptoms in Infected Pregnant Women

Joint and muscle pains: joint pains are often so severe as to make the patient bend over and be unable to walk properly. The ankle, elbow joints and wrists are particularly affected, and the pain is excruciating, especially in the morning. The pain might persist for a week or for more than a month, and at times there might be swelling around the joints.[4]

Fever: high and recurring fever as high as 40°C.

Chills: as with malaria, chikungunya infection causes chills.

Rash: which is maculopapular occurs in 40–50 per cent of cases, two to five days after onset of symptoms.

Headaches: severe headaches accompany chikungunya infection and can be very painful.

Pain in the lower back region: along with a headache, the lower back may also ache.

Nausea, vomiting and diarrhoea: the feeling of having an upset stomach with the sensation of throwing up, followed by vomiting, is symptomatic.

Fatigue: a feeling of tiredness and being low on strength.

The disease can be acute or chronic.[5]

Acute Phase

In the acute phase, there are two stages:

- A viral stage, during which viraemia occurs during the first five to seven days
- A convalescent stage in which symptoms improve and the virus cannot be detected in the blood, lasting approximately 10 days

Chronic Phase

The **chronic phase** of the infection has been poorly described in the obstetric population. Serious complications are uncommon. Mostly infection is mild and may go unrecognised or be misdiagnosed as dengue in areas affected by dengue.

Incubation period is usually between 3 and 7 days but can vary from 1 to 12 days.

Chikungunya is not fatal, but the symptoms can be severe and cause debilitating and long-lasting joint pain.[6]

Effects of Chikungunya Infection on Maternal and Neonatal Outcomes

The effects of chikungunya infection on maternal outcomes are limited.

There is no clear evidence that pregnant women infected with chikungunya have more obstetric complications.

Chikungunya virus is not transmitted to the fetus. However, immunity is transferred to the fetus that may last a few years after the birth.[7]

Vertical Transmission

If the woman becomes infected just before delivery, the virus is vertically transmitted to the fetus during labour.[8] The risk for vertical transmission is increased to 50 per cent when maternal viraemia is present during delivery.[6] In such cases, the neonate can be severely infected during the birth.

The largest study from Latin America at four large regional maternity hospitals in three different centres involving 169 symptomatic newborns suggested that vertical transmission during labour and delivery ranged between almost 27 per cent and 48 per cent and mortality rate was 5 per cent.[8]

Neonatal Implications

- Infected neonates should be treated at a tertiary hospital immediately, as they are at a higher risk of developing morbidities and mortalities. When maternal infection occurs late in pregnancy, serious and life-threatening fetal and neonatal complications can occur such as meningoencephalitis and disseminated intravascular coagulation.[9]
- Caesarean section does not prevent transmission.[10]
- The death rate is not high, but mortality has been observed in large chikungunya outbreaks.[11]
- The most common clinical signs in newborns were fever, irritability, rash, seizures, diffuse limb

oedema, meningoencephalitis and bullous dermatitis.

- Pregnant women with chikungunya should be treated in highly specialised obstetric and neonatal units to prevent adverse outcomes. Once infected, lifelong immunity develops against the disease.[11]
- Congenital infection rate is unrelated to mode of delivery.
- The predominant clinical manifestations in symptomatic newborns are fever (100%), irritability (90%), rash (84%), generalised oedema (86%), hyperalgesia (94%), stiff neck or pain on mobilisation (38%) and hemodynamic instability (52%).[12]

Breastfeeding

There has been no evidence to suggest that the virus spreads through breastfeeding, therefore breastfeeding should be encouraged.[13]

Diagnosis

Serological Tests

Enzyme-linked immunosorbent assays (ELISA) can bedone to confirm the presence of immunoglobin M(IgM) and immunoglobin G (IgG) anti-chikungunya antibodies.

IgM antibody levels are highest three to five weeks after the onset of illness and persist for about two months.[13]

Viral Nucleic Acid

Various reverse transcriptase–polymerase chain reaction (RT–PCR) methods are also available but are of variable sensitivity. Diagnostic results can be available in one to two days.[14]

Virus Isolation

The virus can be isolated from the blood during the first few days of infection.

Virus isolation provides the most definitive diagnosis, but takes one to two weeks for completion and must be carried out in biosafety level III laboratories.

Treatment

- There is no specific antiviral drug treatment for chikungunya.
- Supportive care is recommended to combat the symptoms.[15]

- Treatment is mainly aimed at relieving the symptoms, by rest, antipyretics such as paracetamol, non-steroidal anti-inflammatory drugs such as naproxen and fluids.
- Application of various herbal or medicated oils and creams can reduce the rashes and help in scaling dryness of skin.
- Gentle exercise and physiotherapy is helpful in reducing the joint pain and muscle stiffness.
- Cold compress and Epsom salt bath can give some relief from the joint pain.

There is no chikungunya vaccine available yet.

Prevention and Control

- Chikungunya can spread all year round. It spreads in a similar way to malaria.
- Warm humid weather and stagnant water allow the mosquitoes to breed.
- Prevention and control rely mostly on stopping the mosquitoes breeding by reducing the number of natural and artificial water-filled container habitats.
- To guard against infection, there should be proper disposal of all waste material, and water stagnation should be discouraged especially during monsoons.
- Light-coloured protective clothing should be worn, as dark colours attract mosquitoes.
- The use of insect repellent and mosquito nets is an important precautionary measure.
- Mosquitoes cannot survive in cold temperatures; therefore it is better to stay indoors or in an air-conditioned room if possible.

Summary

Chikungunya can easily be contracted through mosquito bites, and if not treated it could prove fatal to both the mother and the unborn child.

The symptoms of the chikungunya infection show up between three and seven days after the mosquito has bitten.

Early detection of the infection is necessary to cure it without allowing it to have a significant impact on the mother or the child.

References

1. World Health Organization. Chikungunya Fact sheet. 12 April 2017. https://www.who.int/en/news-room/fact-sheets/detail/chikungunya.

2. Hamer DH, Chen LH. Chikungunya: establishing a new home in the Western hemisphere. *Ann Intern Med.* 2014; **161**: 827–8.

3. Yactayo S, Staples JE, Millot V, Cibrelus L, Ramon-Pardo P. Epidemiology of Chikungunya in the Americas. *J Infect Dis.* 2016; **214**(suppl 5): S441–5.

4. Thiberville SD, Moyen N, Dupuis-Maguiraga L et al. Chikungunya fever: epidemiology, clinical syndrome, pathogenesis and therapy. *Antiviral Res.* 2013; **99**(3): 345–70.

5. Powers AM, Logue CH. Changing patterns of chikungunya virus: re-emergence of a zoonotic arbovirus. *J Gen Virol.* 2007; **88**(9): 2363–77.

6. Gérardin P, Couderc T, Bintner M et al. Chikungunya virus-associated encephalitis: a cohort study on La Réunion Island, 2005–2009. *Neurology.* 2016; **86**(1): 94–102.

7. Escobar M, Nieto AJ, Loaiza-Osorio S, Barona JS, Rosso F. Pregnant women hospitalized with Chikungunya virus infection, Colombia, 2015. *Emerg Infect Dis.* 2017; **23**(11): 1777–83.

8. Robillard P-Y, Boumahni B, Gérardin P et al. Vertical maternal fetal transmission of the chikungunya virus. Ten cases among 84 pregnant women. *Presse Med.* 2006; **35**: 785–8.

9. Villamil-Gómez W, Alba-Silvera L, Menco-Ramos A et al. Congenital chikungunya virus infection in Sincelejo, Colombia: a case series. *J Trop Pediatr.* 2015; **61**(5): 386–92.

10. Gérardin P, Barau G, Michault A et al. Multidisciplinary prospective study of mother-to-child chikungunya virus infections on the island of La Réunion. *PLoS Med.* 2008; **5**(3): e60.

11. Caglioti C, Lalle E, Castilletti C, Carletti F, Capobianchi MR, Bordi L. Chikungunya virus infection: an overview. *New Microbiol.* 2013; **36**(3): 211–27.

12. Torres RJ, Falleiros-Arlant LH, Dueñas L, Pleitez-Navarrete J, Salgado DM, Castillo JB-D. Congenital and perinatal complications of chikungunya fever. *Science Direct.* 2016; **51**: 85–8.

13. Campos GS, Albuquerque Bandeira AC, Diniz Rocha VF, Dias JP, Carvalho RH, Sardi SI. First detection of chikungunya virus in breast milk. *Pediatr Infect Dis J.* 2017; **36**(10): 1015–17.

14. Centers for Disease Control and Prevention. Chikungunya Virus. Diagnostic Testing. Last updated 2017. www.cdc.gov/chikungunya/hc/diagnostic.html.

15. Centers for Disease Control and Prevention. Chikungunya Virus. Symptoms, Diagnosis, & Treatment. Last updated 2016. www.cdc.gov/chikungunya/symptoms/index.html.

Chapter 14

Antibiotics during Pregnancy and Methicillin-Resistant *Staphylococcus aureus* (MRSA)

Adel Elkady, Prabha Sinha and Soad Ali Zaki Hassan

Antibiotics are a group of medicines used for treating infections caused by bacteria and certain parasites but are not effective against viral or fungal infection.

They are also called antibacterial or antimicrobials and work by killing the organisms or stopping them from multiplying.[1]

Antibiotics are commonly prescribed during pregnancy; however, the specific medication must be chosen carefully as most antibiotics might be safe while some are not.

Safety depends on various factors, including the type of antibiotic, gestational age, dose and duration of the use of the antibiotics.

They are usually grouped together based on mode of action as each only works against certain types of organisms; therefore, different antibiotics are used for different infections.

Classification of Antibiotics According to Groups

Penicillin – phenoxymethylpenicillin, flucloxacillin and amoxicillin

Cephalosporins – cefaclor, cefadroxil and cefalexin

Aminoglycosides – gentamicin and tobramycin

Macrolides – erythromycin, azithromycin and clarithromycin

Tetracyclines – tetracycline, doxycycline

Clindamycin

Sulfonamides and trimethoprim – co-trimoxazole

Metronidazole and tinidazole

Quinolones – ciprofloxacin, levofloxacin and norfloxacin

Antibiotics Grouping by Mechanism of Action

Cell Wall Synthesis

Penicillins

Cephalosporins

Vancomycin

Beta-Lactamase Inhibitors

Carbapenems

Aztreonam

Polymycin

Bacitracin

Protein Synthesis Inhibitors

Aminoglycosides (gentamicin)

Tetracyclines Inhibit 50s Subunit

Macrolides

Chloramphenicol

Clindamycin

Linezolid

Streptogramins

Folic acid synthesis inhibitors

Sulfonamides

Trimethoprim

DNA Synthesis Inhibitors

Fluoroquinolones

Metronidazole

RNA Synthesis Inhibitors

Rifampin

Mycolic acid synthesis inhibitors

Isoniazid

Guidelines for Prescribing an Antibiotic during Pregnancy

- Antibiotics should only be used if no other treatment option will suffice
- Should be avoided during the first trimester when possible
- Safe medication tested on pregnant women should be chosen
- Monotherapy single prescriptions rather than polypharmacy are preferred when possible
- Lowest possible dose and duration of use proven effective should be given
- Advise patients not to use over-the-counter medications during antibiotic treatment[2]

Antibiotics Used during Pregnancy

Common antibiotics that are generally considered safe during pregnancy include:

- Penicillins (amoxicillin and ampicillin)
- Cephalosporins
- Erythromycin

Penicillins and cephalosporins are the drugs of first choice in pregnancy.[3] The penicillins interfere with cell wall synthesis and are bactericidal.

Tetracyclines are not recommended as they can discolour developing baby's teeth.[4]

Clinical Information and New Antibiotics

Older antibiotics are usually prescribed as they are tested in pregnancy. For newer antibiotics, there is very little clinical information available regarding the effect on pregnancy and fetus as they are not tested. However, in some cases, despite the lack of formula testing and lack of evidence during pregnancy, obstetricians are faced with risks versus benefits choices if there are no other alternatives.

If the benefits of prescribing a new antibiotic during pregnancy outweigh the potential risks, the antibiotic in question is chosen.[5]

When choosing an antibiotic, physicians should consider the effectiveness, risk of adverse effects and resistance rates in the local community.

Regardless of which antibiotic is chosen for initial empiric therapy, the regimen should be revised as necessary after microbial culture susceptibility results are available.

The choice of antibiotic mainly depends on

- How severe the infection is
- Type of infection
- Renal and liver function test
- Dosing schedule
- Other medications used
- Common or even rare side effects
- A history of having an allergy to a certain type of antibiotic

Quinolones, tetracyclines and aminoglycosides should be avoided in pregnancy, unless the infection is severe or life-threatening.[6] (British National Formulary appendix 4: Pregnancy)

Because only a few controlled scientific studies have addressed whether drugs are safe to use during pregnancy, physicians usually rely on data from animal research and from the collective experience in practice to decide. In 1979, the US Food and Drug Administration (FDA) developed a classification system for drugs, including anti-infectives, and their potential harmful effects on an unborn child.

The FDA Drug Category System

The FDA list of pharmaceutical pregnancy categories helps doctors to know the prenatal safety of medications. The categories are A, B, C, D and X. Drugs within category A have been found to be safe for use in pregnant women, whereas drugs within category X have been found to be harmful to fetuses and should not be used by pregnant women.[7]

Antibiotics used during pregnancy should fall into either category A or category B on the FDA list.

Category A

Controlled studies fail to demonstrate a risk to the fetus in the first trimester and no evidence of risk in later trimesters. The possibility of fetal harm appears remote.

Category B

Animal reproduction studies have not demonstrated a fetal risk, but there are no controlled studies in pregnant women. Animal reproduction studies have not shown an adverse effect (other than a decrease in fertility), but which was not confirmed in controlled studies of women in the first trimester (and there is no evidence of risk in later trimesters).

Category C

Animal studies have revealed adverse effects on the fetus, and there are no controlled studies on women and animals available. Drugs in this category should be given only if the potential benefit justifies potential risk to the fetus.

Category D

There is positive evidence of human fetal risk, but the benefits of use in pregnant women may be acceptable despite the risk (serious disease for which safer drugs cannot be used or are ineffective).

Category X

Studies on animals or humans have demonstrated fetal abnormalities, or evidence of fetal risk based on human experience, or both. The drug should not be used by women who are or may become pregnant.

Birth defects associated with antibiotics defined within category X include anencephaly, choanal atresia (a blockage of the nasal passage), transverse limb deficiency, diaphragmatic hernia, eye defects, congenital heart defects and cleft palate.[7]

In general, unborn babies are most likely to be harmed in the first trimester of pregnancy. However, the use of sulfa antibiotics is safe in early pregnancy. Later in pregnancy, it can cause jaundice in the newborns and should not be used.

Effects of Antibiotics during Pregnancy

It is important to remember that the choice of an antibiotic relies on multiple factors, including the targeted organism, the possibility for resistance and the potential for adverse effect on pregnancy.

- Metronidazole is now considered safe in most cases according to the new research.
- Nitrofurantoin may be recommended for recurrent urinary tract infections and should be stopped at 36 weeks (or immediately if labour is

Table 14.1 Antibiotics risks of fetal defects and developmental disabilities

CONSIDERED SAFE IN PREGNANCY	CONSIDERED UNSAFE IN PREGNANCY
Amoxicillin	Bactrim
Ampicillin	Ciprofloxacin
Augmentin	Doxycycline
Penicillin	Furadantin, macrodantin
Cephalexin	Macrobid
Clindamycin	Minocycline, tetracycline
Erythromycin	Septrin

imminent before). There is a small risk of baby's red blood cells destruction if taken within a few days before delivery.
- Trimethoprim should not be used during the first trimester. It blocks the effects of folic acid, which is crucial during pregnancy and preconception as it reduces the risk of developing neural tube and other birth defects.
- Streptomycin can cause hearing loss in the baby, and tetracycline can discolour baby's teeth.

Antibiotics without Known Teratogenic Effects

Cephalosporins, penicillins, erythromycin (except the estolate), azithromycin, clindamycin, augmentin and metronidazole have no known teratogenic effect.

An association between spontaneous abortion and first trimester use of macrolides (excluding erythromycin), quinolones, tetracyclines, sulfonamides and metronidazole was observed in a case control study including over 95 000 pregnant women.[8]

The following antibiotics have been associated with known or potential teratogenic effects:
- **Aminoglycosides** carry a risk of fetal (and maternal) ototoxicity and nephrotoxicity, but not with structural birth defects.
- **Doxycycline** is avoided during pregnancy because other tetracyclines have been associated with transient suppression of bone growth and with staining of developing teeth, but available data do not show teratogenic effects from doxycycline.[9]
- **Fluoroquinolones** are generally avoided during pregnancy and lactation because they are toxic to developing cartilage in experimental animal studies. However, neither adverse effects on cartilage nor an

increase in congenital malformations from use during human pregnancy has been documented.[10]

- **Trimethoprim** is generally avoided in the first trimester because it is a folic acid antagonist and has caused abnormal embryo development in experimental animals.[11]

- **Sulfonamides, nitrofurantoin:**

  o The safest course is to avoid using nitrofurantoin or sulfonamides in the first trimester if another antibiotic that is safe and effective is available.[12]

  o Sulfonamides and nitrofurantoin are contraindicated in patients with glucose-6-phosphate dehydrogenase deficiency.

  o Sulfonamides which may be indicated for urinary tract infection compete with bilirubin for albumin binding sites and may increase the risk of fetal kernicterus at low bilirubin levels if taken during the third trimester.

  o In the National Birth Defects Prevention Study (NBDPS) data, the antibiotics most frequently used by pregnant women are cephalosporins (e.g. Keflex), penicillins and erythromycins.

  o Generally, women who used these medications were not at greater risk for most birth defects.[13,14]

Exposure and Birth Defects

Teratogenesis caused by drugs or other agents is most likely to occur during the first trimester, when organs and nervous systems are forming.

The American College of Obstetricians and Gynecologists (ACOG) reviewed available evidence on maternal use of nitrofurans, sulfonamides and other specific antibiotics during pregnancy and subsequent development of birth defects in the offspring.[15]

- The conclusion of the ACOG recommendations included:

  o 'Commonly used antibiotics, such as penicillins, erythromycin, and cephalosporins, have not been found to be associated with an increased risk of birth defects.

  o The evidence regarding an association between the nitrofurans and sulfonamide classes of antibiotics and birth defects is mixed.

  o Antibiotics should be prescribed for pregnant women only for appropriate indications and for the shortest effective duration.

Table 14.2 Antibiotics And Fetal Side Effects

Antibiotics	Side effects and Comment
Aminoglycosides	Ototoxicity (damage to fetal labyrinth), resulting in deafness
Chloramphenicol	In women or fetuses with G6PD deficiency, causes haemolysis, grey baby syndrome
Fluoroquinolones	Musculoskeletal defects (impaired bone growth)
Nitrofurantoin	In women or fetuses with G6PD deficiency, causes haemolysis. Contraindicated during the first trimester, and at term, during labour and delivery
Sulfonamides	When given after 34 weeks, neonatal jaundice and kernicterus can occur as interference with the bile conjugating mechanism of the neonate (except sulfasalazine, which has minimal fetal risk). Should be avoided if delivery is imminent
Tetracycline	Slows bone growth, enamel hypoplasia, permanent yellowing of the teeth bone, and increased susceptibility to cavities in offspring; when administered intramuscularly (IM), occasionally produces maternal liver failure
Trimethoprim	Increased risk of neural tube defects due to folate antagonism, safe after the first trimester
Metronidazole	Manufacturer advises avoidance of high dose
Streptomycin	May cause fetal auditory nerve damage deafness in baby
Erythromycin	Not known to be harmful

  o Pregnant women should not be denied appropriate treatment because untreated infections can commonly lead to serious maternal and fetal complications.

  o Prescribing sulfonamides or nitrofurantoin in the first trimester is still considered appropriate when no other suitable alternative antibiotics are available.

  o During the second trimester, sulfonamides and nitrofurantoins may continue to be used as first-line agents for the treatment and prevention of urinary tract infections and other infections caused by susceptible organisms.'

- Many other studies corroborate these findings, with no increased risk for birth defects associated

with prenatal exposure to penicillin, ampicillin, amoxicillin/clavulanate, pivampicillin, cephalosporins, gentamicin, oxacillin, erythromycin and metronidazole.
- Untreated infections may cause serious maternal and fetal complications, and pregnant women therefore should not be denied appropriate treatment.

Antibiotics can play a vital role for the health of mother and fetus, but should be used only when definitely indicated and according to the different guidelines controlling its use.

Methicillin-Resistant *Staphylococcus aureus* (MRSA)

MRSA refers to a group of gram-positive bacteria that are genetically distinct from other strains of *Staphylococcus aureus*. Strains of *S. aureus* develop through horizontal gene transfer and natural selection, and develop resistance to most antibiotics including beta lactam antibiotics (penams – penicillin derivatives such as methicillin and oxacillin – and cephems such as the cephalosporins).[16] MRSA is responsible for human infections that are difficult to treat with antibiotics.

β-lactam antibiotics (beta-lactam antibiotics) are a class of broad-spectrum antibiotics. They are all antibiotic agents that contain a beta-lactam ring in their molecular structures, which includes penicillin derivatives penams, cephems, monobactams and carbapenems.

β-lactam antibiotics inhibit cell wall biosynthesis in the bacterial organism and are the most widely used group of antibiotics.

Bacteria often develop resistance to β-lactam antibiotics by synthesising the enzyme β-lactamase, an enzyme that attacks the β-lactam ring. To overcome this resistance, β-lactam antibiotics are often given with β-lactamase inhibitors such as clavulanic acid.

There are other strains of *S. aureus* that have emerged which are resistant to other antibiotics (oxacillin, clindamycin, teicoplanin and erythromycin).

MRSA began as a hospital-acquired infection, but has become community-acquired.

MRSA is common in hospitals, prisons and nursing homes, where people with open wounds, invasive devices such as catheters and weakened immune systems are at greater risk of hospital-acquired infection.

- **A hospital-acquired infection (HAI)**, also known as a nosocomial infection, is an infection acquired in a hospital, nursing home, rehabilitation facility, outpatient clinic or other clinical settings. Infection can spread through health care staff, contaminated equipment, bed linens or air droplets. In some cases the micro-organism originates from the patient's own skin microbiota, becoming opportunistic after surgery or other procedures that compromise the protective skin barrier. Though the patient may have contracted the infection from their own skin, the infection is still considered nosocomial since it develops in the health care setting.[17]

Microbiology of MRSA

Methicillin-resistant *S. aureus* (MRSA) is a gram-positive, spherical (coccus) bacterium that is about 1 micron in diameter.

Prevention of MRSA

- Hand washing: wash hands using soap and water or an alcohol-based sanitiser
- Keep wounds clean and covered
- Avoid contact with other people's wounds
- Avoid sharing personal items such as razors or towels
- Shower before using swimming pools or whirlpools
- Wipe all horizontal surfaces with disinfectant daily
- Restrict antibiotic use

Glycopeptides, cephalosporins and, in particular, quinolones are associated with an increased risk of colonisation of MRSA. Reducing use of antibiotic classes that promote MRSA colonisation, especially fluoroquinolones, is recommended.

Diagnosis of MRSA Infection

Diagnostic microbiology and culture: the bacterium must be cultured from blood, urine, sputum or other body-fluid samples. Because no quick and easy method exists to diagnose MRSA, initial treatment of the infection is often based upon 'strong suspicion' and techniques by the treating physician

Quantitative PCR procedures, quick detection and identifying MRSA strains

Rapid latex agglutination test that detects the PBP2a protein. PBP2a is a variant penicillin-binding protein that imparts the ability of *S. aureus* to be resistant to oxacillin[18]

MRSA in Pregnancy

Prevalence
In a study of 5732 mothers who delivered 5804 infants, genital tract colonisation with MRSA affected 3.5 per cent of pregnant women.

However in this study, such a genital tract colonisation did not predispose to a high risk of early-onset neonatal MRSA infection.[19] [EL 2]

Maternal Clinical Presentation
- Skin and soft tissue infections:
  - In the extremities, buttocks, breasts, vulva or groin, abdomen
  - Multiple and recurrent lesions with a necrotic appearance that patients often refer to as 'spider bites'[20]
- Postpartum infections:
  - Mastitis progressing to breast abscess
  - Furunculosis
  - Cellulitis
  - Wound infection
- Other serious infections:[20]
  - Necrotising pneumonia
  - Pleural empyema
  - Necrotising fasciitis
  - Myositis
  - Fulminant severe puerperal sepsis

MRSA in the Neonate
- Skin and soft tissue infections
- Bacteraemia
- Osteomyelitis
- Myositis
- Empyema

Treatment of MRSA Infections

For empirical coverage of CA-MRSA in outpatients, oral antibiotic options include:[21]
- Clindamycin
- Trimethoprim-sulfamethoxazole (TMP-SMX)
- Linezolid (US FDA pregnancy category: C; potential benefits may warrant use of the drug in

pregnant women despite potential risks), 400 - 600 mg every 12 hours for a duration of 10–28 days

Linezolid is a synthetic antibiotic belonging to a new class of antimicrobials called the oxazolidinones. It disrupts bacterial growth by inhibiting the initiation process of protein synthesis – a mechanism of action that is unique to this class of drugs. It is well absorbed with high bioavailability that allows conversion to oral therapy as soon as the patient is clinically stable. It has been approved for certain gram-positive infections including certain drug-resistant enterococcus, staphylococcus and pneumococcus strains.

It is generally well tolerated, with myelosuppression being the most serious adverse effect.

For hospitalised patients
- Intravenous (IV) vancomycin (category B) at a dose of 250 mg every six hours for 7–10 days [EL 1]
- Oral (PO) or IV linezolid 600 mg twice daily [EL 1]
- Clindamycin 600 mg IV or PO three times a day. Seven to 14 days of therapy is recommended but should be individualised on the basis of the patient's clinical response

Conclusion
MRSA is a serious mainly hospital-acquired infection that is resistant to most antibiotics.

Antibiotic therapy should be given after culture and sensitivity results.

Linezolid (US FDA pregnancy category C) is emerging as an effective treatment.

Isolation of patients is recommended to prevent spread of infection.

References
1. Anderson L. Antibiotics Guide. Reviewed 23 August 2016. Drugs.com. www.drugs.com/article/antibiotics.html.

2. Moore D. Antibiotic Classification & Mechanism. Ortho Bullets. www.orthobullets.com/basic-science/9059/antibiotic-classification-and-mechanism.

3. Royal College of Obstetrics & Gynaecology. RCOG statement on the use of antibiotics in pregnancy and the relative risk of neurological disorders. 2015. www.rcog.org.uk/en/news/rcog-statement-on-the-use-of-antibiotics-in-pregnancy-and-the-relative-risk-of-neurological-disorders/.

4. NHS Forth Valley. Empirical Antimicrobial Guidelines for Forth Valley Hospitals 2013–2015. www.carronbank.co.uk/Clinical_Guidance/FV_Clinical_Guidance/pc-management-of-infection-guidance.pdf.

5. Clinical Information and New Antibiotics. Baby Med. www.babymed.com/medications/safe-antibiotics-during-pregnancy.

6. Use of Quinolones in Pregnancy. UKTIS/Public Health England. (Date of issue: June 2017, Version: 3.1). www.medicinesinpregnancy.org/bumps/monographs/USE-OF-QUINOLONES-IN-PREGNANCY/.

7. FDA Pregnancy Category System. Drugs in Pregnancy and Lactation. www.fda.gov/downloads/Drugs/DevelopmentApprovalProcess/SmallBusinessAssistance/UCM431132.pdf.

8. Muanda FT, Sheehy O, Bérard A. Use of antibiotics during pregnancy and risk of spontaneous abortion. *CMAJ*. 2017; **189**: E625–33.

9. Cooper WO, Hernandez-Diaz S, Arbogast PG et al. Antibiotics potentially used in response to bioterrorism and the risk of major congenital malformations. *Paediatr Perinat Epidemiol*. 2009; **23** (1): 18–28.

10. Hernández-Díaz S, Werler MM, Walker AM, Mitchell AA. Neural tube defects in relation to use of folic acid antagonists during pregnancy. *Am J Epidemiol*. 2001; **153**: 961–8.

11. Newman RD, Parise M, Nahlen B. Folic acid antagonists during pregnancy and risk of birth defects. *N Engl J Med*. 2001; **344**: 934; author reply 934.

12. Klarskov P, Andersen JT, Jimenez-Solem E et al. Short-acting sulfonamides near term and neonatal jaundice. *Obstet Gynecol*. 2013; **122**: 105–10.

13. Nordeng H, Lupattelli A, Romøren M, Koren G. Neonatal outcomes after gestational exposure to nitrofurantoin. *Obstet Gynecol*. 2013; **121**(2 Pt 1): 306–13.

14. Centers for Disease Control and Prevention. The national birth defects study. www.nbdps.org/.

15. American College of Obstetricians and Gynecologists. Committee opinion, Sulfonamides, Nitrofurantoin, and Risk of Birth Defects. Number 717, September 2017. www.acog.org/Clinical-Guidance-and-Publications/Committee-Opinions/Committee-on-Obstetric-Practice/Sulfonamides-Nitrofurantoin-and-Risk-of-Birth-Defects.

16. Centers for Disease Control and Prevention. General Information About MRSA in the Community. 10 September 2013. Retrieved 9 October 2014.

17. Centers for Disease Control and Prevention. Multidrug-resistant organisms (MDRO) Management. 2006. www.cdc.gov/infectioncontrol/guidelines/mdro/index.html.

18. François P, Schrenzel J. Rapid diagnosis and typing of Staphylococcus aureus. In: Lindsay J, ed. *Staphylococcus: Molecular Genetics*. Wymondham: Caister Academic Press; 2008: 71–90.

19. Andrews WW, Schelonka R, Waites K, Stamm A, Cliver SP, Moser S. Genital tract methicillin-resistant Staphylococcus aureus: risk of vertical transmission in pregnant women. *Obstet Gynecol*. 2008; **111**(1): 113–18.

20. Kellie SM. Methicillin-resistant Staphylococcus aureus (MRSA) in pregnancy: epidemiology, clinical syndromes, management, prevention, and infection control in the peripartum and postpartum periods. www.antimicrobe.org/h04c.files/history/MRSA%20and%20pregnancy.pdf.

21. Clinical Practice Guidelines by the Infectious Diseases Society of America for the Treatment of Methicillin-Resistant Staphylococcus aureus Infections in Adults and Children. *Clin Infect Dis*. 2011; **52**(3): e18–55. https://academic.oup.com/cid/article/52/3/e18/306145.

Gonorrhoea, Syphilis and Lymphogranuloma Venereum

Nutan Mishra

Gonorrhoea

Introduction

Gonorrhoea is a common sexually transmitted disease caused by *Neisseria gonorrhoeae*, a gram-negative diplococcus. The primary site of infection is the mucous membranes of the urethra, endocervix, rectum, pharynx and conjunctiva.

Transmission is usually by the direct inoculation of infected secretions from one mucous membrane to the other. Transluminal spread from urethra or endocervix may occur and cause epididymo-orchitis or prostatitis in men and pelvic inflammatory disease (PID) in women. Haematogenous spread may also occur, causing skin lesions, arthralgia, arthritis and tenosynovitis (disseminated gonococcal infection).

Prevalence[1]

The World Health Organization (WHO) estimates that in 2012 there were 78 million new cases, with a global incidence rate of 19 per 1000 females and 24 per 1000 males, with the highest prevalence in the Western Pacific and African Regions.

Co-infection with *Chlamydia trachomatis* is detected in 10–40 per cent of people with gonorrhoea.

Clinical Features

- Infection of the endocervix is asymptomatic in 50 per cent of cases, whereas increased or altered vaginal discharge may be present in another 50 per cent of cases.
- Lower abdominal pain is present in up to 25 per cent of cases, along with the commonest symptoms.[2]
- Rectal and pharyngeal infection are usually asymptomatic.
- Urethral infection may cause dysuria.

- Commonly no abnormal findings are present on examination, but muco-purulent endocervical discharge and easily induced endocervical bleeding and pelvic and lower abdominal tenderness may be present.

Maternal Signs and Symptoms

- Gonococcal infection in pregnancy generally remains asymptomatic. The main complaints are usually a painful or burning sensation when urinating; and/or increased vaginal discharge.

  It may cause acute cervicitis, proctitis, pharyngitis and disseminated infection.

  The rate of pharyngeal gonococcal infection increases during pregnancy due to possible altered sexual practices.

- Disseminated gonococcal infection occurs more frequently in pregnant than non-pregnant women and is characterised by a bacteraemic phase associated with malaise, fever and a pustular haemorrhagic rash and a secondary septic arthritis (usually with symmetrical involvement of the knees, wrists or ankles).[3]
- Rectal infections may either cause no symptoms or cause symptoms in both men and women that may include: discharge; anal itching; soreness; bleeding; painful bowel movements.
- After delivery, mothers are at risk of developing endometritis.

Fetal Risks

- Premature rupture of membranes
- Low birthweight
- Preterm delivery
- Chorioamnionitis

Newborn Implications

- Infants can be infected at delivery, resulting in neonatal conjunctivitis manifesting as purulent ocular discharge and swollen eyelids. Untreated conjunctivitis may lead to corneal ulceration, perforation, scarring and blindness.[4]
- Ophthalmia neonatorum occurs in up to 50 per cent of exposed newborns. A large controlled clinical trial in Nairobi found that the eye infection could be prevented by instilling either 1 per cent silver nitrate solution or 1 per cent tetracycline ointment into the eyes of infants at the time of delivery.
- However, since that study was conducted, the prevalence of the tetracycline-resistant strain of *N. gonorrhoeae* has increased dramatically in many parts of the developing world, and 2.5 per cent povidone–iodine solution appears to be an effective alternative.[4,5]

Diagnosis[6]

The diagnosis of gonorrhoea is established by the detection of *Neisseria gonorrhoeae* at an infected site. The method used to test depends on the clinical setting, storage and transport facility to the laboratory, local prevalence of the infection and the range of tests available in the laboratory. None of the tests for gonorrhoea offers 100 per cent sensitivity and specificity.

N. gonorrhoea can be diagnosed by nucleic acid amplification tests (NAATs), culture or Gram staining.

Nucleic Acid Amplification Tests (NAATs)

- Are highly sensitive and specific diagnostic tests that can be conducted on a wide range of samples, including urine, vulvovaginal, cervical and urethral swabs.
- NAATs have a sensitivity of over 90 per cent; the sensitivity varies by NAAT type and is frequently lower for rectal and pharyngeal samples.
- A drawback of currently available commercial NAATs is their inability to provide information on antimicrobial susceptibility.
- To avoid false-positive diagnoses, all NAATs should be confirmed by supplementary culture.[6] [EL 1]

Bacterial Culture

- Culture is a specific, sensitive and cheap diagnostic test.

- It not only allows a confirmatory test but also helps in guiding treatment due to widespread antimicrobial resistance.
- Swabs should also be taken from the pharynx and rectum in women with genital gonorrhoea. Microbiological cultures have a sensitivity of 85–95 per cent for urethral and endocervical infection.

Gram-Stained Smears

- Provide a presumptive diagnosis of gonorrhoea, especially among symptomatic men with urethritis.
- In low-income settings, Gram stains may provide a less expensive alternative to NAATs for symptomatic men.
- Only 50–70 per cent of asymptomatic infections in men are positive on Gram stain.

Treatment during Pregnancy

First line of treatment is single-dose ceftriaxone 250 or 500 mg intramuscularly (IM), and azithromycin 1 g orally is the recommended treatment for genital or extragenital site.[7,8] [EL 1]. Centers for Disease Control and Prevention (CDC) recommend this dual therapy; ceftriaxone and azithromycin should be administered together on the same day, preferably simultaneously.

Pregnant and breastfeeding women should not be treated with quinolones and tetracycline antimicrobials.

Amoxicillin with probenecid, streptomycin, ceftriaxone and cefixime are equally effective, but because of emerging high levels of resistance, penicillins are not recommended.

Test of Cure

A test of cure is advised at all infected sites due to recent emergence of cephalosporin resistance. Therapeutic regimes should include chlamydial treatment due to high rates of co-infection.

The WHO Sexually Transmitted Infection (STI) guideline recommends that local resistance data should determine the choice of therapy (both for dual therapy and single therapy). In settings where local resistance data are not available, the WHO STI guideline suggests dual therapy over single therapy for people with genital or anorectal infections, oropharyngeal infections and infections in pregnancy.

Women should be closely monitored for complications.[9]

The WHO guideline suggests the following options:[9]

- ## Dual Therapy

  - Ceftriaxone 250 mg (IM) as a single dose PLUS azithromycin 1 g orally as a single dose, or
  - Cefixime 400 mg orally as a single dose PLUS azithromycin 1 g orally as a single dose

- ## Single Therapy (According to Recent Local Resistance Data and Susceptibility to the Antimicrobial)

  - Ceftriaxone 250 mg IM
    or
  - Cefixime 400 mg orally
    or
  - Spectinomycin 2 g IM

In People Who Have Failed Treatment

- If treatment failure occurred with regimen not recommended by WHO, re-treat with a WHO-recommended regimen.
- If treatment failure occurred and resistance data are available, re-treat according to susceptibility, preferably with a WHO-recommended regimen.
- If treatment failure occurred after WHO-recommended single therapy, re-treat with WHO-recommended dual therapy, with one of the following dual therapies:

  - Ceftriaxone 500 mg IM PLUS azithromycin 2 g orally
    or
  - Cefixime 800 mg orally PLUS azithromycin 2 g orally as a single dose
    or
  - Gentamicin 240 mg IM PLUS azithromycin 2 g orally as a single dose.

Treatment for Neonatal Infection[9]

The WHO STI guideline suggests one of the following options for gonococcal conjunctivitis:

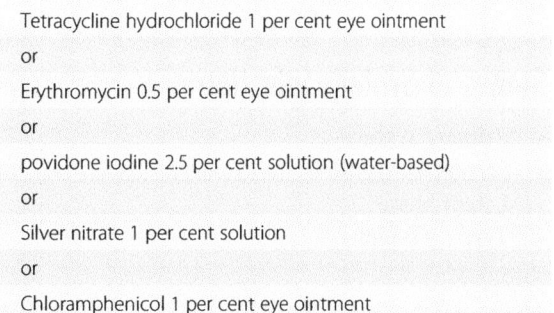

Single-dose ceftriaxone 50 mg/kg (maximum 150 mg) IM

or

Single-dose kanamycin 25 mg/kg (maximum 75 mg) IM

or

Single-dose spectinomycin 25 mg/kg (maximum 75 mg) IM

For the Prophylaxis of Gonococcal and Chlamydial Ophthalmia Neonatorum

WHO STI guideline recommends topical use of the following options to both eyes immediately after birth:

Tetracycline hydrochloride 1 per cent eye ointment

or

Erythromycin 0.5 per cent eye ointment

or

povidone iodine 2.5 per cent solution (water-based)

or

Silver nitrate 1 per cent solution

or

Chloramphenicol 1 per cent eye ointment

Syphilis

Introduction

Syphilis is a sexually transmitted disease caused by spirochaete *Treponema pallidum*.

It is transmitted by direct contact with mucocutaneous syphilitic lesions like chancre or condyloma lata or during pregnancy by vertical transmission from mother to fetus.

Syphilis during pregnancy is rare in the Western world today. It has tremendous consequences for the mother and her developing fetus if left untreated. Most untreated primary and secondary syphilis infections in pregnancy result in severe adverse pregnancy outcomes.

Latent (asymptomatic) syphilis infections in pregnancy also cause serious adverse pregnancy outcomes in more than half of cases.

Fetus can be easily cured with treatment, and the risk of adverse outcomes to the fetus is minimal if the mother receives adequate treatment during early pregnancy, ideally before the second trimester. The cervical changes which occur during pregnancy such as hyperaemia, eversion and friability facilitate the entry of spirochaete and lead to spirochaetaemia. The fundamental histological changes in both congenital and acquired syphilis are vasculitis and its consequences, necrosis and fibrosis.

Prevalence and Incidence

An estimated 350 000 adverse pregnancy outcomes worldwide were attributed to syphilis in 2012. The figures include 143 000 early fetal deaths/stillbirths, 62 000 neonatal deaths, 44 000 preterm/low-birthweight babies and 102 000 infected infants.[10] [EL 1]

Stages of Syphilis Infection

- Primary syphilis
- Secondary syphilis
- Latent phase
- Tertiary syphilis

Clinical Manifestation[11]

Primary Syphilis

- The incubation period is 3–90 days.
- A primary lesion or painless chancre appears at the site of inoculation and often goes unnoticed. Spontaneous resolution occurs within four to six weeks on average if not treated.
- Regional lymphadenopathy associated with primary disease lasts for months after the primary lesion has healed. Lymph nodes are non-suppurative and painless.

Secondary Syphilis

- Occurs six to eight weeks following untreated primary disease.
- Consists of systemic and local mucocutaneous lesions with generalised parenchymal and constitutional manifestations.
- Systemic manifestations include headache, low-grade fever, generalised lymphadenopathy, symmetrically distributed maculopapular rash found on the palms and the soles, the patchy moth-eaten alopecia with follicular scalp lesions, mild hepatitis, nephrotic syndrome and highly infectious condilomalatum found on the genitalia.

Left untreated, secondary syphilis spontaneously resolves within one to six months. Thereafter, the patient enters the latent phase of syphilis.

Latent Phase

- Characterised by the absence of clinical symptoms but positive serologic tests.
- Early latent syphilis is latent disease for less than one year's duration.
- Late latent syphilis is more than a year after infection.
- Except for early latent syphilis, latent disease is not sexually transmitted but can be vertically transmitted.[12]

After years of untreated disease, one-third of adults can develop tertiary syphilis.

Tertiary Syphilis

- Consists of destructive lesions of the aorta, such as aortic aneurysm, regurgitation, central nervous system disorders, meningovascular syphilis, skin and skeletal system manifestations.
- Breastfeeding does not result in transmission of syphilis unless an infectious lesion is present on the breast.

Effect on Pregnancy

Syphilitic stages are not altered because of pregnancy but >50 per cent of infants will be clinically affected in untreated early syphilis and 35 per cent in latent disease.

Pregnancy does not affect the course of syphilis, but syphilis can significantly affect the course of pregnancy.

Mother-to-Child Transmission

- The mother can transmit the infection transplacentally to the fetus or by direct contact with a lesion in birth canal during childbirth.
- Fetal infection occurs in >50 per cent of untreated early syphilis and 35 per cent of untreated latent disease.
- 25 per cent of pregnancies may result in stillbirth, miscarriage or other adverse pregnancy outcome.
- Vertical transmission of syphilis occurs in all stages of syphilis and in each trimester of pregnancy.
- Silver and immunofluorescent staining of the fetal tissue or polymerase chain reaction showed that *T. pallidum* gains access to the fetal compartment as early as nine to ten weeks.

Fetal Implications

Fetal syphilis is a continuum characterised by early hepatic and placental involvement followed by amniotic fluid infection, hematologic dysfunction, and finally ascites and fetal immunoglobulin M (IGM) production. Congenital syphilis is a multisystem infection which can result in stillbirth, neonatal death and long-term disability.

Untreated syphilis during pregnancy can have profound effect on pregnancy outcome, resulting in:

- Spontaneous abortion
- Stillbirth
- Non-immune hydrops fetalis
- Intrauterine growth restriction
- Premature delivery
- Perinatal death
- Serious sequelae in live-born infected children

Imaging for the Diagnosis of Fetal Syphilis

Ultrasound abnormalities suggestive of fetal syphilis can be seen after more than 20 weeks of pregnancy and in all stages of maternal syphilis.

The abnormalities seen on ultrasound scan include:

- Hepatomegaly
- Elevated middle cerebral artery blood flow
- Placentomegaly
- Polyhydramnios
- Ascites and fetal hydrops

Screening in Pregnancy

All pregnant women should be serologically screened for syphilis at the first antenatal care visit.

In women at high risk for infection, serologic testing should also be performed twice during the third trimester (once at 28–32 weeks and again at delivery).

Diagnosis and Testing[12,13]

There are two main diagnostic methods, the direct and the indirect methods.

Direct Methods

- Detection of *T. pallidum* by microscopic examination of fluid or smears from lesions (dark-field microscopy for the detection of *T. pallidum*).

  - On a wet mount under dark-field microscopy, the exudates and fluids from lesions are examined. *T. pallidum* is identified based on the characteristic morphology and motility of the spirochaete.
  - The direct fluorescent antibody test for *T. pallidum* can also be used, instead of dark-field microscopy. It detects antigen and, thus, does not require the presence of motile treponemes.

- Histological examination of tissues

  - It detects *T. pallidum* in tissue sections upon histological staining.

- Nucleic acid amplification methods such as polymerase chain reaction (PCR)

  - For the detection of *T. pallidum* in clinical specimens but these methods are not standardised yet.[13]

Indirect Methods

- Non-treponemal tests

  - Non-treponemal antibodies: rapid plasma reagin (RPR) test and the Venereal Disease Research Laboratory (VDRL) test which detects both IgM and immunoglobulin G (IgG) antibodies against cardiolipin released from host cell damage during infection.

- Treponemal tests

  - These tests can be qualitative or quantitative, with titres that increase with active disease and decrease with therapy.
  - Serum is the specimen of choice for serological testing, although plasma can be used in some non-treponemal serological tests.
  - Cerebrospinal fluid is used to diagnose congenital and tertiary syphilis in the presence of neurological symptoms.[13]

The WHO STI guideline suggests on-site tests and treatment strategy for pregnant women rather than the standard off-site laboratory-based screening in cases of:

- low settings coverage of syphilis screening
- high loss to follow-up of pregnant women or limited laboratory capacity
- in area of low prevalence of syphilis (below 5 per cent), rapid syphilis test (RST) be used to

screen pregnant women (Strategy A) rather than a single on-site RPR test

- in area of high prevalence of syphilis (5 per cent or greater), on-site rapid syphilis test (RST) (duo test for HIV and syphilis) and, if positive,
  - provision of a first dose of treatment and a RPR test, and then,
  - if the RPR test is positive, provision of treatment according to duration of syphilis
  - sequence of tests and treatment rather than a single on-site RST or a single on-site RPR test

Treatment of Syphilis during Pregnancy

Management of syphilis in pregnancy should involve the obstetrician, genitourinary physicians and neonatologist. Women should be assessed clinically to establish the stage of infection. Treatment should be initiated as soon as possible to limit fetal exposure.

If delivery occurs less than 30 days after completion of treatment, the neonate will require empirical treatment.[14]

Benzathene penicillin G (BPG) is highly effective and remains the only recommended treatment for maternal syphilis and prevention of congenital syphilis.

Studies have found an efficacy of 99.7 per cent for eradicating maternal disease and 98.2 per cent for preventing congenital syphilis across all stages of syphilis.

Skin testing should be carried out to avoid the risk of acute allergic reactions.

Approximately 5–10 per cent of pregnant women will have a history of penicillin allergy.

If skin testing is positive, they can undergo intravenous or oral penicillin desensitisation.

No serious reactions have been observed and this method is currently recommended so that all pregnant women with penicillin allergy can receive penicillin treatment.

There is no satisfactory alternative to penicillin for the treatment of syphilis during pregnancy.

Erythromycin is not recommended because it frequently fails to eradicate syphilis in both the mother and the fetus.

Tetracycline is effective, but not recommended because of dental staining and impairment of long bone growth in the fetus. If used intravenously with coexisting renal insufficiency it can cause hepatotoxicity.

Insufficient data exist to recommend erythromycin or ceftriaxone during pregnancy.

WHO guidelines on syphilis screening and treatment of pregnant women. 2017. Recommended management/treatment of syphilis during pregnancy:[14] [EL 2 & 3]

- Test for syphilis at first antenatal visit, third trimester and delivery
- Obtain proper history for all positive test results
- Examination is required to stage the disease
- If a woman is asymptomatic, check if a past infection was adequately treated
- If adequate treatment cannot be confirmed or titre is four-fold or higher, re-treat
- According to the stage of maternal disease (2 doses of BPG in early syphilis) of <1 year for fetal benefit
- Perform thorough fetal anatomy survey with ultrasound if viable fetus
- Commence first dose of BPG in labour/delivery under continuous fetal monitoring for 24 hours
- Consider early delivery with neonatal treatment if signs of fetal compromise or signs of fetal anomaly before term
- Antenatal testing can be considered in third trimester
- Notify neonatologist at delivery for adequate neonatal evaluation
- Send placenta for histopathology examination
- **WHO recommends these treatments for acquired syphilis during pregnancy: [EL 2 & 3]**

Stage of infection	Regimen and duration
1. Primary, secondary or early latent	Single-dose benzathene penicillin G, 2.4 million units IM
2. Late latent (>1 year) or unknown duration	Benzathene penicillin G, 2.4 million units IM weekly × 3 weeks
3. Neurosyphilis	Aqueous penicillin G, 2.4 million units IM every 4 hours × 10–14 days
	Or
	Procaine penicillin G, 2.4 million units IM and probenecid 500 mg orally four times daily × 10–14 days

- **Follow-up for success of treatment**
  Monthly serology is required to monitor treatment response. Indications for further treatment of the mother include:
  - presentation late in pregnancy
  - inadequate treatment response
  - venereal disease reference laboratory / reactive plasma reagin serofast at a titre more than 1:8
  - use of non-penicillin regime
- **Jarisch–Herxheimer reaction:**[15]

  This reaction occurs in up to 45 per cent of patients after treatment for acquired early syphilis. It consists of fever, chills, myalgia, headache, hypotension, tachycardia and transient accentuation of the cutaneous lesions. It begins within several hours of treatment and resolves within 24–36 hours. The release of *T. pallidum* lipoprotein from dead or dying organisms which possess inflammatory activity is implicated as the likely cause of this phenomenon.

  Supportive management of the Jarisch–Herxheimer reaction is offered and includes antipyretics.

  If fetal compromise is already present before treatment and the fetus is viable, then delivery with subsequent treatment of the fetus and mother may result in improved outcome.

Treatment of Neonates

The CDC recommends the following treatment:

Aqueous crystalline penicillin G 100 000–150 000 units/kg/day, administered as 50 000 units/kg/dose IV every 12 hours during the first 7 days of life and every 8 hours thereafter for a total of 10 days

or

Procaine penicillin G 50 000 units/kg/dose IM in a single daily dose for 10 days.[16]

Conclusion

Syphilis infection during pregnancy still presents a worldwide public health problem. Prenatal syphilis screening should be carried out at the first prenatal visit and again at 32–36 weeks. Women who deliver a stillborn infant after 20 weeks' gestation should be tested for syphilis.

Preconception serological tests for syphilis are the key to reduce the incidence of congenital syphilis.

Treatment when carried out properly offers a high chance of cure.

Lymphogranuloma Venereum

Introduction

Lymphogranuloma venereum (LGV) is a genital ulcer sexually transmitted disease. It is characterised by inguinal lymphadenopathy, anogenital lesions and fibrosis with gross distortion of the perineal tissues. It is caused by *Chlamydia trachomatis* serotypes L1, L2, L3. L2 is the most common strain involved.

The course of the disease is not altered with pregnancy, and transmission to the baby does not occur. Infection may be acquired during childbirth through infected birth canal. The obstetrical relevance of LGV lies in the fact that it may be associated with other sexually transmitted diseases and may make labour and delivery of women with stenosing perirectal lesions more difficult. LGV is not known to be associated with direct harm to the fetus.[17]

Prevalence

LGV is most frequently found in tropical and subtropical areas of the world.

Primary Lesion

The incubation period is extremely variable (3–30 days) from time of sexual contact with an infected individual. The primary lesion may be transient and imperceptible, in the form of a painless papule or pustule or shallow erosion or ulcer; it is often found on the after coronal sulcus of penis in men and on the posterior vaginal wall, fourchette or vulva, and occasionally on the cervix of women.

Secondary Lesion

C. trachomatis serovars L1–L3 are lymphotropic, infecting lymphocytes and macrophages. The essential pathological process is thrombolymphangitis and perilymphangitis. Thus, regional dissemination will be characterised by inflammation and swelling of lymph nodes and surrounding tissue. Classically, the most common clinical manifestation of genital LGV amongst heterosexuals is tender inguinal and/or femoral lymphadenopathy that is typically unilateral (two-thirds of cases). The disease process may involve one lymph node or the entire chain, which can become matted with considerable periadenitis and bubo formation. Buboes may ulcerate and discharge pus from multiple points, creating chronic fistulae. When both inguinal and femoral lymph nodes are involved, they may be separated by the so-called 'groove sign', which consists of the separation of these two lymph node systems by the inguinal ligament. Though considered pathognomonic of LGV, the 'groove sign' only occurs in 15–20 per cent of cases. Lymphadenopathy commonly follows the primary lesion by a period of a few days to weeks (10–30 days, rarely months). The systemic spread of *C. trachomatis* may be associated with fever, arthritis, pneumonitis and more rarely abnormal hepatic enzymes and perihepatitis.[18]

Tertiary Stage (or the genito-anorectal syndrome)

The majority of patients recover after the secondary stage without sequelae, but in a few patients the persistence or progressive spread of *C. trachomatis* in anogenital tissues will incite a chronic inflammatory response and destruction of tissue in the involved areas, including: proctitis, proctocolitis mimicking Crohn's disease, fistulae, strictures and chronic granulomatous disfiguring fibrosis and scarring of the vulva with *esthiomene* (Greek word meaning 'eating away'). These conditions occur most frequently in women, reflecting the involvement of retroperitoneal lymphatics (rather than inguinal).

Diagnosis

Diagnosis is based on clinical suspicion, epidemiologic information, and by exclusion of other causes of proctocolitis, inguinal lymphadenopathy, genital or rectal ulcers.

Swabs from the lesions or bubo aspirate can be tested for *C. trachomatis* by culture, direct immunofluorescence or nucleic acid detection. The diagnosis is difficult as there is no characteristic presentation, laboratory procedures for this pathogen are not standardised and serologic tests have low specificity.

For rectal specimens, studies have demonstrated a high sensitivity and specificity using nucleic acid detection.

Commercial molecular diagnostic techniques to detect *C. trachomatis* remain the primary test of choice, with referral of *C. trachomatis*-positive specimens for molecular tests to confirm the presence of LGV-associated DNA.

All patients with LGV should be treated for HIV infection and other sexually transmitted disease.

Treatment

Treatment during the secondary stage will prevent tertiary complications.

Erythromycin

- Pregnant and lactating women are treated with erythromycin 500 mg orally four times a day for 21 days.
- Test of cure is advised in pregnancy if rectal or genital LGV is diagnosed.
- A three-week course of erythromycin 500 mg four times daily orally is recommended. The most common erythromycin side effects are gastrointestinal problems including mild diarrhoea, stomach pain, and nausea and vomiting.
- Late sequelae such as fistulas and stricture may require subsequent surgical repair.
- Patients with both LGV and HIV infection should receive the same regimen as those who are HIV-negative.

Oral thiamphenicol can also be used in the dose of 1.5 g for 21 days, but only in the final trimester of pregnancy.

Drainage of buboes (by surgical incision) is contraindicated, except in cases of intense compression for patient's relief and it should be done with thick bevel needles.

- Late lesions with fibrosis and stenosis in the birth canal may indicate the need for a caesarean section.

References

1. Clinical Effectiveness Group, British Association for Sexual Health and HIV. *UK National Guidelines for the Management of Gonorrhea in Adults, 2011.* London: BASHH; 2011.

2. Centers for Disease Control and Prevention. *Sexually Transmitted Disease Surveillance, 2015.* Atlanta, GA: US Department of Health and Human Services; 2016.

3. Lacey CJ, Milne JD. Preterm labour in association with Neisseria gonorrheae: case reports. *Br J Vener Dis.* 1984; **60**: 123–4.

4. Gul SS, Jamal M, Khan N. Ophthalmia neonatorum. *J Coll Physicians Surg Pak.* 2010; **20**(9): 595–8.

5. Fifer H, Ison CA. Nucleic acid amplification tests for the diagnosis of Neisseria gonorrhoeae in low-prevalence settings: a review of the evidence. *Sex Transm Infect.* 2014; **90**(8): 577–9.

6. *WHO Guidelines for the Treatment of Neisseria Gonorrhoeae.* Geneva: World Health Organization; 2016.

7. Brocklehurst P. Antibiotics for gonorrhea in pregnancy. *Cochrane Database Syst Rev.* 2002; 2: CD000098.

8. Bignell C, Unemo M, European STI Guidelines Editorial Board. 2012 European guideline on the diagnosis and treatment of gonorrhoea in adults. *Int J STD AIDS.* 2013; **24**(2): 85–92. doi:10.1177/0956462412472837.

9. Workowski KA, Bolan GA, Centers for Disease Control and Prevention. STD treatment guidelines 2015. www.cdc.gov/std/tg2015/.

10. Kenyon CR, Osbak K, Tsoumanis, A, Small PLC. The global epidemiology of syphilis in the past century: a systematic review based on antenatal syphilis prevalence. *PLoS Negl Trop Dis.* 2016; **10**(5): e0004711.

11. Centers for Disease Control and Prevention. Syphilis – CDC Fact Sheet. www.cdc.gov/std/syphilis/stdfact-syphilis.htm.

12. Morsheda MG, Singh AE. Recent trends in the serologic diagnosis of syphilis. *Clin Vaccine Immunol.* 2015; **22**(2), 137–47.

13. World Health Organization. WHO guidelines on syphilis screening and treatment of pregnant women. 2017. http://apps.who.int/iris/bitstream/10665/259003/1/9789241550093-eng.pdf.

14. Belum GR, Belum VR, Chaitanya Arudra SK, Reddy BS. The Jarisch-Herxheimer reaction: revisited. *Travel Med Infect Dis.* 2013; **11**(4): 231–7.

15. De Santis M, De Luca C, Mappa I et al. Syphilis infection during pregnancy: fetal risks and clinical management. *Infect Dis Obstet Gynecol.* 2012; **430585**: e461–6.

16. Centers for Disease Control and Prevention. Congenital syphilis. www.cdc.gov/std/tg192015/congenital.htm.

17. Oud EV, de Vrieze NH, de Meij A, de Vries HJ. Pitfalls in the diagnosis and management of inguinal lymphogranuloma venereum: important lessons from a case series. *Sex Transm Infect.* 2014; **90**(4):279–82.

18. Ceovic R, Jerkovic Gulin S. Lymphogranuloma venereum: diagnostic and treatment challenges. *Infect Drug Resist.* 2015; **8**: 39–47.

Mycoplasma, Ureaplasma, Chancroid, Granuloma Inguinale (Donovanosis)

Nutan Mishra

Mycoplasma genitalium

Introduction

Seven mycoplasmal strains have been isolated from the genital tract, of which *Mycoplasma hominis* and *Mycoplasma genitalium* are the commonest.

M. genitalium has an unknown incubation period, but symptoms commonly develop within one to three weeks.

There is an estimated 2–2.5-fold increase in the risk of urethritis, cervicitis, pelvic inflammatory disease, infertility and preterm delivery for women infected with *M. genitalium*.[1]

It can be found in the vagina, cervix and endometrium, and usually the infections are asymptomatic. Most studies have the organism in 10–30 per cent of women with clinical cervicitis.

M. genitalium infection is a sexually transmitted infection.

Clinical Presentations

- Dysuria
- Vaginal discharge
- Urethral discharge
- Pelvic pain
- Possibly proctitis
- Intermenstrual bleeding
- Post-coital bleeding

Complications

- Pelvic inflammatory disease (PID)
- Infertility
- Ectopic pregnancy

Effect on Pregnancy

- Preterm labour
- Miscarriage
- Chorioamnionitis

  o A meta-analysis demonstrated an approximately two-fold increased risk of cervicitis, preterm birth and spontaneous abortion in women infected with *M. gentialium*. [EL 1]

  o *M. hominis* was isolated from blood in approximately 13 per cent of women with postpartum and post-abortion fever.

  o It was found to be an independent risk factor for preterm delivery after 24 weeks of gestation.[2]

Diagnosis

M. genitalium is a slow-growing organism.

Culture can take up to six months, and only a few laboratories in the world are able to recover clinical isolates.

Nucleic acid amplification test (NAAT) is the preferred method for *M. genitalium* detection. It is only available in a few large medical centres and commercial laboratories.

Diagnosis is made by NAAT testing of urine, urethral, vaginal and cervical swabs and through endometrial biopsies, typically using in-house polymerase chain reaction (PCR) or assays intended for research use only.[3]

Treatment

M. genitalium lacks a cell wall, and thus antibiotics targeting cell wall biosynthesis (e.g. beta-lactams including penicillins and cephalosporins) are ineffective against this organism.

Due to diagnostic challenges, treatment of most *M. genitalium* infections occurs in the context of syndromic management for urethritis, cervicitis and PID.[4]

Urethritis and Cervicitis

First-Line Therapy

- Single dose of 1 g azithromycin was more effective than doxycycline in two randomised urethritis treatment trials and is the preferred choice. [EL 1]

  However, resistance to azithromycin appears to be rapidly growing as median cure rate used to be approximately 85 per cent, but in the most recent trial (278) was found to be in only 40 per cent.

- Longer course of azithromycin (an initial 500 mg dose followed by 250 mg daily for four days) might be marginally superior. However, in some settings, approximately 50 per cent of all *M. genitalium* infections are caused by organisms that are already resistant to azithromycin, therefore no regimen has beneficial effect over others.

Second-Line Therapy

- Moxifloxacin, a fourth-generation fluoroquinolone (400 mg daily for 14 days), has been successfully used to treat *M. genitalium* in men and women with previous treatment failures, with cure rates of 100 per cent in initial reports.

- However, it has been used in only a few cases, and the drug has not been tested in clinical trials. Although generally considered effective, studies in Japan, Australia and the United States have reported moxifloxacin treatment failures after the seven-day regimen.[5]

Pelvic Inflammatory Disease

PID unresponsive to the standard treatment should be tested for *M. genitalium* where available. A regimen of moxifloxacin 400 mg/day for 14 days has been effective in eradicating the organism. Nevertheless, no data have been published that assess the benefits of testing women with PID for *M. genitalium*, and the importance of directing treatment against this organism is currently unknown.

- Effective treatment reduces the risks of preterm labour and neonatal complications.[6]
- Because of the increasing resistance among *M. genitalium* for macrolides and quinolones, treatment courses should be short and convenient in order to ensure compliance.
- Patients with *M. genitalium* infection should observe abstinence from unprotected intercourse until both sexual partners have completed the treatment and are symptom-free.
- Both sexual partners should be screened for other STIs.
- If the partner does not get tested, the same treatment is offered as given to the index patient.
- A test of cure should also be performed routinely for all patients, in view of the increasing prevalence of macrolide resistance, which may exist prior to initiation of therapy or can evolve during therapy with a macrolide.[7]

Contact Tracing

- In heterosexuals there is a greater risk of PID and reproductive complications, which suggests a greater need to trace, test and treat infected contacts. The time period for contact tracing is unknown.
- Usual testing method: nucleic acid amplification testing on first-pass urine in men (urethral swab less sensitive) and first-pass urine, high vaginal or cervical swab in women.
- It is sexually transmitted, with possible infection due to oral sex.
- Duration of potential infectivity is unknown, but persistent infection occurs in 25 per cent of cases, which may persist to more than 12 months. Infections up to two to three years have been reported.[8]

Ureaplasma

Ureaplasma parvum (serovars 1, 3, 6 and 14) and *Ureaplasma urealyticum* (serovars 2, 4, 5 and 7–13) lack cell walls, hydrolyse urea to generate adenosine triphosphate (ATP), have limited biosynthetic functions and adhere to human mucosal surfaces of the genitourinary tract in adults and respiratory tract in newborns.

These organisms can be detected in vaginal flora in 40–80 per cent of healthy women, and their presence has been causally linked to infertility and other fetal implications.

Fetal Implications

Vertical transmission from mothers to their infants occurs *in utero* or during delivery.

- Early pregnancy loss
- Stillbirth, preterm birth
- Neonatal morbidities

The clinical history of patients with urogenital or extragenital infections because of *Ureaplasma* species is syndrome-specific, not organism-specific. Usually there are no distinguishing features to indicate the microbiologic aetiology of these infections.[9]

Because of lack of facilities to diagnose *Ureaplasma* infections in many clinical settings, many clinicians are unfamiliar with aetiologic agents. Identification of these organisms may be achieved only as a last resort, especially if initial treatment with ineffective drugs is unsuccessful.

Signs and Symptoms in Adults

- Urethritis
- Pyelonephritis
- Cystitis
- Urinary calculi
- Endometritis or chorioamnionitis
- Infectious arthritis
- Surgical and non-surgical wound infections
- Bacteraemia
- Pneumonia
- Meningitis

Neonatal Implications

Neonates, particularly if preterm, are especially vulnerable to dissemination of infectious organisms (acquired *in utero* or at birth) in the bloodstream and, ultimately, the central nervous system.

Usually there are no characteristic signs and symptoms to predict the type of organism present. Subtle manifestations, such as temperature instability, blood pressure fluctuations, heart rate and respiratory efforts, may be the only signs that an infection is present.

Consider *Ureaplasma* species if signs and symptoms of infection are present; if the neonate does not respond to beta-lactam drugs; and if cultures from blood, the lower respiratory tract and cerebrospinal fluid (CSF) do not reveal a more common microbiological cause.

Radiographic evidence of pneumonitis in the absence of a proven bacterial or viral cause and mononuclear or polymorph nuclear pleocytosis (an abnormal increase in the amount of lymphocytes in the CSF with a negative Gram stain and culture result are consistent with *Ureaplasma* infection.

Although these organisms have been considered of low virulence, in vitro and in vivo experimental models have provided extra evidence that perinatal morbidities in premature babies (such as bronchopulmonary dysplasia, intraventricular haemorrhage and necrotising enterocolitis) do exist.[10]

Diagnosis

Culture Methods

Since *Ureaplasma* species hydrolyse urea and use it for a substrate for ATP generation, the organisms require media containing urea such as 10B broth and A8 agar. In experienced laboratories, the detection limit for culture methods is 100–1000 viable organisms.

For females, urine, cervical swabs or vaginal swabs are acceptable.

Polymerase Chain Reaction, Molecular Techniques (PCR)

This is more sensitive than culture for detection (<100 genome copies) of non-viable as well as viable ureaplasmas.[11]

Antimicrobial Therapy

Erythromycin ethylsuccinate
   Dose: oral 800 mg tablets, eight-hourly for seven days
Clarithromycin
   (USA only) Dose: suspension, 500 mg oral 12-hourly for 7–14 days
Azithromycin
   Dose: 1 g orally in a single dose[12]

Chancroid (*Haemophilus ducreyi* Infection)

Background

Chancroid is a bacterial sexually transmitted disease (STD) caused by *Haemophilus ducreyi* infection. It is characterised by painful necrotising genital ulcers that may be accompanied by inguinal lymphadenopathy. It is a highly contagious but curable disease.

Clinical manifestations include genital ulcers and inguinal lymphadenopathy.[13]

Chancroid was previously highly prevalent in many areas of the world. Because of collaborative efforts and increasing social awareness, along with subsequent changes in sexual practices, improved diagnosis and treatment options, it has been eradicated as an endemic disease in industrialised countries.[14]

- In 2000, the proportion of chancroid among genital ulcerative diseases decreased from 69 per cent to 15 per cent.
- It remains prevalent in certain underdeveloped regions such as Asia, Africa and the Caribbean. In these areas, outbreaks occur in cities among workers in the sex trade.
- Individuals travelling to these high-risk areas are at risk of contracting the disease.
- In addition, individuals from high-risk areas who travel to other countries to work in the sex industry remain a source of outbreaks in the industrialised world.

Bacteriology and Pathophysiology

Haemophilus ducreyi is a small, gram-negative, facultative anaerobic bacillus that is highly infective. It is pathogenic only in humans, with no intermediary environmental or animal host.

H. ducreyi invades the skin through disrupted mucosa with a local inflammatory reaction. It produces a distending toxin that appears to be responsible for its destructive effects on the tissues and consequent aggravation of the ulcers.

The organism has an incubation period of one day to two weeks, with a median time of five to seven days.[15]

Clinical Features

- The incubation period is short: three to five days after sexual intercourse with an infected person.
- Usual presentation is the development of a tender erythematous papule, mostly on the prepuce and frenulum in men and on the vulva cervix and perineal area in women.
- Infection starts as a papule, which quickly progresses to a pustule and subsequent ulcer formation.

- Painful inguinal lymphadenopathy with subsequent ulceration, usually unilateral, develops in approximately 50 per cent of patients within one to two weeks.
- The ulcer is a soft chancre because it is not indurated, as opposed to the indurated syphilitic chancre.
- The lesion begins as erythematous tender papules that pustulate and later erode to form an extremely painful and deep ulcer.
- Ulcers may be single or multiple, and as many as 10 ulcers have been reported on a single patient.[15]
- Men more commonly present with single ulcers, whereas women typically have multiple lesions. 'Kissing ulcers' occur when one ulcer spreads the infection to the opposite skin surface. Kissing ulcers can form on the lips of the labia majora.
- Individual ulcers vary in size from 1 to 20 .
- In circumcised men, lesions are most commonly found on the coronal sulcus. In uncircumcised men, the lesions are commonly found on the prepuce.
- In women, lesions are most commonly found on the fourchette, labia, vestibule, clitoris, cervix and anus. Women may not have external sores but may present with dysuria, dyspareunia and vaginal or rectal discharge.[16]

Differential Diagnosis

- Herpes simplex
- Syphilitic ulcers

Diagnostic Considerations

Clinical

The combination of a painful genital ulcer and tender suppurative inguinal adenopathy suggests the diagnosis of chancroid.

For both clinical and surveillance purposes, a probable diagnosis of chancroid can be made if all of the following criteria are met:

- The presence of one or more painful genital ulcers.
- Appearance of genital ulcers with regional lymphadenopathy are typical for chancroid.
- The patient has no evidence of *T. pallidum* infection by dark-field examination of ulcer exudate or by a serologic test for syphilis. performed at least seven days after onset of ulcers
- A negative herpes simplex virus PCR test.

95

Ulcer Biopsy and Histologic Findings of the Ulcer Exudate

A Gram stain of the ulcer exudates may show short, plump, gram-negative rods in the classic picture of fish appearance.

Ulcer biopsy should reveal three distinct zones:

- The most superficial zone contains erythrocytes, fibrin, necrotic tissue and neutrophils.
- The next zone consists of marked endothelial cell proliferation and many thrombosed new blood vessels.
- The deepest layer is characterised by a dense infiltrate of plasma and lymphoid cells.[17]

Culture and Isolation of *H. ducreyi*

Isolation of *H. ducreyi* on special media is the definitive diagnosis, but such tests are not readily available in many centres. Also, lesion culture is inaccurate owing to the excessively particular, critical nature of the organism, with a sensitivity of less than 80 per cent.[18]

Polymerase Chain Reaction

The role of PCR in rapid detection of *H. ducreyi* is promising and may supersede culture in diagnosis.[19]

Treatment

- Successful treatment for chancroid cures the infection, resolves the clinical symptoms and prevents transmission to others. In advanced cases, scarring can result despite successful therapy.
- Patients presenting with suspected or diagnosed chancroid should undergo complete evaluation for any sexually transmitted infections and receive appropriate antimicrobial therapy for the eradication of *H. ducreyi* and the treatment of other more common STDs.

Recommended regimens (according to the CDC's 2015 Sexually Transmitted Diseases Treatment Guidelines and the UK National Guideline for the management of chancroid) [EL 2 & 3]

Azithromycin 1 g orally in a single dose

or

Ceftriaxone 250 mg intramuscularly (IM) in a single dose

or

Ciprofloxacin 500 mg orally twice a day for three days

or

Erythromycin base 500 mg orally three times a day for seven days

- Azithromycin and ceftriaxone offer the advantage of single-dose therapy.[20]
- Ceftriaxone is the treatment of choice in pregnant women.
- Ciprofloxacin presents a low risk to the fetus during pregnancy, with potential toxic effects during breastfeeding.
- Sexual partners of patients with chancroid should be examined and treated regardless of the presence of symptoms if they had sexual contact within 10 days preceding the onset of symptoms.
- Men who are uncircumcised and with HIV infection do not respond as well to treatment as patients who are circumcised or HIV-negative.
- Patients should be tested for HIV infection at the time chancroid is diagnosed. If the initial test results were negative, a serologic test for syphilis and HIV infection should be performed three months after the diagnosis of chancroid.[20]
- Patients should abstain from unprotected sexual intercourse while undergoing treatment.

Follow-Up

Patients should be re-examined three to seven days after initiation of therapy.

Ulcers usually improve symptomatically within three days and objectively within seven days after therapy.

Clinical resolution of fluctuant lymphadenopathy is slower than that of ulcers and might require needle aspiration or incision and drainage, despite otherwise successful therapy.

Effect on Pregnancy

No adverse effects of chancroid on pregnancy outcome have been reported. Use of drugs such as ciprofloxacin presents a low risk to the fetus during pregnancy, with a potential for toxicity during breastfeeding. Alternate drugs like erythromycin and ceftriaxone should be used during pregnancy and lactation.

Granuloma Inguinale (Donovanosis)

Granuloma inguinale is a genital ulcerative disease caused by the intracellular gram-negative bacterium *Klebsiella granulomatis*.[21]

The molecular structure of the causative organism is similar to *Klebsiella* gram-negative pleomorphic bacillus *Klebsiella granulomatis* species.[21]

Modes of Transport

Primarily occurs through sexual contact; however, it has low infectious capabilities because repeated exposure is necessary for clinical infection to occur.[22]

Granuloma inguinale may also be obtained through the faecal route.[22]

Vertical transmission through passage through an infected birth canal.

Clinical Picture

Clinically, the disease is commonly characterised as painless, progressive ulcerative lesions without regional lymphadenopathy. The incubation period is about 50 days.

There are four main types of cutaneous lesions:

1. **Nodular**: the initial lesion is a papule or nodule that arises at the site of inoculation. The nodule is soft, often pruritic and erythematous, and eventually ulcerates.
2. **Ulcerovegetative** (most common): these granuloma inguinale lesions start as nodular lesions and then create large, usually painless, expanding, suppurative ulcers. The ulcers have clean, friable bases with distinct, raised, rolled margins and have a tendency to bleed easily. The ulcers are 'beefy red', slowly expanding centrifugally, eventually becoming more granulomatous with serpiginous borders. Ulcers often become secondarily infected with other types of bacteria and emit a putrid odour.
3. **Cicatricial**: dry ulcers evolve into cicatricial plaques and may be associated with lymphedema growing into a vegetating mass, which may resemble genital warts.
4. **Elephantiasis-like** swelling of the external genitalia is a frequent complication and is found most often in infected females in the late stage of granuloma inguinale.

Lymphadenopathy is not a direct result of the primary infection with *Klebsiella granulomatis*, but it occurs from secondary bacterial infections.[23]

Complications

- Carcinoma is the most serious complication. It occurs in 0.25 per cent of patients. This includes squamous cell carcinoma and basal cell carcinoma.
- Extensive fibrosis, stricture formation and Pharoses (the inability to retract the skin), leading to significant deformity and functional disability.
- Elephantiasis of the genitals may develop secondary to lymphatic destruction.
- Auto-amputation of the penis has been reported in a man with long-standing granuloma inguinale associated with underlying HIV-2 infection.

Differential Diagnoses

- Dermatologic manifestations of chancroid
- Dermatologic manifestations of herpes simplex
- Dermatologic manifestations of Lymphogranuloma venereum

Diagnosis

Culture and Recovery of the Organism

The organism is extremely fastidious. Culture is beyond the capability of most laboratories.

Smears from the Base of the Ulcer

Smears of the base of the ulcer are the easiest method to visualise the organism. The organisms are seen within the cytoplasm of histiocytes. Characteristically, they exhibit bipolar staining, which has been likened to a safety-pin appearance, and are referred to as Donovan bodies.

Special Stains to Demonstrate the Donovan Bodies

Alternatively, a crush preparation can be performed. A small piece of tissue should be obtained from the ulcer edge or base via punch biopsy, curettage or a thin wedge resection. A Wright–Giemsa, Warthin–Starry, toluidine blue, or Leishman stain may be used to demonstrate Donovan bodies.

A Tissue Biopsy Specimen

The biopsied tissue is stained with haematoxylin and eosin. Thin, paraffin-embedded sections stained with Giemsa's or silver stain may facilitate identification of the rod-shaped, encapsulated organisms within the macrophages.

Polymerase Chain Reaction

These may be may be more sensitive; however, they are currently only used for scientific research.

Papanicolaou Smears

These may identify Donovan bodies in patients undergoing routine cervical cytological screening.

Effect on Pregnancy

Lesions tend to grow more rapidly during pregnancy.

Transmission may occur during vaginal delivery, and careful cleansing of neonates born to infected mothers is recommended.

Rarely, disseminated Donovanosis with spread to bone and liver may occur and is usually associated with pregnancy and cervical infection.

Treatment

- Prolonged therapy is usually required to permit granulation and re-epithelialisation of the ulcers. Relapse can occur 6–18 months after apparently effective therapy.
- Pregnancy is a relative contraindication to the use of sulfonamides.
- Pregnant and lactating women should be treated with the erythromycin regimen, and consideration should be given to the addition of a parenteral aminoglycoside (e.g. gentamicin).
- Azithromycin might prove useful for treating granuloma inguinale during pregnancy, but published data are lacking. Doxycycline and ciprofloxacin are contraindicated in pregnant women.
- During pregnancy, erythromycin 500 mg four times daily for at least three weeks is used.
- Therapy should be continued for at least three weeks and until all lesions have completely healed. Some specialists recommend the addition of an aminoglycoside (e.g. gentamicin 1 mg/kg IV every eight hours) to these regimens if improvement is not evident within the first few days of therapy.

CDC Recommended Regimen[24]

Azithromycin: 1 g orally once per week or 500 mg daily for at least three weeks and until all lesions have completely healed

Or

Alternative Regimens

Doxycycline: (contraindicated in pregnancy) 100 mg orally twice a day for at least three weeks and until all lesions have completely healed

Or

Ciprofloxacin: (category C) 750 mg orally twice a day for at least three weeks and until all lesions have completely healed

Or

Erythromycin base: 500 mg orally four times a day for at least three weeks and until all lesions have completely healed

Or

Trimethoprim–sulfamethoxazole: (category D, contraindicated in pregnancy) one double-strength (160 mg/800 mg) tablet orally twice a day for at least three weeks and until all lesions have completely healed

Follow-Up

Patients should be followed clinically until signs and symptoms have resolved.

Management of Sex Partners

Persons who have had sexual contact with a patient who has granuloma inguinale within the 60 days before onset of the patient's symptoms should be examined and offered therapy. However, the value of empiric therapy in the absence of clinical signs and symptoms has not been established.

References

1. Australian Sexual Health Alliance. Australian STI management guidelines. Mycoplasma genitalium. 2018. www.sti.guidelines.org.au/xually-transmissible-infections/mycoplasma-genitalium#contact-tracing.

2. Latino MA, Botta G, Badino C et al. Association between genital mycoplasmas, acute chorioamnionitis and fetal pneumonia in spontaneous abortions. *J Perinat Med.* 2017; 25 May: 0305.

3. Le Roy C, Pereyre S, Bébéar C. Evaluation of two commercial real-time PCR assays for detection of

Mycoplasma genitalium in urogenital specimens. *J Clin Microbiol.* 2014; **52**(3): 971–3.

4. Sethi S, Zaman K, Jain N. Mycoplasma genitalium infections: current treatment options and resistance issues. *Infect Drug Resist.* 2017; **10**: 283–92.

5. Jernberg E, Moghaddam A, Moi H. Azithromycin and moxifloxacin for microbiological cure of Mycoplasma genitalium infection: an open study. *Int J STD AIDS.* 2008; **19**(10): 676–9.

6. Vouga G, Greub G, Prod'hom C et al. Treatment of genital mycoplasma in colonized pregnant women in late pregnancy is associated with a lower rate of premature labour and neonatal complications. *Clin Microbiol Infect.* 2014; **20**(10): 1074–9.

7. Jensen JS, Cusini M, Gomberg M, Moi H. 2016 European guideline on Mycoplasma genitalium infections. *J Eur Acad Dermatol Venereol.* 2016; **30**(10): 1650–6.

8. Australian Sexual Health Alliance. Australian STI management guidelines. Mycoplasma genitalium. The Australian Contact Tracing Manual. 2018. contacttracing.ashm.org.itions/when-contact-tracing-is-recommended/mycoplasma-genitalium.

9. Waites, KB. Ureaplasma Infection Clinical Presentation. Medscape. https://emedicine.medscape.com/article/231470-clinical.

10. Waites KB, Katz B, Schelonka RL. Mycoplasmas and ureaplasmas as neonatal pathogens. *Clin Microbiol Rev.* 2005; **18**(4): 757–89.

11. Kokkayil P, Dhawan B. Ureaplasma: current perspectives. *Indian J Med Microbiol.* 2015; **33**(2): 205–14.

12. Centers for Disease Control and Prevention. 2015 Sexually Transmitted Diseases Treatment Guidelines. 2015. www.cdc.gov/std/tg2015/urethritis-and-cervicitis.htm.

13. Buensalido JAL, Francisco CN. Chancroid. Medscape. Drugs & Diseases > Infectious Diseases. 2015. https://emedicine.medscape.com/article/214737-overview.

14. World Health Organization. Richard Steen. Eradicating chancroid. www.who.int/bulletin/archives/79(9)818.pdf.

15. Health line. Chancroid. www.healthline.com/health/chancroid.

16. Medical Encyclopedia. Chancroid. https://medlineplus.gov/ency/article/000635.htm.

17. Alfa M. The laboratory diagnosis of Haemophilus ducreyi. *Can J Infect Dis Med Microbiol.* 2005; **16**(1): 31–4.

18. Lewis. DA. Diagnostic tests for chancroid. *BMJ.* 2000; **76**(2): 137–41.

19. Glatz M, Juricevic N, Altwegg M et al. A multicenter prospective trial to assess a new real-time polymerase chain reaction for detection of Treponema pallidum, herpes simplex-1/2 and Haemophilus ducreyi in genital, anal and oropharyngeal ulcers. *Clin Microbiol Infect.* 2014; **20**(12): O1020-7.

20. O'Farrell N, Lazaro N. UK National Guideline for the management of Chancroid 2014. *Int J STD AIDS.* 2014; **25**(14): 975–83.

21. Anderson K. The cultivation from granuloma inguinale of a microorganism having the characteristics of Donovan bodies in the yolk sac of chick embryos. *Science.* 1943; **97**(2529): 560–1.

22. Satter EK. Granuloma Inguinale (Donovanosis). Drugs & Diseases > Dermatology. Medscape. Updated 23 January 2017. http://emedicine.medscape.com/article/1052617-overview#a5.

23. Velho PE, Souza EM, Belda W Jr. Donovanosis. *Braz J Infect Dis.* 2008; **12**(6): 521–5.

24. Centers for Disease Control and Prevention. 2015. Sexually Transmitted Diseases Treatment Guidelines. www.cdc.gov/std/tg2015/donovanosis.htm.

Genital *Chlamydia trachomatis* and Bacterial Vaginosis

Adel Elkady, Prabha Sinha and Soad Ali Zaki Hassan

Introduction

Chlamydia trachomatis genitourinary infection is a sexually transmitted infection affecting the uterus, the salpinges, the cervix, the urethra and the epididymis.

The infection is the most commonly reported bacterial sexually transmitted disease (STD) in the United States and a leading cause of infertility in women.

It can cause several sequelae, including chronic pelvic pain, pelvic inflammatory disease (PID) and tubal factor infertility.

Chlamydia trachomatis is commonly diagnosed in pregnancy. It has been linked to several pregnancy complications (premature rupture of membranes (PROM), preterm labour and birth, low birthweight, intrauterine growth retardation and postpartum endometritis).

In infected pregnant women, infants are at risk for acquiring *C. trachomatis* pneumonitis, conjunctivitis and nasopharyngeal infection.

Bacteriological Background

Genera *Chlamydia* bacteria (*Chlamydia trachomatis, Chlamydophila pneumoniae* and *Chlamydophila psittaci*) are microscopic unicellular prokaryotic organisms characterised by the lack of a membrane-bound nucleus and membrane-bound organelles.[1]

Chlamydiae are small, aerobic, gram-negative obligate intracellular micro-organisms that need oxygen to grow.[2] Chlamydia depend on the host cell for intermediates, including adenosine triphosphate (ATP).

C. trachomatis has 18 serologically variant strains (serovars based on monoclonal antibody-based typing assays).

These serovars are associated with different medical disorders.

- Serovars A, B, Ba and C cause a serious eye disease (trachoma) characterised by chronic conjunctivitis which if untreated may lead to blindness.
- Serovars D–K cause genital infections; in women they are a common cause of cervicitis, urethritis, endometritis, salpingitis and perihepatitis.[2]
- Serovars L1–L3 cause genital ulcers (Lymphogranuloma venereum (LGV)).[3]

Incidence and Prevalence of Chlamydia Infection during Pregnancy

Worldwide prevalence studies of *C. trachomatis* in pregnant women suggest similar if not higher rates than in non-pregnant women. In Africa, prevalence in pregnant women is up to 31.1 per cent,[3] and in Asian countries the reported prevalence rates varied between 4.9–14 per cent and 41–44 per cent.[4]

Certain groups of women are at increased risk: those receiving care at public health clinics, young women and those with multiple sexual partners.

In a study in the USA, of a prospective cohort of 125 pregnant adolescents (12–18 years), 19 per cent were diagnosed at booking for prenatal care. Nine per cent had a recurrent infection, and 4 per cent were diagnosed with new *C. trachomatis* only on repeat testing. This study also shows that the infection may arise *de novo* during pregnancy.[5] [EL 2]

Risk Factors for Chlamydia Infection during Pregnancy

Age <25 Years

The young sexually active population is consistently associated with increased risk of chlamydial infection.[6]

Twenty-nine of 34 studies of females and five of seven studies of males have shown a significant relationship between age and chlamydial infection in a multivariate analysis.[7] [EL 1]

The increased prevalence in adolescents may also often be attributed to differences in sexual behaviours, multiple premarital relations, multiple sexual partners and unsafe sex practices.[8]

Marital Status

Chlamydia infection rates tend to be highest in women who are single and have had multiple sexual partners.[9]

Race, Ethnicity and Social Status

In the United States, data show higher rates of reported STDs among some racial or ethnic minority groups when compared with the white population.

Sexual Partners

- Two-thirds of partners of people testing positive for chlamydia will also test positive.
- Two or more sexual partners in the preceding year increases the risk.
- The length of time between partnerships ('gap') is an important determinant of the overall transmission of STD.
- A rapid recent change in sexual partners (a positive gap) who may have had an undiagnosed or untreated chlamydia infection also plays a role in increasing the risk of infection.[10]

Infection with Another Sexually Transmitted Infection (STI)

Other risk factors include having an STI in the past or currently.

Maternal Implications

- As many as 85–90 per cent of infected men and women are asymptomatic.
- *C. trachomatis* has been implicated with maternal infections in the post-abortal, post-caesarean section, puerperal sepsis and PID.
- These complications are particularly relevant to elective termination surgery. In a study in Denmark, in women undergoing elective termination of pregnancy, 15 out of 23 chlamydia-infected women (65.20 per cent) developed acute PID.[11] [EL 2]
- A recent meta-analysis of 22 studies concluded that women infected with *C. trachomatis* have a higher risk of cervical cancer. Six studies

suggested that co-infection of human papillomavirus (HPV) and *C. trachomatis* was related to a higher risk of uterine cervix cancer (OR = 4.03), thus stressing the need for screening and treatment of women with chlamydia infection, particularly those with HPV infection. [EL 1][12]

Signs and Symptoms

Symptomatic women may describe vaginal discharge and dysuria (always consider chlamydia as a cause of sterile pyuria, which is the presence of 6–10 or more neutrophils per high-power field of unspun, voided mid-stream urine).

They may describe vague lower abdominal pain or fever. Dyspareunia, intermenstrual or post-coital bleeding has also been reported.

Physical examination may reveal:

- A friable, inflamed cervix, sometimes with a follicular or 'cobblestone' appearance, with contact bleeding and/or mucopurulent endocervical discharge.
- Abdominal pain.
- Pelvic adnexal tenderness or cervical excitation may be elicited on bimanual palpation. Sometimes, chlamydial infection in women is suggested by inflammatory changes in their cervical cytology report and this may require follow-up.[13]

Non-genital chlamydia may present with a reactive arthritis, Reiter's syndrome (urethritis, arthritis and conjunctivitis). In perihepatitis (Fitz-Hugh Curtis syndrome), upper abdominal pain is a presenting feature.

Symptoms in a male partner of any pregnant woman are an indication for STI screening of the couple.

Male partners may complain of urethritis with dysuria and urethral discharge or epididymo-orchitis presenting as unilateral testicular pain and/or swelling. Fever may also be a presenting feature in men.

Fetal Implications

The pathogenesis of *C. trachomatis* is still not well understood. Adverse pregnancy outcomes may be due to stimulating a fetal immunogenic response with cytokine release or causing an excessive maternal immunogenic response due to the homology of the human and chlamydial 60 kDa heat shock proteins (CHSP-60).[14]

Ectopic Pregnancy (EP)

Chlamydia infection can cause tubal damage (salpingitis, peritubal adhesions and intramural fibrosis) which predisposes to ectopic pregnancy and has been suggested by several studies.[15] [EL 3]

Miscarriage

One study performed in Switzerland found that women with positive chlamydial serology had a 2.3 odds ratio for miscarriage compared to the control group. [EL 2]

Stillbirth

Data are scarce, but a few studies have shown a relation between stillbirth and chlamydia infections.

The odds ratio in one Australian study was estimated at 1.40.

C. trachomatis immunoglobulin (IgG) antibodies are frequently detected in sera from mothers with stillbirth.

Preterm Birth and/or Premature Rupture of Membranes

- Preterm birth before 37 completed weeks is an important element of neonatal mortality and morbidity, with long-term adverse consequences for health. It occurs in 9.6 per cent of all births worldwide. Late sequelae of preterm births include cerebral palsy, sensory deficits, learning disabilities and respiratory illnesses, psychological and economic costs.
- A US population-based cohort study raised the possibility that C. trachomatis is an important factor associated with PROM and preterm delivery, in women with C. trachomatis infection compared with those without infection.[16] [EL 2]
- A more recent Dutch study found that C. trachomatis detected by nucleic acid amplification tests (NAATs) was significantly associated with prematurity before 35 weeks of pregnancy, with a higher risk if infection occurs before 32 weeks.

Low Birthweight and Small for Gestational Age

Low birthweight is defined as weight below 2500 g; small for gestational age (SGA) is defined as birthweight less than 2 standard deviation scores (SDSs) below the mean for gestation.

A population-based, non-interventional, prospective cohort study showed that neonates born to chlamydia-positive women had, on average, a lower birthweight (<2500 g), especially when prematurely born. However, the difference did not reach statistical significance.

Neonatal Chlamydia

Neonatal chlamydial infection is a significant cause of neonatal morbidity.

Following passage through an infected birth canal, neonates have a significant risk of acquiring C. trachomatis ophthalmia neonatorum (ON) and conjunctivitis (18–50 per cent), pneumonitis (3–18 per cent) and nasopharyngeal infection (15–20 per cent).[17]

Neonatal infection occurs because of vertical transmission from an infected mother at the time of delivery.

The mother-to-child vertical transmission rate is higher after vaginal birth and can be as high as 50–60 per cent.

Vertical transmission can occur with caesarean section if there has been prolonged rupture of membranes, and rarely with intact membranes, indicating either a transmembrane or a transplacental transmission.

Diagnosis of Neonatal Chlamydia Infection

- Clinical suspicion.
- NAAT should be effective in the diagnosis of neonatal infections.
- In conjunctivitis, specimens should be obtained from the everted eyelid using a dacron-tipped swab or the swab specified by the manufacturer's test kit.

Treatment of Neonatal Chlamydia Infection

Oral erythromycin for two weeks is the recommended treatment of neonatal chlamydia or pneumonia, and additional topical therapy is unnecessary. A repeat oral course of antibiotics may be required in approximately 20–30 per cent of infants.[18]

Pathophysiology of Female Genital *Chlamydia trachomatis* Infection

In the female, *C. trachomatis* infection affects the cervix, urethra, salpinges and the uterus. Epithelial cells, through a release of cytokines and interferons, initially respond to infection by a neutrophilic infiltration, followed by lymphocytes, macrophages, plasma cells and eosinophilic invasion.[19]

Chlamydial organisms infection causes a humoral cell response, with the production of circulatory immunoglobulin M (IgM), immunoglobulin A (IgA) and IgG antibodies.[19]

Infectivity of *Chlamydia trachomatis*

- The bacterium is usually spread to sexual partners through all forms of sexual activity via unprotected vaginal, oral or anal sexual intercourse
- The incubation period is usually 7–21 days
- An infected male has a 25 per cent chance per sexual encounter of transmitting the infection
- Approximately 50 per cent of infected males and 80 per cent of infected females are asymptomatic[20]
- In women with PID, 5–10 per cent develop perihepatitis (i.e. Fitz-Hugh–Curtis syndrome)
- Fitz-Hugh–Curtis syndrome is characterised by acute right upper abdominal pain; clinical diagnosis is apparent if it is associated with other chlamydia signs or symptoms

If untreated, chlamydial infection may persist for years.

Diagnosis

- Nucleic acid amplification test
  - NAAT is a molecular technique to detect the genetic material (nucleic acid) of a particular pathogen (virus or bacterium) in a blood, other body-fluid or tissue specimen. It yields rapid results and accurate diagnosis.
  - NAATs can be performed on different body fluids (endocervical, urethral, vaginal, pharyngeal, rectal or first-void urine (FVU) samples).

  - The accuracy of NAATs on urine samples is nearly identical to that of samples obtained directly from the cervix or urethra. [EL 1]
  - Vaginal, introital or vulvar swabs from women are excellent specimens and can be self-obtained for the detection of *C. trachomatis* by NAAT tests. For self-taking of vaginal swabs, the swab is inserted about 5 cm into the vagina and rotated gently for 10–30 seconds.
  - For FVU testing, the first 10–30 mL of urine is collected for testing. Specimens should ideally be obtained between two and six hours after the last micturition. It is not necessary, and may not be advantageous, to obtain the first urine specimen passed in the morning.
  - The Centers for Disease Control (CDC) currently recommend using NAAT as the standard laboratory test, as it allows prompt treatment and therefore reduction of disease transmission. [EL 1]

- Serum specimens are not recommended for the diagnosis of acute chlamydia infections as the immune responses that can be detected are usually short-lived or are present due to past infections. The only two exceptions where serology may be helpful are chlamydial neonatal pneumonia (high IgM) or chlamydial tubal factor infertility (high IgG). A clotted specimen should be submitted.[21]

  Fresh samples are preferred, but frozen material (−70°C) is acceptable.

- Cytological testing is relatively insensitive when diagnosing adult conjunctival and genital tract infections.

- Isolation in cell culture and microbiological examination
  - Most, if not all, chlamydiae appear to be able to grow in cell culture. This is the only method to confirm the presence of viable bacteria because other diagnostic methods (antigen/antibody testing or the NAAT) can show positive results in the absence of viable infectious particles.
  - Either immunofluorescence or a fluorescent microscope is required.
  - It can take a few days for the bacteria to multiply to sufficient numbers to be identified by culture.
  - Vaginal swabs are the preferred specimen for screening women for genital chlamydia infection.

○ Rectal and oropharyngeal specimens are preferred for those at risk of extragenital tract infections.

Differential Diagnosis

Differential diagnosis of *Chlamydia trachomatis* infection includes a long list of diseases, which may produce similar symptoms:

- Gonorrhoea (although co-infection is relatively common)
- Herpes simplex
- *Trichomonas vaginalis* infection
- Urinary tract infection
- Bacterial vaginosis
- Candidiasis
- Urethral/vaginal foreign body
- A periurethral abscess may also cause similar symptoms

Work-Up Considerations to Help Reach a Diagnosis

First, it is important to exclude pregnancy as it modifies the treatment and management (pregnancy is a contraindication for the use of doxycycline and ofloxacin).

Laboratory work-up should include NAAT of endocervical, urethral, rectal or oropharyngeal specimens as indicated by the history of the patient's sexual practices. This will also differentiate gonorrhoeal infection.

Patients should be tested for HIV as co-infection is common.

Cervical smear screening should be carried out because of the association with cervical squamous cell carcinoma.

Contact tracing and screening of sexual partners if any STD is diagnosed.

Ultrasound and/or computed tomography (CT) are useful diagnostic adjuncts in cases of suspected pelvic pathology, e.g. sequelae of PID (tubovarian abscess or hydrosalpinx), endometriosis or ectopic pregnancy.

Antenatal Screening

The availability of NAATs as a rapid test result has allowed for expansion in methods of screening.

The United States Preventive Services Task Force (USPTF), the American College of Obstetricians and Gynecologists (ACOG) and the American Academy of Family Physicians (AAFP) recommend screening pregnant women:

- All pregnant women under 25 years of age
- Pregnant women aged 25 and older at increased risk:
  ○ If the sexual partner has proven or suspected chlamydia
  ○ If she has had chlamydia treatment in the past three months
  ○ If she has had unprotected sexual contact or had the occasional relation with a stranger
  ○ If she has had more than one sexual partner in the past year
- Retest during the third trimester for women under 25 years of age or at risk
- Pregnant women with chlamydial infection should have a test of cure three to four weeks after treatment and be retested within three months[22]
- If a pregnant woman is presenting for termination of pregnancy, she should be primarily screened for *Neisseria gonorrhoeae* and *Chlamydia trachomatis*. Screening for other STI depends on her risk assessment

Centers for Disease Control and Prevention, Sexually Transmitted Diseases Treatment Guidelines, 2015

First-Line Therapy

Azithromycin (US Food and Drug Administration (FDA) category B for pregnancy: Animal reproduction studies have failed to demonstrate a risk to the fetus and there are no adequate and well-controlled studies in pregnant women). 1 g orally in a single dose is the recommended first-line regimen.

- A meta-analysis of 12 randomised clinical trials of azithromycin versus doxycycline in non-pregnant women, for the treatment of urogenital chlamydial infection, demonstrated that the treatments were equally efficacious, with microbial cure rates of 97 per cent and 98 per cent, respectively.[23] [EL 1]
- Azithromycin can cause nausea, vomiting, stomach pain or mild to severe diarrhoea.

- Azithromycin is contraindicated in patients with a history of cholestatic jaundice/hepatic dysfunction. There may be a need to follow up with liver functions tests.

Breastfeeding

Azithromycin is not expected to cause adverse effects in breastfed infants. However, infants should be monitored for possible effects on the gastrointestinal flora, such as diarrhoea and candidiasis (thrush, diaper rash). Unconfirmed epidemiologic evidence indicates that the risk of hypertrophic pyloric stenosis in infants might be increased by maternal use of macrolide antibiotics during breastfeeding.

Alternative Regimens

Erythromycin base 500 mg orally four times a day for seven days

    or

Erythromycin ethylsuccinate 800 mg orally four times a day for seven days

    or

Levofloxacin (category C for pregnant women) 500 mg orally once daily for seven days

    or

Ofloxacin (category C for pregnant women) 300 mg orally twice a day for seven days

In unscreened women undergoing elective surgical termination of pregnancy, there is no need to wait until the result of screening, but a prophylactic of 1 g azithromycin + metronidazole 800 mg orally or 1 g rectally should be administered prior to or at the time of surgery.[24] [*Grade A, C recommendation*]

Treatment of the Infected Neonate

- Oral erythromycin treatment is 50 mg/kg/day in four divided doses for 14 days
- Azithromycin 20 mg/kg/day orally, one dose daily for three days
- Mothers of infants with chlamydial infection should be tested and treated

Test of Cure (TOC)

- An NAAT TOC in pregnant women, after three to four weeks of completion of treatment is recommended if there was any doubt about compliance, if symptoms persist or if she had a re-exposure.[23]
- If chlamydia is detected during the first trimester, repeat testing for reinfection should also be performed within three to six months, or in the third trimester.
- In England, the national screening programme recommends that young people under the age of 25 who have tested positive for chlamydia should have a repeat test three months later. A second positive result after treatment may be due to poor compliance, or reinfection from an untreated or new partner.[25]

Contact Tracing and Treatment of Sexual Partners

Partners of infected pregnant women should be notified of infection, and referred for evaluation and treatment.

All sexual partners should be offered, and encouraged to undergo, full STI screening, including HIV and hepatitis B testing. Hepatitis B vaccination should be offered when indicated.[22]

Reinfection and Repeat Testing

In practice, it may be difficult to differentiate between failure of treatment and reinfection. Reinfection usually occurs within two to five months of a previous infection.

Medico-Legal Cases

If the pregnancy is a result of suspected sexual abuse, and if there is a need for medico-legal cases, a NAAT should be taken from all the sites where possible penetration may have occurred. Cell culture is no longer recommended because of low sensitivity (60–80 per cent), longer time to produce results and lack of availability in many centres.[26]

Prevention of Chlamydia Infection during Pregnancy

The main preventive policies should include screening as explained above, a proactive health education, early diagnosis, timely treatment and barrier contraception.

The most reliable way to avoid transmission is to abstain from oral, vaginal and anal sex or to be in a long-term, mutually monogamous relationship with a partner known not to be infected.

Pregnant patients who are under treatment, or if the partner is undergoing treatment, should be counselled to encourage abstinence from any sexual contact until completion of the entire course of medication and a TOC is positive.

Male condoms made of latex or polyurethane, when used consistently and correctly, can reduce the risk of transmitting the infection.

However, 2–6 per cent of condoms break or fall off during intercourse even with perfect use.

Key Issues

- *Chlamydia trachomatis* is a prevalent sexually transmitted infection caused by genera *Chlamydia* (*Chlamydia trachomatis*)
- It can be asymptomatic in around half of cases
- Antibiotic treatment is available in oral forms and is effective in 95 per cent of cases
- Prevention is possible via screening, contact tracing, health education and the correct use of barrier contraception

Bacterial Vaginosis

Bacterial vaginosis (BV) is a clinical syndrome caused by excessive growth of bacteria that may normally be present in the vagina.

Aetiology

It is polymicrobial in nature; *Gardnerella vaginalis*, *Lactobacillus*, *Bactericides*, *Peptostreptococcus*, *Fusobacterium*, *Eubacterium* and anaerobes being the prominent associated organisms.

When these multiple species of bacteria that normally reside in the vagina become unbalanced, a woman can have a vaginal discharge with a foul odour (non-specific vaginitis or bacterial vaginosis).

Signs and Symptoms

- Women with bacterial vaginosis may be asymptomatic.
- There may be an unpleasant abnormal vaginal discharge.

- The discharge has unpleasant fish-like odour, especially after sexual intercourse.
- The discharge is generally white or grey.
- Women may experience burning during urination or itching around the vagina.

Diagnosis

Microscopic Examination of the Discharge

Demonstrating three of the following four Amsel's criteria:

Clue cells (vaginal epithelial cells that have bacteria adherent to their surfaces. The edges of the squamous epithelial cells, which normally have a sharply defined cell border, become studded with bacteria. The epithelial cells appear to be peppered with coccobacilli) **on a saline smear**

A pH greater than 4.5

A positive whiff test result (i.e. a fishy odour to the vaginal discharge before or after the addition of 10 per cent potassium hydroxide solution)

Characteristic discharge appearance is thin, grey and homogeneous[27]

The Amsel criteria are:[29]

- Increased homogeneous thin vaginal discharge
- pH of the secretion greater than 4.5
- Amine odour when potassium hydroxide 10 per cent solution is added to a drop of vaginal secretions
- Presence of clue cells in wet preparations

Fetal Implications

- Premature labour unresponsive to tocolytic therapy[30]
- Low birthweight
- Intrauterine fetal death infection is transmitted via the placenta

Management

All women with BV should be tested for HIV and other STDs, Medications:

- **Clindamycin** (category B) 300 mg PO q 12 h for 7 days. Use during the first trimester is not recommended unless clearly needed.
- **2 per cent vaginal cream** formulation (one full applicator (5 g) intravaginally at bedtime for seven days). This inhibits bacterial growth, by blocking dissociation of peptidyl transfer ribonucleic acid

(tRNA) from ribosomes, causing RNA-dependent protein synthesis to arrest.Both have an 85 per cent cure rate. [EL 3]

- **Oral metronidazole** dose for pregnant women500 mg PO twice daily (BID) × 7 days, or250 mg PO three times daily (TID) × 7 days.

  o Metronidazole crosses the placenta. In multiple cross-sectional and cohort studies of pregnant women there was no evidence of teratogenicity or mutagenic effects in infants exposed to metronidazole treatment. [EL 2]

  o Metronidazole is secreted in breastmilk. With maternal oral therapy, breastfed infants receive metronidazole in doses that are less than those used to treat infections in infants.

- Routine treatment of sexual partners is not recommended.[31,32]

Follow-up

- Women should be advised to return for re-evaluation if symptoms recur.
- For women who have a recurrence, a different recommended treatment regimen can be considered; however, re-treatment with the same recommended regimen is an acceptable option.
- If the woman complains of multiple recurrences after completion of a recommended treatment, 0.75 per cent metronidazole gel twice weekly for four to six months has been shown to reduce recurrences.
- Limited data suggest that an oral nitroimidazole (metronidazole or tinidazole 500 mg twice daily for seven days) followed by intravaginal boric acid 600 mg daily for 21 days and then suppressive 0.75 per cent metronidazole gel twice weekly for four to six months for those women in remission might be another option for women with recurrent BV.[32] [EL 3]
- Monthly oral metronidazole 2 g administered with fluconazole 150 mg may be attempted as suppressive therapy.[33]

References

1. The Columbia Electronic Encyclopedia™ Copyright © 2013, Columbia University Press. Licensed from Columbia University Press. All rights reserved. www.cc.columbia.edu/cu/cup/.

2. Prescott LM, Harley JP, Klein DA. *Microbiology*, 3rd ed. Dubuque, IA: Wm. C. Brown Publishers; 1996: 130–1.

3. CDC Grand Rounds. Chlamydia prevention: challenges and strategies for reducing disease burden and sequelae. *MMWR*. 2011; **60**: 370–3.

4. World Health Organization. Global incidence and prevalence of selected curable sexually transmitted infections – 2008. http://apps.who.int/iris/bitstream/10665/75181/1/9789241503839_eng.pdf.

5. World Health Organization. *Global Strategy for the Prevention and Control of Sexually Transmitted Infections: 2006–2015*. Geneva: World Health Organization; 2007.

6. Public Health England. Sexually transmitted infections and chlamydia screening in England 2015 – Infection Report, July 2016. www.gov.uk/government/uploads/system/uploads/attachment.2017.

7. Navarro C, Jolly A, Nair R, Chen Y. Risk factors for genital chlamydial infection. *Can J Infect Dis*. 2002; **13**(3): 195–207.

8. Waris Qidwai P, Ishaque S, Shah S, Maheen Rahim, EUS. Adolescent lifestyle and behaviour: a survey from a developing country. *PLoS ONE*. 2010. www.ncbi.nlm.nih.gov/pmc/articles/PMC2946339/.

9. Centers for Disease Control and Prevention. Sexually transmitted infections. STDs in Racial and Ethnic Minorities. Sexually Transmitted Disease Surveillance 2014. cdc.gov/std/stats14/default.htm.

10. Kraut-Becher JR, Aral SO. Gap length: an important factor in sexually transmitted disease transmission. *Sex Transm Dis*. 2003; **30**: 221–5.

11. Møller BR, Ahrons S, Laurin J, Mårdh PA. Pelvic infection after elective abortion associated with Chlamydia trachomatis. *Obstet Gynecol*. 1982; **59**(2): 210–13.

12. Madeleine MM, Anttila T, Schwartz SM et al. Risk of cervical cancer associated with Chlamydia trachomatis antibodies by histology, HPV type, and HPV cofactors. *Int J Cancer*. 2007; **120**(3): 650–5.

13. NHS choices. Chlamydia complications. nhs.uk/Conditions/Chlamydia/.

14. Adachi K, Nielsen-Saines K, Klausner JD. Chlamydia trachomatis infection in pregnancy: the global challenge of preventing adverse pregnancy and infant outcomes in sub-Saharan Africa and Asia. *Biomed Res Int*. 2016; **2016**: 9315757.

15. Mejuto P, Boga JA, Leiva PS. Chlamydia trachomatis infection in pregnant women: an important risk to maternal and infant health. *The Grant Medical Journal*. 2017; **2**(1): 001–011 iog/16/1620/gmj.

16. Centers for Disease Control and Prevention. STDs during Pregnancy – CDC Fact Sheet, 2017. www .cdc.gov/std/pregnancy/stdfact-pregnancy-detailed.htm.

17. American Academy of Pediatrics. Prevention of Neonatal Ophthalmia. In: Pickering LK, ed. *American Academy of Pediatrics. Red Book: 2012 Report of the Committee on Infectious Diseases*, 29th ed. Elk Grove Village, IL: American Academy of Pediatrics.

18. World Health Organization. Giddiness for treatment of chlamydia. 2016. http://apps.who.int/iris/bitstream/10665/246165/1/9789241549714-eng.pdf.

19. British Medical Journal. BMJ best practice. Pathophysiology of chlamydia trachomatis. 2016. best practice.bmj.com/best-practice/monograph/basics/pathophysiology.html.

20. Cook RL, Hutchison SL, Østergaard L, Braithwaite RS, Ness RB. Systematic review: noninvasive testing for Chlamydia trachomatis and Neisseria gonorrhoeae. *Ann Intern Med.* 2005; **142**(11): 914–25.

21. Mishori R, McClaskey EL, Winklerprins J. Chlamydia trachomatis infections: screening, diagnosis, and management. *Am Fam Physician.* 2012; **22–86**(12): 1127–32.

22. Centers for Disease Control and Prevention. Screening Recommendations and Considerations Referenced in Treatment Guidelines and Original Sources. 2015. cdc .gov/std/tg2015/screening.

23. Centers for Disease Control and Prevention. Sexually Transmitted Diseases Treatment Guidelines. 2015. Chlamydial Infections. www.cdc.gov/std/tg2015/chlamydia.htm.

24. Royal College of Obstetricians and Gynaecologists. The care of women requesting induced abortion. Clinical guidelines number 7, 2011.

25. Public Health England. National Chlamydia Screening Programme (NCSP). 2017. www.gov.uk//collections/national-chlamydia-screening-programme.

26. British Association for Sexual Health and HIV. Chlamydia trachomatis UK Testing Guidelines Clinical Effectiveness Group. Date of writing: 2010. www.bashh.org/documents/3352.pdf.

27. Girerd PH. Bacterial vaginosis. 2017. Medscape. http://emedicine.medscape.com/article/254342-workup.

28. Amsel R, Totten PA, Spiegel CA, Chen KC, Eschenbach D, Holmes KK. Nonspecific vaginitis. Diagnostic criteria and microbial and epidemiologic associations. *Am J Med.* 1983; **74**(1): 14–22.

29. Nelson DB, Macones NG. Bacterial vaginosis in pregnancy: current findings and future directions. *Epidemiol Rev.* 24(2): 102–8.

30. Flynn CA. Bacterial vaginosis in pregnancy and the risk of prematurity: a meta-analysis. *J Fam Pract.* 1999; **48**(11): 885–92.

31. Brocklehurst P, Gordon A, Heatley E, Milan SJ. Antibiotics for treating bacterial vaginosis in pregnancy. *Cochrane Database Syst Rev.* 2013; **1**: CD000262.

32. Centers for Disease Control and Prevention. 2015. Sexually Transmitted Diseases Treatment Guidelines. www.cdc.gov/std/tg2015/bv.htm.

33. Reichman O, Akins R, Sobel JD. Boric acid addition to suppressive antimicrobial therapy for recurrent bacterial vaginosis. *Sex Transm Dis.* 2009; **36**: 732–4.

Streptococcal Infection

Rachana Dwivedi and Shabnum Sibtain

Introduction

- Group B *Streptococcus* (GBS) is a harmless opportunistic commensal bacterium but has the potential to cause severe infections.
- In adults, streptococcal A infections can cause necrotising fasciitis (Group A) or meningitis.[1]
- In neonates, GBS causes early- or late-onset neonatal infection. GBS is the common cause of life-threatening infections in neonates.[2]
- GBS is also known to cause urinary tract infection, intra-amniotic infection and invasive disease during pregnancy and postpartum endometritis.

Prevalence and Incidence for Neonatal Infections

According to research led by the London School of Hygiene and Tropical Medicine, out of the 410 000 cases of GBS detected globally every year, 147 000 end in stillbirth or infant death. In 2015 Africa had the highest incidence of maternal and fetal morbidity and mortality, including infant death. The research found GBS was present all over the world, with an average of 25 per cent of pregnant women colonised with the bacteria (ranging from 11 per cent in eastern Asia to 35 per cent in the Caribbean).[3]

Since active prevention began in the mid-1990s, the rate of group B strep disease among newborns in the first week of life has declined by 80 per cent.

- In the USA, where GBS is the leading infectious cause of morbidity and mortality among infants, the rate of early-onset infection has decreased from 1.7 cases per 1000 live births (1993) to 0.24 cases per 1000 live births in 2014.[4]
- In the UK, the incidence of early-onset GBS (EOGBS) disease in 2015 was 0.57/1000 births (517 cases), a significant increase in incidence since previous surveillance undertaken in 2000 (0.48/1000).[5]

Microbiology

GBS has a bacterial capsule composed of polysaccharides and sub-classified into 10 serotypes (Ia, Ib, II–IX) depending on the immunologic reactivity of their polysaccharide capsule. Five of nine capsular serotypes, III, Ia, V, Ib and II, cause 95 per cent of invasive disease (in decreasing frequency). The most important virulent part of GBS is capsular polysaccharide which is rich in sialic acid and β-haemolysin and probably the key virulence factor.[6]

Pathophysiology

GBS is a gram-positive cocci identified by its β-haemolytic nature. GBS infection during pregnancy is associated with increased rates of preterm and neonatal complications. The precise pathophysiology is unknown. It has been possible to isolate numerous virulence factors that are required to overcome the local host defence, vaginal flora and invade the amniotic cavity.

GBS is thought to be transmitted from person to person via multiple routes, including faecal–oral, sexual and vertical transmission but it is not classified as a sexually transmitted disease (STD).

GBS normally colonises the intestine, vagina or rectum of healthy women. Due to the female anatomy, the proximity of the vagina and rectum allows for easier trafficking of the intestinal flora. Once the bacteria enter the vagina they are overcome by the hostile environment, including the physical mucus and epithelial barriers, low pH of the vagina, local immune factors including antimicrobial peptides and antibodies, as well as a vaginal microbiome dominated by lactobacilli.[7,8]

Once GBS has reached the amniotic sac, it adheres to the epithelial cell, inducing secretion of pro-inflammatory chemokines including TNFa, IL-1B and IL-6. While preterm birth is usually associated with severe microbial invasion, the induction of cytokines in the absence of invasive disease is sufficient to induce labour and fetal lung injury. GBS bacteraemia results when there is a failure in epithelial barrier function and immunological clearance, resulting in septicaemia and related consequences. Invasive disease of the fetus *in utero* can cause direct tissue damage, pneumonia, meningitis, sepsis and fetal death.

Adult Beta *Streptococcus* Infections: Signs and Symptoms

- In adults, GBS is present in the bowels, vagina and lower urogenital tract (30–40 per cent) without any symptoms. This is 'colonisation' and the woman is then a 'carrier'.
- These women are asymptomatic and generally do not have problems and do not require treatment.
- However, GBS colonisation may cause serious invasive illnesses:
  - ○ Bloodstream infection (septicaemia)
  - ○ Skin and soft tissue infection
  - ○ Bone and joint infection
  - ○ Pneumonia
  - ○ Urinary tract infection
  - ○ Meningitis

The rate of serious invasive group B strep disease among non-pregnant adults is about 10 cases out of every 100 000 non-pregnant adults.

Neonatal Transmission[4]

- GBS is present in the bowel flora of 20–40 per cent of adults (colonisation).
- During pregnancy, GBS colonisation is asymptomatic and generally does not cause problems and does not require treatment.
- Vertical transmission occurs during intrapartum/labour from the time of membrane rupture to delivery of the baby.[7]

Neonatal Infection

GBS infection is the leading cause of neonatal infections; EOGBS neonatal infection or late streptococcal infection.

Early-Onset (EOGBS) in Neonates

EOGBS infection occurs before age seven days (mean age at presentation is age 13 hours). Clinically, it manifests as non-focal sepsis (80–85 per cent), pneumonia (10–15 per cent) or meningitis (5–10 per cent).

Signs and Symptoms of EOGBS

- Poor feeding
- Grunting and tachypnea
- Lethargy
- Hypotension
- Hypoglycaemia
- Irritability
- Blotched skin
- Pain in neck and back
- Stiff neck
- Stupor to coma
- Petechial rash
- Diagnosis is by CSF culture

It can be fatal in 10 per cent of cases.

Those who survive may end up with long-term disability such as quadriplegia, cerebral palsy, hearing and sight problems.

Intrapartum antibiotics have reduced the incidence of EOGBS, with no changes in late-onset GBS.

Late-Onset GBS

Late-onset GBS is defined when infection occurs between a week and three months of life. It is uncommon after one month and rare after three months.

Signs of Late-Onset GBS Infection[11,12]

- Irritability with high pitched/whimpering cry, or moaning
- Blank, staring or trance-like expression
- Floppy and fretful
- Tense or bulging fontanelle
- Involuntary stiff body or jerking movements
- Meningitis and septicaemia

Previously, mortality rate was as high as 50 per cent, which has recently dropped to 10 per cent because of intrapartum antibiotic prophylaxes (IAP) and improved neonatal care.

Amongst the survivors 50 per cent may sustain neuro-disability.

A Cochrane review concluded that IAP for colonised mothers reduced the incidence of EOGBS disease (relative risk 0.14; 95 per cent CI 0.04–0.74), although the numbers of deaths were too small to assess the impact of the intervention on mortality. [EL 1]

Late-onset GBS, however, is not preventable with IAP.

Risk Factors for EOGBS

- Previous baby with GBS infection:If a woman has had a previous baby infected with GBS, she has a 10 times higher risk
- Urinary tract infection or colonisation:The risk is four times higher if GBS is found in a woman's urine during the current pregnancy
- Raised temperature during labour:
  There is a four times higher risk if a woman's temperature is raised during labour (37.5°C or higher)
- Colonisation in a rectal or vaginal swab:
  The risk is three times higher if found on a vaginal or rectal swab during the current pregnancy
- Premature rupture of membranes:
  The risk is three times higher if PROM occurs more than 18 hours before delivery[11]
- Preterm labour in known GBS carrier:
  There is a three times higher risk of preterm labour in a known GBS carrier
- A classic prospective cohort study conducted during the 1980s revealed that pregnant women with GBS colonisation were >25 times more likely than pregnant women with negative prenatal cultures to deliver infants with EOGBS disease[12] [EL 2]
- In the absence of any intervention, an estimated 1–2 per cent of infants born to colonised mothers develop EOGBS infections

Investigations during Pregnancy

Standard Low Vaginal and Rectal Swabs

These are easily available and routinely used to test any vaginal infection. They detect a wide range of microorganisms but have low sensitivity and specificity for GBS.[12,13]

Urine Test

GBS is found in the urine of 2–7 per cent of pregnant women. Studies have shown that bacteriuria in pregnancy increases the likelihood of colonisation. Even in the absence of negative vaginal culture at 35–37 weeks, bacteriuria in antenatal period is a recognised risk factor for EOGBS disease.

Enriched-Medium Swabs – Perianal Swabs

In the laboratory, the cells from the swab(s) are incubated in an enriched culture medium specifically designed to encourage the growth of GBS and so enhance its detection. The result takes between 24 and 72 hours to establish the diagnosis.

The Centers for Disease Control (CDC) guideline recommends that specimens should undergo 18- to 24-hour incubation at 35–37°C in an enriched broth medium to enhance recovery from GBS.

Swabbing both the lower vagina and rectum (through the anal sphincter) increases the culture yield substantially compared with sampling the cervix or the vagina.

Polymerase Chain Reaction (PCR)

This DNA amplification has a shorter incubation time. It has the potential to be used as a point-of-care test; however, the expensive equipment is a limitation. It is Food and Drug Administration (FDA)–approved in the USA and Canada but is not validated in the UK.

Screening and Prevention

Risk-Based Prevention

In November 2003, the Royal College of Obstetricians and Gynaecologists recommended that women with selected risk factors for EOGBS infection in their babies should be offered intrapartum antimicrobial prophylaxis (IAP).

It had been expected that a risk-based prevention would reduce the rate of EOGBS infection by 50 per cent.

Screening- and Testing-Based Prevention

Most developed countries with a GBS prevention strategy offer a screening test to all pregnant women for the carrier status.

IAP is then offered to those who are positive and also to the women who do not have a test result but present with high-risk factors.

In these countries, the rate of EOGBS infection has fallen significantly. In the USA, guidelines on preventing EOGBS disease were issued in 1996 and revised in 2002 and 2010.[14]

The recommendation was to offer screening tests to all women, at 35–37 weeks' gestation.

One study found that 85 per cent of pregnant women were screened for GBS. Among those screened, 98 per cent had results available at delivery. Eighty-five per cent of women with an indication for IAP received treatment.

Systematic review in 2010 has concluded that optimum timing for screening is at 35–37 weeks [EL 1]; however this is limited by the fact that 6 per cent of women may be negative in antenatal cultures.

CDC recommends screening all women at 35–37 weeks to reduce EOGBS.

In the USA, CDC's 2010 guidelines for GBS prevention were updated to recommend universal culture-based screening to determine which women should receive intrapartum GBS chemoprophylaxis.

In support of their recommendation, a large population-based study conducted during 1998–99 demonstrated the superiority of culture-based screening over the risk-based approach to prevention of EOGBS disease. The study found that culture-based screening resulted in the identification of a greater proportion of women.

UK Screening Policies

Universal bacteriological screening is not recommended. [*Grade D recommendation*]

The UK's National Institute for Health and Care Excellence (NICE) does not recommend routine testing for GBS, because evidence of its changing colonisation, clinical benefit and cost effectiveness remains uncertain:

- Many women carry the bacteria, and, in the majority of cases, babies are born without developing an infection.
- Screening all women late in pregnancy cannot accurately predict which babies will develop GBS infection.
- Between 17 per cent and 25 per cent of women who have a positive swab at 35–37 weeks of gestation will be GBS-negative at delivery.
- Between 5 per cent and 7 per cent of women who are GBS-negative at 35–37 weeks of gestation will be GBS-positive at delivery.

- Many babies severely affected by GBS infection are born prematurely, prior to the suggested GBS screen at 37 weeks.

Treating all carriers of GBS with IAP means that a very large number of women would receive treatment that do not need it. This may increase adverse outcomes to mother and baby.

Intrapartum Antibiotic Prophylaxes (IAP)

IAP aims to reduce the risk of neonatal morbidity and mortality from GBS neonatal infection.

In the United States, there is widespread acceptance that IAP reduces vertical transmission of GBS infections in high-risk women and has resulted in a significant decline in rates of EOGBS infection.[15] [EL 1]

Indications for IAP

- Women who have GBS in their urine should be treated as per sensitivity. They should receive IAP to prevent EOGBS disease.
- Women with GBS colonisation with preterm labour.
- Women with known GBS colonisation with preterm rupture of membrane after 34 weeks.
- Women with GBS colonisation (detected in this pregnancy) and in labour. There is no contraindication for membrane sweep.
- Women with pyrexia (38°C and above) in labour.
- Women with term rupture membrane and known GBS carrier.
- Women with a previous baby with EOGBS should be offered IAP.
- Women with GBS urinary tract infection (growth of greater than 105 cfu/mL) during pregnancy. In addition to IAP, urinary tract infection should be treated during pregnancy.

Neonatal Care

- Babies with clinical signs of EOGBS disease should be treated with penicillin and gentamicin within an hour of the decision for treatment.
- In women with known GBS colonisation who decline IAP, the baby should be very closely followed and monitored for 12 hours after birth. They should be discouraged from seeking very early discharge.

IAP Treatment Options

- Benzylpenicillin 3 g intravenously (IV) loading dose followed by 1.5 g IV every four hours. The aim is to achieve adequate drug levels in the fetal circulation and amniotic fluid while avoiding neurotoxicity.
- Women who are allergic to penicillin should be considered for cephalosporin.
- If the reaction was severe then vancomycin is the drug of choice. The drug should be administered at least four hours prior to delivery.

Potential Adverse Effects of IAP

- Maternal anaphylaxis.
- Effect on neonatal bowel flora, causing reductions in colonisation with lactobacilli or bifidobacterium. [EL 2]
- Theoretical risk of long-term sequelae: e.g. allergy, obesity or diabetes.[16]

Vaccines to Prevent GBS Disease

Although an effective GBS vaccine would be a powerful tool against GBS disease, no licensed vaccine is yet available.

Conclusion

Group B *Streptococcus* (GBS) is a harmless opportunistic commensal bacterium but can occasionally cause severe infections. In adults, it rarely causes symptoms or complications.

In the neonates, GBS causes early- or late-onset neonatal infection and is a common cause of life-threatening infections and complications.

Maternal carrier status, past history of an infected baby, preterm rupture of the membranes and premature labour or GBS urine infection is the highest risk for the newborn.

Screening policies for the maternal carrier status vary according to different countries.

IAP is the cornerstone for the prevention of neonatal disease.

References

1. Depani SJ, Ladhani S, Heath PT et al. The contribution of infections to neonatal deaths in England and Wales. *Pediatr Infect Dis J.* 2011; **30**: 345–7.

2. Regan JA, Klebanoff MA, Nugent RP. The epidemiology of group B streptococcal colonization in pregnancy. Vaginal Infections and Prematurity Study Group. *Obstet Gynecol.* 1991; **77**: 604–10.

3. Liu L, Johnson HL, Cousens S et al. Global, regional, and national causes of child mortality: an updated systematic analysis for 2010 with time trends since 2000. *Lancet.* 2012; **379**(9832): 2151–61.

4. Centers for Disease Control and Prevention. Group B Strep Infection in New-borns. 2016. www.cdc.gov/groupbstrep/about/newborns-pregnant.html.

5. Group B streptococcus support, 2.18. https://gbss.org.uk/health-professionals-2s-incidence/.

6. Maisey, HC, Doran KS, Nizet V. Recent advances in understanding the molecular basis of group B Streptococcus virulence. *Expert Rev Mol Med.* 2009; **10**: 1–16.

7. Campbell JR, Hillier SL, Krohn MA, Ferrieri P, Zaleznik DF, Baker CJ. Group B streptococcal colonization and serotype-specific immunity in pregnant women at delivery. *Obstet Gynecol.* 2000; **96**(4): 498–503.

8. McKenna DS, Matson S, Northern I. Maternal group B streptococcal (GBS) genital tract colonization at term in women who have asymptomatic GBS bacteriuria. *Infect Dis Obstet Gynecol.* 2003; **11**(4): 203–7.

9. Edmond K, Kortsalioudaki S, Schrag S et al. Group B streptococcal disease in infants aged younger than 3 months: systematic review and meta-analysis. *Lancet.* 2012; **379**: 547–56.

10. Dudek CJ, Shah C, Zayas J, Rathore MH. The many faces of Late Onset Group B Streptococcus. *J Pediatr Infect Dis.* 2016; **1**: 14.

11. Royal College of Obstetricians and Gynaecologists. Prevention of Early-onset Neonatal Group B Streptococcal Disease. Green-top Guideline No. 36. 2017. doi: 10.1111/1471-0528.14821.

12. Yancey MK, Schuchat A, Brown LK, Ventura VL, Markenson GR. The accuracy of late antenatal screening cultures in predicting genital group B streptococcal colonization at delivery. *Obstet Gynecol.* 1996; **88**: 811–15.

13. Kovavisarach E, Sa-adying W, Kanjanahareutai S. Comparison of combined vaginal-anorectal, vaginal and anorectal cultures in detecting of group B streptococci in pregnant women in labor. *J Med Assoc Thailand* [Chotmaihet thangphaet]. 2007; **90**: 1710–14.

14. Centers for Disease Control and Prevention. 2010 Guidelines for the Prevention of Perinatal Group B Streptococcal Disease. www.cdc.gov/groupbstrep/guidelines/guidelines.html.

15. Verani JR, McGee L, Schrag SJ. Division of Bacterial Diseases, National Center for Immunization and Respiratory Diseases, Centers for Disease Control and Prevention (CDC). *MMWR Recomm Rep.* 2010; 59(RR-10): 1–36.

16. Corvaglia L, Tonti G, Martini S et al. Influence of intrapartum antibiotic prophylaxis for group B streptococcus on gut microbiota in the first month of life. *J Pediatr Gastroenterol Nutr.* 2016; **62**: 304–8.

Enterococci and Bacterial Infections

Varsha S. Puranik

Introduction

Pregnant women are generally healthy but, as with non-pregnant women, are at risk of developing some infections. Some of these may be exacerbated by pregnancy and some are specific to pregnancy.[1]

Gram-Positive and Gram-Negative Bacteria

Gram stain is an important bacteriological technique that provides a rapid and presumptive identification of pathogens, giving important clues about the pathogen in the specimen.

This helps in dividing bacterial species into two large groups:

- Those that take up the basic dye, crystal violet, are gram-positive bacteria.
- Those that allow the primary stain to be washed with decoloriser alcohol are gram-negative bacteria.[2,3]

Bacterial Infections in Pregnancy

Infections Specific to Pregnancy[4]

- Chorioamnionitis
- Endometritis (with or without the products of conception)
- Surgical site infection (wound infection post-caesarean section)
- Perineal infection
- Lactational mastitis

Chorioamnionitis

This is the inflammation of the membranes and chorion of the placenta which may extend up to the umbilical cord. It is strongly associated with spontaneous rupture of membrane (SROM).

Associated Pathogens:

The majority of the infections are polymicrobial due to ascending colonisation from the genital flora.

The most common species include genital mycoplasmas – *Ureaplasma* and *Mycoplasma* species.

Enteric gram-negative bacilli (E. coli, *Klebsiella* spp., *Enterobacter* spp.), group B *Streptococci*.

Endometritis

This is the infection of the decidua in the uterine cavity which occurs postpartum. This condition may occur within a normally sterile uterine cavity or with associated adnexal infection.[5]

Associated Pathogens:

- Aerobic gram-positive cocci (GPC): group B *Streptococci*, *Staphylococcus aureus*, *Enterococci*
- Anaerobic GPC: *Peptococci* and *Peptostreptococci*
- Anaerobic gram-negative bacilli (GNB): *Bactericides* and *Prevotella* spp.
- Aerobic GNB: E. coli, *K. pneumoniae* and *Proteus* spp.

Surgical Site Infection (Wound Infection Post-Caesarean Section)

This is the most common complication of caesarean section, leading to maternal sepsis.

In a UK study across 14 hospitals it was found that 9.6 per cent developed post-caesarean infection of which 0.6 per cent required readmission.

Associated Pathogens:

Staphylococcus aureus is the most common pathogen followed by coagulase-negative *Staphylococcus aureus* (CONS), *Enterococcus* spp. gram-negative bacilli like E. coli.

The common microbial source of pathogens comprises skin and vaginal flora that colonise the wound and cause surgical site infection (SSI).[6]

Preoperative practices and management of co-morbidities (like diabetes mellitus), hair removal, skin preparation and antibiotic prophylaxis reduce the chances of post-caesarean section wound infection.

Perineal Infection

During childbirth the stretching of the perineum makes the tissue thinner to the extent that it might lead to a tear.

Most perineal wounds heal well; however, it sometimes leads to complications like:

- Haematoma: which interferes with the wound healing, having the following signs and symptoms – intense pain, inability to sit on the wound directly, difficulty in walking[7]
- Wound infection: the wounds are at high risk due to their location, and the infection sets in from three to five days

Common signs and symptoms include feverish feeling, increasing pain, offensive odour from the wound, yellowish discharge/pus from the wound, difficulty in walking.

Associated Pathogens:

Common pathogens include group B *Streptococci*, *G. vaginalis*, *M. hominis*, E. coli.

Lactation Mastitis

Mastitis is clinically defined as localised, painful inflammation of the breast occurring with flu-like symptoms (fever, malaise etc.). If the condition occurs at the time of lactation then it is termed as lactation mastitis.

Common signs and symptoms include pain, redness, swelling, tenderness in the area of the breast.

Fever, malaise, enlarged axillary lymph nodes and well-defined fluctuant lump in the affected breast are the other features.

Nursing mothers are most vulnerable to breast abscess at two stages:

- During the first month of lactation due to inexperience, inadequate hygiene when the nipples are more likely to be traumatised.
- During the time of weaning when the breasts are likely to be engorged and the trauma caused by the baby's teeth increases the likelihood of nipple trauma.

Associated Pathogens:

Staphylococcus aureus, Staphylococcus epidermidis, methicillin-resistant *Staphylococcus aureus* (MRSA), *Streptococcus* species.

Antibiotics that are alkaline and which concentrate well in the breastmilk are preferred, e.g. erythromycin.

β-lactamase–resistant penicillins like fucloxacilin, dicloxicillin and cloxacillin are also used.

In case of allergy to penicillin, cephalexin or clindamycin may be used.

Infections Arising during Pregnancy

- Pneumonia
- Listeriosis
- Urinary tract infection (including pyelonephritis)
- Genital tract infections

Pneumonia

- Community-acquired pneumonia (CAP) is the most frequent cause of non-obstetric infection. The widely reported causes for development of pneumonia include decreased lymphocyte proliferation in second and third trimesters, decrease in circulating helper T cell and reduced lymphocyte activity
- The difficulty in diagnosis during pregnancy is mainly due to the complexity of distinguishing symptoms related to physiological changes of pregnancy and the symptoms of pneumonia
- Common signs and symptoms include fever, cough, sputum, dyspnoea, pleuritic chest pain
- Chest X-ray
- Common X-ray changes include pulmonary infiltrate, atelectasis, pleural effusion, pneumonitis, pulmonary oedema, and about 42 per cent of chest X-rays will show no changes in pregnant women
- Most X-ray diagnostic procedures expose the embryo to less than 50 mSv. This level of radiation exposure will not increase reproductive risks (either birth defects or miscarriage). A much higher dose above 200 mSv is associated with an increased incidence of birth defects or miscarriage

- Laboratory investigations include: complete blood picture, total leucocyte count (TLC), haemoglobin concentration, fasting and postprandial blood sugar, liver function tests (alanine aminotransferase (ALT), angiotensin sensitivity test (AST), alkaline phosphatase, direct bilirubin – total proteins, and kidney function tests like urea and creatinine.

Other investigations include direct smear with Gram and Ziehl–Neelson (ZN) stain, aerobic culture for bacteria, polymerase chain reaction (PCR)/nucleic acid amplification to detect nucleic acid for chlamydia, pneumoniae and mycoplasma pneumonia.

Associated Pathogens:

Streptococcus pneumoniae, H. influenzae, Mycoplasma pneumoniae, Staphylococcus, Chlamydophila pneumoniae, Legionella pneumophila, Klebsiella pneumoniae, Pseudomonas aeruginosa.[8]

Listeria Infection[9]

Please refer to Chapter 20.

Urinary Tract Infection

Please refer to Chapter 21.

Genital Tract Infections

With signs and symptoms of:

- Purulent vaginal discharge
- Lower abdominal pain/tenderness

Associated Pathogens:

Frequently isolated species

Enterococcus faecalis

Enterococcus faecium

Enterococcus gallinarum

Enterococcus casseliflavus

E. faecalis is the most commonly isolated species followed by *E. faecium*. *E. faecium* is on the rise among hospitals, probably due to acquisition of resistance to vancomycin and other antibiotics.

Infections Incidental to Pregnancy

- Sexually transmitted diseases
- Tuberculosis
- Endocarditis

Enterococcal Infections

The genus *Enterococcus* includes all the members that were previously classified with group D *Streptococci*.[2]

These organisms are gram-positive cocci which are the normal residents of the gastrointestinal tract and biliary tract and in lower numbers are known to colonise the vagina and male urethra.

The organisms under this genus are important because they are increasingly becoming agents of human disease because of their resistance to many antimicrobials to which most *Streptococci* are susceptible.

Enterococcus species are a component of the human intestinal flora and may be found in the birth canals of women.

They are one of the most common causes for hospital-acquired urinary tract, wound and bloodstream infection. This organism is most commonly isolated from women with post-caesarean endometritis and wound infections.

Microbiology of *Enterococci*

These are a group of gram-positive cocci that have been distinguished from *Streptococci* based on the following properties:

- Ability to grow at 10°C and 45°C
- Growth in presence of 6.5 per cent NaCl
- Growth at pH 9.6
- Ability to hydrolyse esculin in presence of 40 per cent bile
- Production of pyrrolidonyl arylamidase (PYR)

Risk Factors for Enterococcal Bacteraemias

- Advanced age
- Immunosuppression
- Underlying diseases
- Prematurity of baby
- Genitourinary tract instrumentation
- Usage of broad-spectrum antibiotics with little or no enterococcal activity (e.g. cephalosporins)

Common Infections Caused by *Enterococci*

- Urinary tract infections (UTIs) and asymptomatic bacteriuria (ASBU)
- Genitourinary tract infection
- Neonatal enterococcal sepsis
- Enterococcal meningitis in neonates

- Puerperal sepsis
- Pneumonia
- Wound and soft tissue infections

Drug Resistance in *Enterococci*

- *Enterococci* display intrinsic, low-level resistance to aminoglycosides and lincosamides.
- They have relatively high minimum inhibitory concentrations (MICs) for penicillin and cephalosporins due to diminished binding of cell wall penicillin-binding proteins (PbP) to these agents.
- They are resistant to the action of sulfonamides in vitro.
- They are still able to block folate synthesis.
- Low-level aminoglycoside resistance is due to decreased penetrability of enterococcal cell wall.
- Serious infections with low-level resistance to aminoglycosides can be treated with a combination of penicillin/ampicillin with an aminoglycoside.
- High-level aminoglycoside resistance has emerged due to transposons and this is easily transmitted to other organisms.
- High-level aminoglycoside resistance has been documented in various strains like *E. faecalis, E. faecium, E. gallinarum, E. pullorum* etc. Such infections cannot be treated with a combination of β-lactam agent and aminoglycoside antibiotic.
- Since the 1980s there has been a huge change in the pattern of susceptibility of *Enterococci* to vancomycin and ampicillin, leading to the emergence of vancomycin-resistant *Enterococci* (VRE).[10]

Epidemiology of Bacterial Infections in Pregnancy

- In a study conducted by Ettore Cincinelli et al., it was found that *E. faecalis* contributed to 22.9 per cent of positive cultures among patients with endometritis who had miscarriages in the past.
- A study undertaken by S Ahmed et al. on aerobic bacterial pattern puerperal sepsis found that *E. faecalis* contributed to 4.76 per cent of the total aerobic isolates isolated from cases of puerperal sepsis.
- According to K Fisher and C Phillips, in the year 2005 in the UK there were a total of 7066 cases of

enterococcal bacteraemias, 63 per cent of which were due to *E. faecalis* and 28 per cent to *E. faecium*.
- A study conducted by R Colgan et al. on asymptomatic bacteriuria in adults observed that healthy persons with ASBU will be likely to be infected with E. coli, whereas a person with indwelling catheter is more likely to be infected with multidrug-resistant organisms like *Enterococci*.[11]
- A Cochrane systematic review found that treatment of ASBU in pregnancy decreases the risk of subsequent pyelonephritis from a range of 20–35 per cent to a range of 1–4 per cent.[12] [EL 1]

Signs and Symptoms

Signs and symptoms vary according to the site of infection (pneumonia, UTI, endometritis, chorioamnionitis, endocarditis, puerperal sepsis etc.).

Work-Up in Bacterial Infections

Specimens to be cultured are

- Blood culture
- Serous/purulent discharge from episiotomy wounds
- Swab of purulent drainage
- Tissue biopsy

Maternal Implications of *Enterococcus* Infection

- Maternal *Enterococci* bacteraemia may lead to shock or disseminated intravascular coagulation
- *Enterococcus* infection may lead to endocarditis, especially in pregnant women with cardiac valve prosthesis
- A common aetiology in UTI during pregnancy
- Postpartum endometritis
- Puerperal sepsis
- Pneumonia

Fetal Implications of *Enterococcus* Infection

- Intrauterine infection triggers an inflammatory response believed to result in preterm labour (PTL) and injury to the developing fetal lung and brain. Pro-inflammatory cytokines and chemokines, small immunologic proteins, likely play a central role in the pathogenesis of infection-associated with preterm birth and fetal injury.

- Intrauterine infection and inflammation is frequently associated with adverse fetal outcomes. In many studies of all preterm births, the incidence of positive amniotic fluid and chorioamniotic culture was as high as 40 per cent. In many cases, infection is largely subclinical.
- Micro-organisms may gain access to the amniotic cavity and fetus through ascending infection from the vagina and cervix; haematogenous dissemination through the placenta (transplacental infection); retrograde seeding from the peritoneal cavity through the fallopian tubes; and inadvertent introduction of infective agents at the time of invasive procedures (amniocentesis, percutaneous fetal blood sampling, chorionic villous sampling or shunting).[13]

Bacterial *Enterococcus* infection is associated with:

- High perinatal mortality rate
- Low birthweight
- Preterm labour
- Injury to the developing fetal lung and brain

Treatment

Monotherapy

Ampicillin is the first choice for monotherapy of susceptible *E. faecalis* infection.

Vancomycin is used for patients with penicillin allergy or infections with strains that have high-level penicillin resistance.

Nitrofurantoin is effective in the treatment of enterococcal UTIs, including many caused by VRE strains.

Linezolid, daptomycin or tigecycline may be used to treat *E. faecium* and *E. faecalis* strains, including VRE.[14]

Polytherapy

- Ampicillin, vancomycin and an aminoglycoside (e.g. gentamicin category C) are considered the standard treatment for *E. faecalis*, particularly in native valve endocarditis. At least four weeks of therapy is recommended. Consideration should be given to limiting the aminoglycoside component

to two weeks in order to avoid nephrotoxic vestibular and ototoxic complications.
- Ceftriaxone plus ampicillin, given as intravenous ampicillin 2 g every four hours plus intravenous ceftriaxone 2 g every 12 hours.[15]

Conclusion

Enterococci are gram-positive cocci which normally reside in the gastrointestinal tract and biliary tract and in lower numbers are known to colonise the vagina and male urethra. During pregnancy they may cause serious infections affecting the health of the mother and baby.

Treatment options include either monotherapy of any of these agents (ampicillin, vancomycin, nitrofurantoin, linezolid, daptomycin or tigecycline) or polytherapy of a combination of two or more antibiotics.

Bacterial Infection in Food Poisoning

Food-borne bacterial infection can be worse during pregnancy and may lead to miscarriage or premature delivery. It can also lead to death or severe health problems in newborn babies. Some food-borne infections (e.g. *Listeria*, *Toxoplasma gondii*, E. coli and *Salmonella*) can infect the fetus even if the mother does not feel sick.

The commonest pathogens are:

- *Listeria*
- E. coli
- *Salmonella*
- *Campylobacter*
- *Toxoplasma gondii*

Signs and Symptoms

- Stomach cramps
- Vomiting
- Diarrhoea

Vomiting and diarrhoea may lead to serious dehydration and death if not treated properly.

Diagnosis of Food Poisoning

History

Eating and travel history may offer a clue to the diagnoses.

Clinical Examination

Signs of hydration include dry, tenting skin, sunken eyes, dry mouth, and lack of sweat in the armpits and groin. There may be a low-grade fever and low blood pressure.

Stool Samples

These may show *Salmonella*, E. coli or other organisms.

Treatment of Bacterial Food Poisoning

- Maintaining good hydration is the first step. Hospitalisation is indicated if the patient is dehydrated or if there is clinical or laboratory evidence of fluid or electrolyte imbalance in their body.
- Medications may be prescribed to control nausea and vomiting.
- Medications to decrease the frequency of diarrhoea may be indicated, e.g. loperamide (Imodium).
- Antibiotics

Antibiotics are not routinely indicated in cases of food poisoning. Except for specific infections, antibiotics are not prescribed in the treatment of most food poisoning. Decision should be based on multiple factors (the intensity of the disease symptoms, if there is serious response to infection (sepsis)).

A pregnant woman suspected of having listeriosis will likely be treated with intravenous antibiotics because of the effect of the infection on the fetus.

Prevention of Food Poisoning during Pregnancy[16]

- Avoid raw and smoked seafood.
- Avoid unpasteurised juice or cider.
- Avoid unpasteurised milk and milk products, which may cause brucellosis.
- Avoid soft cheese.
- Only consume well-cooked eggs, because undercooked eggs may contain *Salmonella*.
- Avoid undercooked meat and poultry.
- Avoid or reheat hot dogs and luncheon meats.
- Be cautious with meat spreads or pâté (risk of *Listeria* infection).
- Avoid mercury-containing fish (king mackerel, marlin, shark, swordfish and tilefish).

References

1. Institute of Obstetricians and Gynaecologists, Royal College of Physicians of Ireland and the National Clinical Programme in Obstetrics and Gynaecology. 2015. Clinical Infections Practice guideline; bacterial Infections Specific to Pregnancy.

2. Winn WC Jr, Koneman EW. *Koneman's Color Atlas and Textbook of Diagnostic Microbiology*, 6th ed. Philadelphia: Lippincott Williams; 2006.

3. Tille P. *Bailey & Scott's Diagnostic Microbiology*, 13th ed. St Louis, MO: Mosby; 2013.

4. Baron S, Salton MR, Kim KS. Structure. In: Baron S, Salton MR, Kim KS. *Baron's Medical Microbiology*, 4th ed. Galveston: University of Texas Medical Branch; 1996.

5. Higgins RD, Saade G, Polin RA et al., for the Chorioamnionitis Workshop Participants. Evaluation and management of women and newborns with a maternal diagnosis of chorioamnionitis: summary of a workshop. *Obstet Gynecol*. 2016; **127**(3): 426–36.

6. Owens CD, Stoessel K. Surgical site infections: epidemiology, microbiology and prevention. *J Hosp Infect*. 2008; **70**(suppl 2): 3–10.

7. Sharma RK, Parashar A. The management of perineal wounds. *Indian J Plast Surg*. 2012; **45**(2): 352–63.

8. Goodnight WH, Soper DE. Pneumonia in pregnancy. *Crit Care Med*. 2005; **33**(suppl 10): S390–7.

9. American College of Obstetricians and Gynecologists. Listeria and Pregnancy. PFS013, January 2017. www.acog.org/Patients/FAQs/Listeria-and-Pregnancy.

10. Miller, WR, Munita JM, Arias CA. Mechanisms of antibiotic resistance in enterococci. *Expert Rev Anti Infect Ther*. 2014; **12**(10): 1221–36.

11. Cormican M, Murphy AW. Akke Vellinga. Interpreting asymptomatic bacteriuria. *BMJ*. 2011; **343**: d4780.

12. Smaill FM, Vazquez JC. Antibiotics for bacterial infection in the urine in pregnancy when there are no symptoms. 2015 Cochrane review.

13. Adams Waldorf KM, McAdams, RM. Influence of infection during pregnancy on fetal development. *Reproduction*. 2013; **146**(5): R151–62.

14. Plosker GL, Figgitt DP. Linezolid: a pharmacoeconomic review of its use in serious Gram-positive infections. *Pharmacoeconomics*. 2005; **23**(9): 945–64.

15. Kristich CJ, Rice, LB, Arias CA. Enterococcal Infection – Treatment and Antibiotic Resistance. 2014. www.ncbi.nlm.nih.gov/books/NBK190424/.

16. US Department of Health and Human Services. Food Safety for Pregnant Women. 2017. www.fda.gov/food/foodborneillnesscontaminants/peopleatrisk/ucm312704.htm.

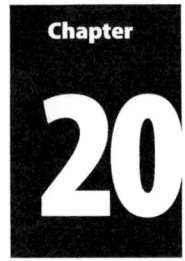

Listeriosis

Adel Elkady, Prabha Sinha and Soad Ali Zaki Hassan

Prevalence and Incidence

In the general population, *Listeria* infection is relatively uncommon, with a prevalence of approximately 4 per million in Canada, 0.27 per million in the USA and between 0.1 and 11.3 per million population in different parts of Europe.[1]

Pregnant women have a 12- to 18-fold increased risk in pregnancy (12/100 000), compared with the non-pregnant population.

Out of all infections with *Listeria*, 16–27 per cent occur in pregnant women.[2]

The exact cause of its higher prevalence in pregnancy is not known. Immunosuppression associated with pregnancy results in suppression of cell-mediated immunity in the placenta, due to high concentration of maternal hormones and other unknown mechanisms.

Approximately 20 per cent of *Listeria* infections involve neonatal infection with potentially severe complications, therefore it is important to stop the outbreaks in pregnant woman and the unwanted consequences for their unborn fetuses.

Microbiology, Organism and Epidemiology

Out of seven *Listeria* species, only *Listeria monocytogenes* is an important pathogenic for humans. Morphologically, they are indistinguishable from diphtheroids, and they are therefore mistaken for contaminants. They can mimic *Streptococci*, as coccoid forms are often seen in cultures or smears from infected tissue.

L. monocytogenes is a small, facultative anaerobic, gram-positive, flagellated, linear motile rod, which is non-spore-forming.[3] It can survive for many months in soil and can be detected in the faeces of animals and humans.

It is mainly acquired by the ingestion of food products, such as meat (hot dogs, deli meat), dairy products, unwashed raw vegetables, seafood, soft cheeses, unpasteurised milk and dairy products, that have been contaminated.

Outbreaks usually occur due to contaminated food, often commercially produced, as the source of infection.[4]

Even refrigerated food can be contaminated, proving to be the source in around 11 per cent of cases.[5]

Many aspects of the epidemiology of listeriosis are unclear because of

- Lack of a sensitive method for strain identification
- Incubation period is very short for gastroenteritis (6 hours to 10 days) but longer for invasive listeriosis (11 to 70 days, with a mean of 28 days)
- Mild or asymptomatic nature of infection
- Variant sources of infection; infecting organism is found in dust, soil, water, sewage, decaying vegetation
- Many species of wild and domestic mammals, avian species, crustaceans, pond trout, ticks and flies harbour *Listeria*
- Milk products (particularly soft cheese) and uncooked vegetables, fish and shellfish, ready-to-eat meat products, ground beef and poultry have all been found to contain the organism
- Up to 70 per cent of the human population harbour the organism in their gastrointestinal tract for short periods (6–16 per cent human faeces)

Listeria infection occurs primarily in elderly people, in pregnant women and their newborn infants, and in immunocompromised patients including patients with cancer, AIDS, organ transplant recipients or patients on corticosteroid therapy.[6]

Signs and Symptoms

The majority of people exposed to *Listeria* are either asymptomatic or have subclinical infection. Twenty-five per cent of culture-positive women report no symptoms. [EL 2]

- Mild flu-like symptoms, fever.
- Self-limiting febrile gastroenteritis. The fever is usually low-grade or may be significant, ranging from 36.5°C to 40.1°C.
- Watery diarrhoea, nausea, vomiting.
- Headache, backache and pain in joints and muscles.
- Bacteraemia, meningitis and meningoencephalitis occur in 20, 40 and 39 per cent of cases, respectively.

Signs and symptoms usually lasts for two days followed by complete recovery.

In a series of 191 cases of listeriosis in pregnancy, 32 per cent suffered flu-like illness and 65 per cent had a fever. Other symptoms included backache (21.5 per cent) (which may be mistaken for a urinary tract infection), headache (10.5 per cent), vomiting/diarrhoea (7 per cent), muscle pains (4 per cent) and sore throat (4 per cent). Approximately 29 per cent of the women were asymptomatic.[6,7] [EL 2–]

Invasive infection is rare in healthy populations but tends to affect the immunocompromised, pregnant or older population.

Diagnosis[8]

In the Pregnant Woman

- **Blood cultures** are the standard and only reliable method for diagnosis in cases of fever and symptoms consistent with listeriosis
- **Gram stain**: the presence of short, gram-positive rods found by Gram stain in maternal blood, urine or faecal matter
- **Fetal placental** or cerebrospinal fluid (CSF) specimens support a presumed diagnosis of listeriosis, but the organism is easily confused with *Streptococci*, diphtheroids and even *Haemophilus*
- **Stool culture**: the American College of Obstetricians and Gynecologists maintains the stool culture has not been validated as a screening tool and it is not recommended for the diagnosis of listeriosis as it may have low sensitivity[8]
- **Serologic tests** are not diagnostically reliable
- **Blood cultures** are mandatory in case of bacteraemia or sepsis, and CSF culture where meningitis is suspected
- **Vaginal and rectal cultures** should also be obtained in symptomatic patients

In Perinatal Listeriosis

Culture can be obtained from

- Blood
- Urine
- Meconium, amniotic fluid, placenta or fetal membranes
- Pus from skin lesions
- Tissue obtained at autopsy
- Cerebrospinal fluid
- Pleural fluid, respiratory tract and gastric aspirate
- Histopathology and culture of rash
- Culture of other infected tissues (joint, pericardial fluid)

CT scanning or MRI may be useful in detecting abscesses in the brain or liver.

Effect of Listeriosis on Pregnancy

During pregnancy, cellular immunity is reduced because of increased progesterone making pregnant women particularly susceptible to intracellular micro-organisms like *L. monocytogenes*. Vertical cell-to-cell transmission permits *L. monocytogenes* to infect the uterus and placenta.

Listeriosis is rarely serious for the pregnant woman herself and symptoms generally resolve after delivery with or without antibiotic therapy. *Listeria* infection in the pregnant woman rarely causes severe maternal complications such as

- Meningitis
- Adult respiratory distress syndrome
- Endocarditis

Past infection does not offer immunity against reinfection.

Fetal Implications

During pregnancy, fetal infection (90 per cent) can occur via transplacental transmission. Vertical transmission can also occur via passage through an infected birth canal or ascending infection after ruptured amniotic membranes [EL 2]. Once the placenta is infected, it becomes a reservoir for reinfection,[6] and placental micro-abscesses may be histologically evident.

- **First Trimester** – miscarriage in 10–20 per cent of cases
- **Second Trimester** – premature labour in 50 per cent of cases if infection occurs after 20 weeks

- **Stillbirth** in almost all cases if infection occurs before 20 weeks

Third Trimester:
- Stillbirth
- Intrauterine death
- Intrauterine growth retardation
- Reduced fetal movements
- Pathological cardiotocography (CTG)
- Non-immune hydrops
- Intracranial calcification
- Chorioamnionitis[9]

In a retrospective case series study of 222 pregnant women, there were 11 *Listeria* infections. Nine of those 11 women developed the infection in their third trimester. There were six preterm deliveries (54 per cent) [EL 2]. All six had shown evidence of neonatal *Listeria* infections. Two of 11 pregnancies (18 per cent) resulted in fetal death because of spontaneous abortion and birth of a fetus that died immediately after birth.

The above figures indicate the serious neonatal risks of *Listeria* infections.

Ultrasound Imaging in Fetal *Listeria* Infections[10]

Ultrasound imaging may reveal mild fetal ascites, dilated gall bladder and small bowel loop dilatation, non-immune hydrops, intracranial calcifications, or intrauterine fetal demise.

Fetal surveillance is recommended according to the gestational age.

However, there is no study or data available to suggest the best plan for fetal surveillance and its frequency.

Neonatal Implications

- Listeriosis in the neonate has two different presentations (early or late) depending on the timing of infection.
- Neonatal infection occurs in almost 68 per cent of cases of maternal infection, with complete recovery in approximately 70 per cent of cases, and long-term sequelae in 12.7 per cent of cases.
- Neonatal death can occur in up to 22 per cent of cases of maternal infection.

Early Onset

Early-onset disease occurs within the first seven days of life or soon after birth. The majority of affected infants have poor prognosis due to prematurity as a result of intrauterine infection (chorioamnionitis). Neonatal early-onset listeriosis is non-specific and difficult to distinguish from early-onset group B streptococcal or any other bacterial infection. However, signs of chorioamnionitis without rupture of the membranes should raise suspicion of *Listeria* infection and may prompt laboratory diagnosis.[11]

Clinical features of neonatal infections include:

- Newborns generally pass meconium *in utero* and show fetal compromise on intrapartum fetal heart rate (FHR) tracings.
- Respiratory distress or pneumonia in 38 per cent, with rapid breathing, and grunting which may include cyanotic episodes.
- Poor feeding and fever are common presenting symptoms.
- Septicaemia and meningitis are the most common clinical manifestation.
- Severe infection causes skin lesions (slightly elevated, 1 to 2 mm pale patches on a bright erythematous base) mostly seen on the infant's back and lumbar area called granulomatosis infantisepticum.
- Disseminated granuloma abscesses involve the liver, spleen, adrenal glands, lungs, oesophagus, the posterior pharyngeal wall and placenta.
- Neutropenia is more characteristic of severe infection. Thrombocytopenia sometimes occurs and anaemia is common, most likely secondary to the haemolysin listeriolysin.

On chest X-ray, non-specific pneumonia is common.

Late Onset

Late-onset neonatal infection occurs from one to eight weeks of life and typically affects full-term infants whose mothers had uncomplicated pregnancies.

The infants are usually healthy at birth and symptoms manifest at a mean of 14 days of life, strongly suggesting acquired horizontal postpartum infection at delivery from the maternal genital tract or through nosocomial infection (delivery rooms or nurseries).

Late-onset infection carries a better prognosis for the newborn (mortality rate of 0–20 per cent).

Laboratory features do not distinguish from other causes of bacterial meningitis.[12]

In more than 95 per cent of late-onset cases, babies do not appear seriously ill.

Severe and serious neonatal illness may appear as:

- Fever and septicaemia
- Meningitis presenting with fever and irritability
- Micro-abscesses or granulomas granulomatosis infantisepticum similar to early-onset infection

Mortality is low, except in severe disease or when diagnosis and treatment are delayed. Morbidity and long-term sequelae are not common in treated cases.

Serious Lifelong Health Sequelae of Neonatal Infection (12.7 per cent)

- Intellectual disability, mental retardation
- Hydrocephalus
- Blindness
- Paralysis, seizures
- Impairments of the brain, kidney or heart[13]

Diagnosis of Neonatal Infection

History of a maternal infection or clinical suspicion of neonatal *Listeria* infection is an indication for diagnostic evaluation:

- Culture of blood, cervix and amniotic fluid (if available) of febrile pregnant woman
- Culture of meconium, gastric aspirate, blood, CSF
- Culture of any grossly diseased parts of the placenta
- Infected tissues of sick neonate (micro-abscesses or granulomas granulomatosis infantisepticum)
- Culture of the mother's lochia
- Cultures of the maternal exudates from cervix and vagina

Management

Early treatment with antibiotics may prevent fetal infection and perinatal death and improve neonatal outcome. It also eradicates asymptomatic carriage in the mother as *Listeria* can persist in cervical/vaginal secretions for several weeks after perinatal listeriosis.

Treatment Principles

Asymptomatic Women

The American College of Obstetricians and Gynecologists does not recommend any testing or treatment of asymptomatic pregnant woman with presumptive exposure to *Listeria*. It does, however, recommend close observation. Patients are instructed to report if they develop symptoms of listeriosis within two months of the presumptive exposure. It does not recommend any modifications of fetal surveillance in asymptomatic women with known or presumptive exposure to *Listeria*.[14]

Women with Mild Symptoms

In a woman who is afebrile with mild symptoms with no strong suggestion of listeriosis infection, expectant management is recommended.

If there is a high suspicion of *Listeria* infection, blood cultures should be sent with clear clinical history and a request of suspicion of listeriosis to avoid a mistaken diagnosis of contaminants.

Some clinicians would withhold therapy unless *L. monocytogenes* is isolated. Others would initiate therapy while awaiting blood culture results. If blood cultures yield *L. monocytogenes*, standard therapy with intravenous (IV) ampicillin should be started.

Women with Fever with or without Other Symptoms Consistent with *Listeria*

- If other causes of fever have been ruled out, pregnant women with fever higher than 38°C should be investigated and treated for *Listeria* infection. Blood and placental culture (if delivered) should be obtained.
- If culture is negative and antibiotics have already been started, then continuation of antibiotics depends on the clinical ground in conjunction with a microbiologist and fetal–maternal medicine specialist.
- In women on immunosuppressive therapy (e.g. renal transplant) if there is delayed response, the immunosuppressive drug dose should be decreased. [*Grade 2C recommendation*]
- There is no consensus on the duration of treatment. In case reports, duration of therapy varied from two weeks to continuous treatment until delivery.[15,16]

- Even if the patient shows clinical improvement, a short course of antibiotic treatment may not be sufficient for a complete bactericidal effect, particularly in immunosuppressed patients.[17,18]
- Relapses have been reported after two weeks of penicillin treatment. In pregnancy, the placenta has the potential of ongoing infection of the fetus. Placental infection may not be clinically apparent and could progress once antibiotic therapy is stopped. For this reason, some experts recommend at least three to four weeks of treatment in pregnancy.[19,20]
- Placental infection may not be clinically apparent and could progress once antibiotic therapy is stopped. For this reason, some experts recommend at least three to four weeks of treatment in pregnancy.
- If there is central nervous system (CNS) involvement, treatment should be continued for six to eight weeks. Oral ampicillin 2 to 3 g per day continued once maternal and amniotic fluid cultures become negative.[21]
- If no clinical improvement or failure to eliminate the bacteria from CSF, additional drug therapy may be contemplated (guided by culture and sensitivity)
- Trimethoprim is contraindicated in the first trimester of pregnancy for possible teratogenic effect (neural tube defect). Sulfamethoxazole can cause sulfur allergy and kernicterus, and can also cause haemolytic anaemia in male infants due to glucose-6-phosphate deficiency, if used in the third trimester.
- Imipenem and meropenem are recently approved for paediatric meningitis in resistant cases as proven very effective in vitro.[22,23]

Antibiotic Therapy

First-Line Therapy

Most experience is available on the use of penicillin and ampicillin.

Ampicillin (6 g daily) is recommended as a first-line therapy in women who are not allergic to penicillin, and continuing it for two weeks is the preferred choice as it provides good host cell penetration without any significant change in pH or concentration and crosses.

- Gentamicin (with gentamicin (3 mg/kg eight-hourly) in three divided doses in serious infection) can be used as a synergistic bactericidal. [*Grade 2C recommendation*]

Second-Line Therapy

Trimethoprim–sulfamethoxazole (TSM-SMX) is a bactericidal that crosses placenta and reaches adequate CSF levels and therefore can be used in cases of meningitis and patients with penicillin allergy. It inhibits bacterial growth by inhibiting synthesis of dihydrofolic acid.

Erythromycin, chloramphenicol, vancomycin and cephalosporins (which bind poorly to *Listeria*'s penicillin-binding protein 3) are less effective.

Management of Chorioamnionitis due to *Listeria* Infection

In other causes of chorioamnionitis, induction of labour is the standard of care. However, in cases where the cause of chorioamnionitis is due to maternal listeriosis, antibiotic treatment and delay of delivery can result in the birth of a healthy infant at term. Amniotic fluid cultures change from positive to negative with appropriate antibiotic therapy. Success of *in utero* therapy and resolution should be documented by demonstrating negative amniotic fluid cultures.

Treatment Options for *Listeria* Infections in the Mother

Bacteraemia in pregnancy: first-line: ampicillin 2 g, four-hourly, IV daily [*Grade 2C recommendation*] for 7–14 days (longer duration if fetus is alive and in early pregnancy)

Meningitis: treat with ampicillin and gentamicin – 3 mg/kg eight-hourly daily, IV for 14–21 days

In poor responders continue for up to 21 days. Stop gentamicin when clinical improvement *or* toxicity

If penicillin allergy, sulfamethoxazole 5 mg/kg (avoid in the last month of pregnancy). *Or* trimethoprim 25 mg/kg every eight hours, IV (avoid in first trimester) for 10–14 days

Endocarditis, meningitis: vancomycin 15–20 mg/kg (around 250 mg; usual maximum: 2 g/dose initially) every 8–12 hours, IV for 10–14 days

If allergy to penicillin, Second-line: erythromycin 4 g/daily IV for 7–14 days (with longer duration if required) *or* trimethoprim *or* meropenem 2 g IV, eight-hourly

Monitoring after Therapy is Completed

The patient is monitored for signs of relapse or poor response such as the recurrence or the continuation of fever and other signs and symptoms after completing the course of therapy.

If there is a suspicion of recurrence or poor response, blood and CSF cultures (to exclude meningitis) should be undertaken. Ultrasound and MRI should be performed for any congenital anomalies.

Time and Mode of Delivery

An extensive literature search did not reveal any recommendations for fetal surveillance, time or mode of delivery.

Consequently, we recommend proper counselling of the pregnant women about the possible risks of stillbirth, preterm birth and other fetal problems, close surveillance, prediction and aggressive management of threatened preterm labour. Each individual case should be managed according to its merits, with proper antenatal care, and in accordance with obstetric guidelines. [EL 4]

Therapy in Neonates

Use of antibiotics such as ampicillin combined with an aminoglycoside is the preferred choice for early-onset neonatal listeriosis. Drug doses and frequency intervals are adjusted by age and weight of the infant.

Ampicillin:
- Infant <7 days and <2 kg: ampicillin 100 mg/kg divided in 2 doses. Infant <7 days and >2 kg: 150 mg/kg divided in 3 doses
- Infant 8–30 days and <2 kg: ampicillin150 mg/kg divided in 4 doses. Infant >2 kg: ampicillin 200 mg/kg divided in 4 doses

Gentamicin:
- Infant <7 days: 2.5mg/kg every 12 hours
- Infant 8–30 days and weighing 1.2–2 kg: 2.5 mg/kg every 8–12 hours; and weighing >2 kg: 2.5 mg/kg eight-hourly

Treatment is recommended for 14 days; however, longer course is required in early-onset infection with meningitis.

Imipenem and meropenem are recently approved for paediatric meningitis in resistant cases, as they are effectively proven in vitro.

Meningitis is the usual presentation in late-onset listeriosis where the organism is generally more difficult to eradicate. Lumbar punctures should be performed daily to monitor therapy.

If the CSF does not become negative after two days, additional drug therapy may be considered based on culture and sensitivity. Further MRI investigation to identify CNS parenchymal involvement is recommended. If an abscess is present, surgical drainage should be carried out.

Therapeutic Options for *Listeria* Infections in Neonates

Bacteraemia: ampicillin with aminoglycoside. Dose and frequency depend on age and weight. Intravenous for 14 days (longer duration if early onset with meningitis)

Meningitis: ampicillin and gentamicin. Ampicillin, 200–400 mg/kg per day in four to six doses in combination with gentamicin. Intravenous. Stop gentamicin after one week or when clinical improvement

Resistant cases, second-line: imipenem and meropenem. Discuss dose with microbiologist. Up to 120 mg/kg, intravenous eight-hourly if culture remains positive after two days

Management of Pregnant Women during an Outbreak

- In the event of an outbreak of listeriosis, women should be advised to eat only thoroughly cooked meat, properly washed vegetables, pasteurised milk/dairy products, and avoid soft cheese.
- A low threshold should exist and body fluid (blood, vaginal and rectal swabs) for culture should be obtained so that an early diagnosis is made and treatment can be initiated as early as possible.
- Where infection is suspected, CSF or amniotic fluid cultures should also be taken.
- Symptomatic women should be treated after culture is obtained.
- Asymptomatic culture-positive women should also be treated.

- Asymptomatic culture-negative women should be observed and another culture should be performed in case of longer incubation period.
- Local health department officials should be notified if *L. monocytogenes* is recovered or a food source has been identified.
- Pregnant women should be informed about the outbreak and the food in question.[23]

Prevention

The American College of Obstetricians and Gynecologists and the Centers for Disease Control and Prevention (CDC) recommend that all pregnant women should be advised to avoid eating the following foods: unpasteurised milk or any foods made with unpasteurised milk; hot dogs; refrigerated pâté; and refrigerated smoked seafoods. Luncheon meats, cold cuts and meat spreads should be heated until steaming hot just before serving. All unwashed raw produce such as fruits and vegetables should be washed thoroughly before use. The recommendations also include advice on how to cook, preserve and chill food products.

Conclusion

Listeriosis is a rare food-borne infection caused by the consumption of contaminated food. It is about 18 times more common in pregnant women than in the general population. Pregnant women with co-morbidities are at increased risk due to compromised cell-mediated immunity. Maternal illness is usually mild, but neonatal disease carries a 20--30 per cent mortality rate. Early diagnosis and treatment reduces fetal and neonatal morbidity and mortality.

Listeria infection causes potentially severe consequences for unborn fetuses, therefore it is important that practising obstetricians are familiar with the diagnosis, treatment, neonatal consequences and prevention of the disease.

Pregnant women should be taught to avoid high-risk foods and to follow routine hygienic measures.

High-dose ampicillin is the treatment of choice with or without gentamicin depending on clinical indication.

All febrile episodes occurring during pregnancy should not be underestimated and need to be investigated if diagnosis is unclear and the woman remains febrile and symptomatic.

References

1. de Valk H, Jacquet C, Goulet V et al. Surveillance of listeria infections in Europe. *Euro Surveill.* 2005; **10**(10): 251–5.

2. Prevention CfDCa. Preliminary FoodNet data on the incidence of infection with pathogens transmitted commonly through food – 10 states, 2007. *MMWR.* 2008; **57**: 366–70.

3. Preliminary FoodNet data on the incidence of infection with pathogens transmitted commonly through food – 10 states, 2009. *MMWR Morb Mortal Wkly Rep.* 2010; **59**(14): 418–22.

4. Lamont RF, Sobel J, Mazaki-Tovi S et al. Listeriosis in human pregnancy: a systematic review. *J Perinat Med.* 2011; **39**(3): 227–36.

5. Okada Y, Ohnuki I, Suzuki H, Igimi S. Growth of Listeria monocytogenes in refrigerated ready-to-eat foods in Japan. *Food Addit Contam Part A Chem Anal Control Expo Risk Assess.* 2013; 29 April.

6. Imanishi M, Routh JA, Klaber M et al. Estimating the attack rate of pregnancy-associated listeriosis during a large outbreak. *Infect Dis Obstet Gynecol.* 2015; **2015**: 201479.

7. Mylonakis E, Paliou M, Hohmann EL et al. Listeriosis during pregnancy: a case series and review of 222 cases. *Medicine* (Baltimore). 2002; **81**: 260.

8. Centers for Disease Control and Prevention. Listeria (Listeriosis). Diagnosis and Treatment. www.cdc.gov/listeria/diagnosis.html.

9. Hasbun J, Sepulveda-Martinez A, Haye MT, Astudillo J, Parra-Cordero M. Chorioamnionitis caused by Listeria monocytogenes: a case report of ultrasound features of fetal infection. *Fetal Diagn Ther.* 2013; **33**(4): 268–71.

10. Haye MT, Astudillo J, Parra-Cordero M. Chorioamnionitis caused by Listeria monocytogenes: a case report of ultrasound features of fetal infection. *Fetal Diagn Ther.* 2013; **33**(4): 268–71.

11. Ross DS, Rasmussen SA, Cannon MJ et al. Obstetrician/gynecologists' knowledge, attitudes, and practices regarding prevention of infections in pregnancy. *J Women's Health.* (Larchmont, NY) 2009; **18**: 1187–93.

12. Bortolussi R, Schlech WF. Listeriosis. In: Remington JS, Klein JO, eds. *Infectious Diseases of the Fetus and Newborn Infant.* Philadelphia: WB Saunders; 2001: 1157–77.

13. Caserta MT. Neonatal Listeriosis. MSD Manual, October 2015. www.msdmanuals.com/professional/pediatrics/neonatal-listeriosis.

14. American College of Obstetricians and Gynecologists. Guideline Committee on Obstetric Practice Management of Pregnant Women with Presumptive Exposure to Listeria monocytogenes. Number 614, December 2014.

15. Janakiraman V. Listeriosis in pregnancy: diagnosis, treatment, and prevention. *Rev Obstet Gynecol.* 2008; **1**(4): 179–85.

16. Lorber B. Listeria monocytogenes. In: Mandell GL, Bennett JE, Dolin R, eds. *Principles and Practice of Infectious Diseases*, 7th ed. Philadelphia: Churchill Livingstone; 2010: 2707.

17. Edmiston CE Jr, Gordon RC. Evaluation of gentamicin and penicillin as a synergistic combination in experimental murine listeriosis. *Antimicrob Agents Chemother.* 1979; **16**: 862–3.

18. Grant MH, Ravreby H, Lorber B. Cure of *Listeria monocytogenes* meningitis after early transition to oral therapy. *Antimicrob Agents Chemother.* 2010; **54**: 2276–7.

19. Scheer MS, Hirschman SZ. Oral and ambulatory therapy of Listeria bacteremia and meningitis with trimethoprim-sulfamethoxazole. *Mt Sinai J Med.* 1982; **49**: 411–14.

20. Tessier F, Bouillie J, Daguet GL, Barrat J. Listeriosis in obstetrical environment. Report on 10-year experience in a maternity hospital in Paris. *J Gynecol Obstet Biol Reprod.* (Paris) 1986; **15**: 305–13.

21. Bortolussi R, Mailman TL. Listeriosis. In: Remington JS, Klein JO, Wilson CB et al., eds. *Infectious Diseases of the Fetus and Newborn Infant*, 7th ed. Philadelphia: Elsevier Saunders; 2011: 470.

22. Zach T. Listeria infection medication: antibiotics. Medscape. 2015. www.emedicine.com/ped/topic1319.htm.

23. American College of Obstetricians and Gynecologists. Listeria and Pregnancy. January 2017. www.acog.org/Patients/FAQs/Listeria-and-Pregnancy.

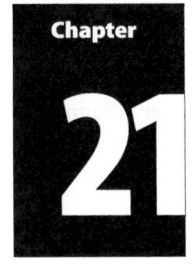
Urinary Tract Infection

Ashok Kumar

Introduction

Urinary tract infection (UTI) is more common during pregnancy because the hormonal and mechanical changes in the urinary tract make women more vulnerable starting from 6 weeks through 24 weeks.

Urinary tract infection in pregnancy involves

- Urethra
- Bladder
- Ureter
- Kidneys

Most of the infections are limited to the bladder and urethra but can lead to kidney infection.

Predisposing Pregnancy Factors

- Women are eight times more likely to get urinary tract infections, due to proximity of the genital tract and the rectum where E. coli are found in faecal matter.
- Progesterone hormonal changes promote urinary stasis and vesicoureteral reflux. Progesterone may also induce smooth muscle relaxation in the ureter.
- Short urethra and difficulty with hygiene due to a distended pregnant abdomen makes women more prone to have UTIs.
- Physiological and structural changes in the urinary tract organs.
- Compression from uterine enlargement and relative dextrorotation.
- Compression from the right ovarian venous plexus that crosses over the ureter, and finally bladder pressure and capacity are also altered due to decreased tone.[1]
- In addition, the immunosuppression of pregnancy may contribute as mucosal interleukin-6 levels and serum antibody responses to E. coli antigens appear to be lower in pregnant women.[2]

- Easier contamination because of the proximity of the anal orifice to the urethra.
- UTIs are associated with risks to both the fetus and the mother, including pyelonephritis, preterm birth, low birthweight and increased perinatal mortality.

Signs and Symptoms

- Pain or burning (dysuria), frequency, urgency, nocturia
- Blood or mucus in the urine
- Cramps or pain in the lower abdomen
- Pain during sexual intercourse
- Chills, fever, sweats, leaking of urine (incontinence)
- Change in amount of urine, cloudy, smells foul or unusually strong
- Pain, pressure or tenderness in the suprapubic area of the bladder

Asymptomatic Bacteriuria

- Asymptomatic bacteriuria is the presence of more than 100 000 organisms/mL in two consecutive urine samples in the absence of declared symptoms.
- Untreated, it is a risk factor for acute cystitis (40 per cent) and pyelonephritis (25–30 per cent) in pregnancy.[3]
- The United States Preventive Services Task Force as well as several other international medical societies recommend screening for and treatment of asymptomatic bacteriuria. Screening and treatment of asymptomatic bacteriuria is cost-effective, especially in populations where its incidence is greater than 2 per cent. If untreated, up to 30 per cent of cases will progress to pyelonephritis.
- With proper treatment of asymptomatic bacteriuria, the number needed to treat to prevent one episode of pyelonephritis is only seven, and

the rate of hospitalisation for pyelonephritis is reduced to 1.4 per cent.

- A review of randomised trials comparing antibiotic treatment versus no antibiotic treatment of asymptomatic bacteriuria resulted in a greater decrease in both pyelonephritis and low-birthweight babies. The rates of preterm delivery, however, were not affected by treatment. [EL 1]
- In a meta-analysis of 19 studies, among women without bacteriuria, the risks of preterm birth and a low-birthweight infant were one-half and two-thirds respectively the risks among women with asymptomatic bacteriuria.[4] [EL 1]
- Other pregnancy complications have also been associated with bacteriuria. A case control study of over 15 000 pregnant women found an increased risk of pre-eclampsia with either asymptomatic bacteriuria or symptomatic UTI.[5] [EL 2]

Asymptomatic bacteriuria during pregnancy increases the risk of pyelonephritis and has been associated with adverse pregnancy outcomes, therefore antibiotic therapy should be given according to the culture and sensitivity.

Acute Cystitis

- Involves only the lower urinary tract
- Is characterised by inflammation of the bladder
- Affects approximately 1 per cent of pregnant patients
- Signs and symptoms include haematuria, dysuria, suprapubic discomfort, frequency, urgency and nocturia
- Acute cystitis is complicated by upper urinary tract disease (i.e. pyelonephritis) in 15–50 per cent of cases[6] Acute cystitis occurs in 1–2 per cent of pregnancies[7]

Symptoms of Acute Cystitis

Urinary frequency, dysuria and urgency; however no correlation has been clearly established between acute cystitis of pregnancy and increased risk of low birth-weight, preterm delivery or pyelonephritis, perhaps because pregnant women with symptomatic lower UTI usually receive treatment, contrary to asymptomatic bacteriuria where it may pass unnoticed as it is an asymptomatic condition.

Treatment of cystitis is the same as that for asymptomatic bacteriuria.

A Cochrane review of nine studies showed that no single treatment regimen for cystitis in pregnancy was superior to another. If symptoms persist with negative urine cultures, consideration of other diagnoses, including cervicitis, vaginitis and especially urethritis, should be considered and other cultures taken appropriately.

Acute Pyelonephritis

- Is the most common urinary tract complication in pregnant women, occurring in approximately 2 per cent of all pregnancies
- Is characterised by fever, flank pain and tenderness in addition to significant bacteriuria
- Other symptoms may include nausea, vomiting, frequency, urgency and dysuria
- Women with additional risk factors (e.g. immunosuppression, diabetes, sickle cell anaemia, neurogenic bladder, recurrent or persistent UTIs before pregnancy) are at an increased risk for a complicated UTI[8]

Pyelonephritis also complicates 1–2 per cent of pregnancies.[9]

- Symptoms and signs of pyelonephritis include symptoms of cystitis, chills, flank pain, nausea, vomiting, fever and costovertebral angle tenderness.
- The diagnosis is made by urine culture. One to two bacteria per high-power field (hpf) on an unspun urine sample or greater than 20 bacteria per hpf on a spun urine sample correlates with 100 000 cfu/mL. The presence of white blood cell casts on urinalysis can confirm the diagnosis as well.
- Bacteraemia is present in 10–20 per cent of patients with pyelonephritis. Standard treatment is administration of intravenous (IV) antibiotics until the patient remains afebrile for at least 48 hours.
- If bacteraemia is present, IV treatment should be extended to a period of at least five to seven days. As with cystitis, E. coli is cultured in 70–81 per cent of cases.
- More serious complications of pyelonephritis include septic shock and pulmonary insufficiency in 10 per cent of cases.
- Furthermore, suppressive antibiotic therapy is recommended for the remainder of the gestation, with a common choice being nitrofurantoin 100 mg orally, at bedtime.

- In non-compliant patients, monthly urine cultures should be obtained to screen for recurrent bacterial growth.

Recurrent Pyelonephritis

- Recurrence rate is approximately 20 per cent.
- Most cases of pyelonephritis occur during the second and third trimesters but can occur in the postpartum period as well.[10]

  As a result, low-dose antimicrobial suppressive therapy with an agent to which the original organism is susceptible is warranted for the remainder of the pregnancy; reasonable options include nitrofurantoin (50–100 mg orally at bedtime) or cephalexin (250–500 mg orally at bedtime).

- Monthly cultures are not necessary if preventive therapy is administered; however, at least one culture, later, at the start of the third trimester, to ensure preventive therapy is working should be done.

Obstetric management: pyelonephritis is not itself an indication for delivery. If induction of labour or caesarean delivery is required for obstetrical indications, it is advisable to wait until the patient is afebrile, as long as delaying the delivery is relatively safe for the mother and fetus.

Tocolysis should not be used when pyelonephritis triggers preterm labour. Risk of pulmonary oedema and acute respiratory distress syndrome (ARDS) may be exacerbated by administration of tocolysis with or without corticosteroids.

Bacteriology of UTI during Pregnancy

Bacteria are the commonest cause of UTI infections but other organisms, including fungus, parasites and protozoa, can cause UTIs.[11]

Escherichia coli, known as E. coli, is responsible for about 80 per cent of urinary tract infections.[12]

In a retrospective study in Norway reviewing 849 urine culture samples, *Staphylococcus saprophyticus* represented 6–17 per cent. Of the causative organisms, this is second to E. coli. [EL 2]

Diagnosis of UTI during Pregnancy

Diagnostic studies for UTI consist of dipstick, urinalysis and culture

Dipstick

A positive leucocyte esterase dipstick test suffices in most instances to indicate urine infection and start further tests.[13]

Urine Microscopy

- If clinical findings suggest UTI, urine microscopy may be indicated even if the leucocyte esterase dipstick test is negative.
- Pyuria is most accurately measured by counting leucocytes in unspun fresh urine using an emocytometer chamber; more than 10 white blood cells (WBCs)/mL is abnormal.
- Microscopic haematuria is found in about half of cystitis cases.
- Low-grade proteinuria is common.

Urine Culture

Remains the gold standard for the diagnosis of UTI. It should be considered in the following circumstances:

- Immunosuppression.
- Recent urinary tract instrumentation.
- Recent exposure to antibiotics.
- Recurrent infection.
- Advanced age.
- Any amount of uropathogen grown in culture from a suprapubic aspirate should be considered evidence of a UTI. A mid-stream sample of urine should be collected after separating the labia.
- Urine specimens may be obtained by suprapubic aspiration or catheterisation.[14]

Management of UTI during pregnancy.
Starting oral therapy with an empirically chosen antibiotic that is effective against gram-negative aerobic coliform bacteria (e.g. *Escherichia coli*) is the first choice and the principal treatment intervention in patients with cystitis.

Antibiotic choices

1. Cephalexin (Keflex) (category B) 250 mg six-hourly

2. Erythromycin (category B) 250–500 mg six-hourly

3. Nitrofurantoin (Macrodantin) (category B) 50–100 mg six-hourly

4. Sulfisoxazole (Gantrisin) (category C), avoid during first trimester and at term, 1 g six-hourly

5. Amoxycillin–clavulanic acid (Augmentin) (category B) 250 mg six-hourly

6. Trimethoprim–sulfamethoxazole (Bactrim) (category C), avoid first trimester and at term, 160/180 mg twice daily[15]

Duration of antibiotic treatment for uncomplicated acute cystitis:

- TMP-SMX is given for three days
- Fosfomycin is given in a single dose
- Nitrofurantoin monohydrate/macrocrystals is given for five to seven days
- β-lactam agents are given for three to seven days

Most women with UTI can be treated as outpatients.

Indications for hospital admission:

- Structural abnormalities (e.g. calculi, tract anomalies, indwelling catheter, obstruction)
- Metabolic disorders (diabetes, renal insufficiency)
- Impaired host defences (HIV infection, current chemotherapy, underlying active cancer)

Effect on Pregnancy

In an 18-year retrospective study of over 500 000 singleton pregnancies in the United States, the rate of preterm birth between 33 and 36 weeks was higher among the 2894 women who had pyelonephritis during pregnancy (10.3 versus 7.9 per cent among those who did not, or 1.3.[9] [EL 2]

Maternal morbidity and obstetric outcomes with pyelonephritis do not appear to differ by trimester.[16]

Maternal Complications

- Hypertension
- Pre-eclampsia
- Anaemia
- Chorioamnionitis
- Symptomatic acute cystitis and acute pyelonephritis
- Higher chance of caesarean deliveries

Fetal Implications

- Intrauterine growth retardation
- Intrauterine death
- Low birthweight
- Prematurity of baby

Prevention of UTI

- Oral hydration with six to eight glasses of water each day and unsweetened cranberry juice

regularly and avoid refined foods, fruit juices, caffeine, alcohol and sugar.
- Vitamin C (250–500 mg), β-carotene (25 000–50 000 IU per day) and zinc (30–50 mg per day) helps in reducing infection.
- It is important to regularly fully empty bladder when feels full.
- It is advisable to urinate before and after intercourse.
- Avoidance of intercourse while being treated for a UTI.
- After urinating, the genital area should be clean and dry and should be wiped from the front to the back.
- Strong soaps, douches, antiseptic creams, feminine hygiene sprays and powders should be avoided.
- Loose cotton underwear and pantyhose should be worn and changed every day.
- Wearing tight-fitting pants should be avoided.[17] [EL 4]

Conclusion

Infections of the urinary tract are commonly encountered in pregnancy, typically during early pregnancy. Asymptomatic bacteriuria can lead to pyelonephritis in 30–40 per cent of cases and adverse pregnancy outcomes if left untreated.

Acute cystitis should be suspected in pregnant women who complain of new-onset dysuria, frequency or urgency.

Acute pyelonephritis during pregnancy is suggested by the presence of flank pain, nausea/vomiting, fever (>38°C), and/or costovertebral angle tenderness, with or without the typical symptoms of cystitis, and is confirmed by urine culture.

Pyelonephritis should be treated in hospital, with intravenous antibiotics, adequate hydration and antipyretics until symptoms and fever subside. Patients must be closely monitored for the development of rare complication of pyelonephritis to sepsis and pulmonary oedema or adult respiratory distress syndrome. This should be treated aggressively at the first sign of such conditions.

Finally, patients with asymptomatic or symptomatic bacteriuria should be monitored for recurrent infection during the remainder of pregnancy, and those with pyelonephritis require daily therapy for the remainder of their gestation.

References

1. Sweet RL. Bacteriuria and pyelonephritis during pregnancy. *Semin Perinatol.* 1977; **1**: 25.

2. Petersson C, Hedges S, Stenqvist K et al. Suppressed antibody and interleukin-6 responses to acute pyelonephritis in pregnancy. *Kidney Int.* 1994; **45**: 571.

3. Smaill F. Asymptomatic bacteriuria in pregnancy. *Best Pract Res Clin Obstet Gynaecol.* 2007; **21**(3): 439–50.

4. Romero R, Oyarzun E, Mazor M, Sirtori M, Hobbins JC, Bracken M. Meta-analysis of the relationship between asymptomatic bacteriuria and preterm delivery/low birth weight. *Obstet Gynecol.* 1989; **73**: 57619.

5. Minassian C, Thomas SL, Williams DJ, Campbell O, Smeeth L. Acute maternal infection and risk of pre-eclampsia: a population-based case-control study. *PLoS ONE.* 2013; **8**: e73047.

6. Glaser AP, Schaeffer AJ. Urinary tract infection and bacteriuria in pregnancy. *Urol Clin North Am.* 2015; **42**(4): 547–60.

7. Gilstrap LC III, Ramin SM. Urinary tract infections during pregnancy. *Obstet Gynecol Clin North Am.* 2001; **28**: 581.

8. Hill JB, Sheffield JS, McIntire DD, Wendel GD Jr. Acute pyelonephritis in pregnancy. *Obstet Gynecol.* 2005; **105**(1): 18–23.

9. Wing DA, Fassett MJ, Getahun D. Acute pyelonephritis in pregnancy: an 18-year retrospective analysis. *Am J Obstet Gynecol.* 2014; **210**: 219.e1.

10. American College of Obstetricians and Gynecologists. Antimicrobial therapy for obstetric patients. *ACOG Educational Bulletin* 245. Washington, DC; 1998.

11. Harvard Medical School, Urinary tract infection in women. In: *Harvard Medical School Health Topics A–Z.* Boston, MA: Harvard Health Publications; 2013. /content/entry/hhphealth/urinarytractinfectioni.

12. Bollestad M, Vik I, Grude N, Blix HS, Brekke H, Lindbaek M. Bacteriology in uncomplicated urinary tract infections in Norwegian general practice from 2001–2015. *BJGP Open.* 2017; 2017-0239.

13. Little P, Turner S, Rumsby K et al. Dipsticks and diagnostic algorithms in urinary tract infection: development and validation, randomised trial, economic analysis, observational cohort and qualitative study. *Health Technol Assess.* 2009; **13**(19): iii–iv, ix–xi, 1–73.

14. Lane DR, Takhar SS. Diagnosis and management of urinary tract infection and pyelonephritis. *Emerg Med Clin North Am.* 2011; **29**(3): 539–52.

15. Infectious Diseases Society of America. Guidelines for Antimicrobial Treatment of Acute Uncomplicated Cystitis and Pyelonephritis in Women. *Clin Infect Dis.* 2011; **52**: e103–20. www.idsociety.org/Guidelines/Patient_Care/IDSA_Practice_Guidelines/Infections_by_Organ_System/Genitourinary/.

16. Archabald KL, Friedman A, Raker CA, Anderson BL. Impact of trimester on morbidity of acute pyelonephritis in pregnancy. *Am J Obstet Gynecol.* 2009; **201**: 406.e1.

17. Schneeberger C, Geerlings SE, Middleton P, Crowther CA. *Cochrane Database Syst Rev.* 2012; **11**: CD009279. doi: 10.1002/14651858.CD009279.pub2.

Chapter 22

Infections and Preterm Labour

Christine Helmy Samuel Azer

Introduction

Preterm labour is defined as the delivery of the fetus when birth occurs between 20 and 37 completed weeks.

Preterm labour is one of the major causes of neonatal mortality (1–5 per cent) and morbidity (necrotising enterocolitis; retinopathy of prematurity, intraventricular haemorrhage; chronic lung disease; cerebral palsy, blindness and learning difficulties; and developmental delay).

It is estimated that 40 per cent of preterm labours are due to infections that can be prevented if detected and treated early. The earlier the preterm birth, the more it is due to infection. Preterm birth is the most frequent cause of infant death in the United States, accounting for at least one-third of infant deaths in 2002.[1]

In many cases, the reasons for preterm labour are largely unknown. In other instances, preterm labour can have a variety of different causes, e.g. infection, an 'incompetent' or weak cervix, multiple pregnancy, history of certain types of surgery on the uterus or cervix, lifestyle factors such as low pre-pregnancy weight, obesity, smoking during pregnancy and substance abuse.[2]

This chapter will focus on inflammatory and infectious conditions.

Pathophysiology

Inflammatory Conditions

Inflammation is a localised reaction that produces redness, warmth, swelling and pain as a result of irritation, injury, infection or disease that are not primarily infective (e.g. asthma, rheumatoid arthritis).

Inflammation promotes the secretion of pro-inflammatory cytokines including tumor necrosis factor α (TNF-α) and interleukin (IL) 1β from the cells composing the uteroplacental unit. Initial pro-inflammatory stimuli by TNF-α and IL-1β trigger production of IL-8 and prostaglandins (PGE2 and PGF2α) in the decidua and the placenta, impairing the tissue integrity of fetal membranes, and leading to prostaglandin release. This causes ripening of the cervix, membrane injury and preterm labour.[3]

Infections

Intrauterine or extrauterine infections produce inflammatory reaction in the form of Toll-like receptors (TLRs). TLRs initiate immune response, inducing pro-inflammatory factors involving cytokines, chemokines, prostaglandins and other effector molecules that result in complications of labour, e.g. rupture of fetal membranes.[4]

There is an abundance of evidence on the relation between infection and preterm labour:

- The amniotic fluid in preterm labour has higher rates of microbial colonisation and levels of inflammatory cytokines than that of preterm patients not in labour.
- Extrauterine maternal infections (pyelonephritis, pneumonia and periodontal disease) or subclinical intrauterine infections have been implicated in preterm labour.

Infections and Preterm Labour

Infectious causes of preterm labour can be either:
- Bacterial
- Viral
- Bacterial vaginosis
- *Chlamydia trachomatis*

These four infectious conditions precipitate chorioamniotitis which in turn initiates preterm labour (as explained in the Pathophysiology section above).

Bacterial Infections

Intrauterine infections caused by bacteria are the leading cause of infection-associated preterm labour. Forty per cent of preterm labours are associated with intrauterine infections.

Ascending cervical and vaginal flora through the cervical canal is the most common pathway to infection of the membranes and chorion (chorioamnionitis).

Uncommonly, chorioamnionitis may occur via haematogenous spread as a result of maternal bacteraemia (e.g. *Listeria monocytogenes*), or via contamination of the amniotic cavity as a result of an invasive procedure (e.g. amniocentesis, fetoscopy).[5]

Viral Infections

Viruses are not a common cause, although adenovirus, cytomegalovirus and enterovirus DNA have been isolated from the amniotic fluid of some low-risk patients that had preterm delivery.

Evidence suggests that viral entry into trophoblast cells induces apoptosis inflammatory reaction, with preterm birth.[6]

Bacterial Vaginosis

There are strong associations between bacterial vaginosis and both histologic and clinical chorioamnionitis infection. *Ureaplasma urealyticum* and *Gardnerella vaginalis* are the micro-organisms most frequently identified by cultivation.

Bacterial vaginosis is associated with increased concentrations of bacterial endotoxins, proteases, mucinases and sialidases.

In two epidemiologic studies (one in a high-risk group of women in labour and another in a lower-risk group of antepartum women), the presence of bacterial vaginosis has been associated with the development of chorioamnionitis. Multiple logistic regression analysis has shown a relationship between isolation of organisms from the chorioamnion and bacterial vaginosis.[7]

Chlamydia trachomatis

Chlamydia trachomatis is the most common sexually transmitted infection worldwide. Starting as cervicitis, chlamydial infection may ascend and infect the placenta or amniotic fluid, which may subsequently lead to preterm delivery.

In a prospective, observational and non-interventional study on 320 pregnant women,
histological evidence of placental inflammation was present in 40 per cent of women who had early preterm delivery.[8]

In a population-based prospective cohort study by Rours G.I.J.G. et al. involving 4055 women, *C. trachomatis* infection contributed significantly to early premature delivery.[9]

Chorioamnionitis

Chorioamnionitis or intra-amniotic infection is an acute infection of the membranes and chorion of the placenta, usually due to ascending bacterial infection which is commonly associated with rupture of membranes.

Chorioamnionitis is associated with as many as 40–70 per cent of preterm births with premature membrane rupture.

Preterm labour may result from a fetal and/or maternal response to chorioamnionitis.

Clinical chorioamnionitis, ruptured membranes

Among women with preterm premature rupture of membranes (PPROM), the rate of positive amniotic fluid cultures at admission is 32.4 per cent. However by the time labour begins, as many as 75 per cent will have microbial infection of the amniotic cavity, which is enhanced by removal of the physical barrier of the membranes after they rupture.[10]

or

Microbiological histopathologic chorioamnionitis with intact membranes

The amniotic cavity is normally sterile. The isolation of bacteria in the amniotic fluid with intact membranes is a pathologic finding, known as microbial invasion of the amniotic cavity and/or the chorioamnion. Most cases are subclinical and are undetectable without amniotic fluid culture. In patients with preterm labour with intact membranes, the rate of positive amniotic fluid cultures is 12.8 per cent.

Diagnosis of Chorioamnionitis

Ideally, an early diagnosis of intra-amniotic infection (IAI) is important for timely treatment and intervention. Usually, early diagnosis is difficult because the clinical signs and symptoms of IAI occur late and are neither sensitive nor specific. To avoid a delay in diagnosis, a high index of clinical suspicion with appropriate laboratory tests may speed diagnosis.

Clinical Diagnosis

- Maternal tachycardia (>100 bpm).
- Fever (> 38°C) is the first sign of suspected chorioamnionitis. It is mediated by the effect of pyrogenic cytokines, interferon-gamma (IFN-γ) and tumour necrosis factor-alpha (TNF-α).
- Uterine tenderness.
- Foul-smelling amniotic fluid if there is rupture of membranes.
- Fetal tachycardia (>160 bpm).
- Other cardiotocography changes (diminished or absent variability, tachycardia or sinusoidal pattern) suggesting fetal distress.

Laboratory Diagnosis of Chorioamnionitis

Leucocytosis (WBC >12 000/mm^3 or >15 000/mm^3) in 70–90 per cent of cases.

Isolated leucocytosis in the absence of the above clinical signs and symptoms has limited value because it may be induced by several other conditions.

High levels of C-reactive protein (CRP), lipopoly-sacharide-binding protein (LBP), soluble intercellular adhesion molecule 1 (sICAM 1) and interleukin-6 (which may be raised) do not offer any clinical value and should not be used to diagnose or monitor chorioamnionitis.[11] [EL 1]

The role of amniocentesis in PPROM to diagnose clinical or subclinical chorioamnionitis membranes remains unclear. It is associated with a delay of at least 48–72 hours for cultures, with no evidence of predictive value for potential maternal and neonatal outcomes. There is a paucity of good-quality trials to demonstrate its role in reducing either maternal or neonatal morbidity.

Differential Diagnosis of Chorioamnionitis

Other conditions causing similar signs and symptoms should be considered in the differential diagnosis of chorioamnionitis.

- Epidural analgesia may cause intrapartum low-grade fever but without maternal tachycardia or other clinical signs of intrauterine infection.
- Extrauterine infections (urinary tract infection (pyelonephritis), influenza, appendicitis and pneumonia) can cause fever and abdominal pain, either during or in the absence of labour.

- In the absence of fever, non-infectious conditions that are usually associated with abdominal pain include thrombophlebitis, round ligament pain, colitis, connective tissue disorders and placental abruption.

Bacteriology of Chorioamnionitis

Cultured specimens in clinical chorioamnionitis most often reveal a polymicrobial infection. The commonest bacteriological aetiology is: *U. urealyticum*, *G. vaginalis* gram-negative anaerobe and *M. hominis* and *Bacteroides bivius*. Fungal organisms, including several species of *Candida* (*Candida albicans*, *Candida tropicalis* and *Candida glabrata*), have also been implicated.

Although viruses have been isolated and implicated in cases of chorioamnionitis, supportive evidence of actually causing chorioamnionitis is very limited.[12]

Risk Factors for Chorioamnionitis

- Long duration of membrane rupture (relative risk (RR): ≥12 hours, 5.8; > 18 hours, 6.9)
- Prolonged labour (active labour >12 hours, RR 4.0; second stage >2 hours (RR 3.7)
- Frequent multiple vaginal examinations (≥3 exams, RR 2–5)
- Meconium-stained liquor (RR 1.4–2.3)
- Fetal scalp electrodes for internal fetal monitoring (RR 2.0)
- Vaginal colonisation with *Ureaplasma* or group B *Streptococcus* and/or bacterial vaginosis
- Immunocompromised conditions and sexually transmitted infections

Maternal Outcomes

Chorioamnionitis is related to a significantly increased risk of maternal blood transfusion, uterine atony, postpartum transfusion and wound/perineal infection or endometritis, septic pelvic thrombophlebitis and pelvic abscess.[13] [EL 2]

Neonatal Outcomes

There is a strong relation between chorioamnionitis and neonatal outcomes, a low 5-minute APGAR ≤3, neonatal sepsis, and seizures, neonatal mechanical ventilation within 24 hours of birth, intraventricular haemorrhage (IVH) and retinopathy.

Adverse neonatal events were significantly associated with chorioamnionitis duration.[14] [EL 2]

Apart from the risk of direct fetal infection and sepsis, fetal inflammatory reaction may induce cerebral white matter injury, resulting in cerebral palsy and other short- and long-term neurological sequelae:

- Perinatal death, asphyxia.
- Early-onset neonatal sepsis.
- Septic shock.
- Pneumonia.
- Intraventricular haemorrhage (IVH).
- Cerebral white matter damage, and long-term disability including cerebral palsy (CP). Chorioamnionitis is associated with a four-fold increase in CP. [EL 2]

Routes of Infection

Chorioamnionitis is caused by the passage of infectious organisms to the umbilical cord.

- The commonest route is by retrograde or ascending infection from the lower genital tract (cervix and vagina).
- Haematogenous/transplacental passage also causes infection.
- Iatrogenic infections complicating amniocentesis or chorionic villous sampling are less common routes of infection.
- Pelvic infection causing anterograde infection from the peritoneum via the fallopian tubes has also been postulated.

Treatment of Chorioamnionitis

- Treatment of acute chorioamnionitis includes immediate administration of antimicrobial agents, antipyretics, expedition of delivery and management of additional symptoms.
- Several randomised controlled trials (RCTs) have used intravenous (IV) ampicillin 2 g six-hourly to cover gram-positive organisms, IV gentamicin 1.5 mg/kg every eight hours for gram-negative bacteria and IV clindamycin 900 mg every eight hours to cover anaerobes, particularly for abdominal delivery.[15] [EL 1]
- Clindamycin provides coverage against *Mycoplasma hominis*.
- Currently there are no published trials suggesting any specific coverage against *Ureaplasma*.

- The frequency of neonatal sepsis is reduced by up to 80 per cent with intrapartum antibiotic treatment.
- Supportive therapeutic measures include antipyretics (acetaminophen or paracetamol) and administration of a single IV additional dose of antibiotics after delivery.
- Further oral antibiotic treatment is not beneficial in most cases.

Prevention

- The main strategy for prevention of chorioamnionitis and its maternal and neonatal sequelae is the correct and timely management of premature rupture of membranes.
- Prophylactic use of antibiotics in PPROM resulted in a significant reduction in the risk of chorioamnionitis, reductions of neonatal infection, use of surfactant, oxygen therapy and abnormal cerebral ultrasound finding prior to discharge. [EL 1]
- Different meta-analyses of grouped studies with different antibiotic regimens did not provide guidance for selecting a drug of choice.
- The ORACLE trial showed improved neonatal outcomes in women treated with erythromycin alone, with prolonged rupture to delivery intervals, a decrease in the number of positive blood cultures and a trend to an improved neonatal composite score.[16] [EL 1]
- Amoxicillin/clavulanate antibiotic combinations should be avoided for PPROM because of a potential association with an increased risk of necrotising enterocolitis.
- Induction of labour and expedition of delivery for PPROM after 34 weeks' gestation is preferred because, compared to expectant management, it is associated with reduced maternal infection and need for neonatal intensive care without any increase in perinatal morbidity and mortality. [EL 2]

Conclusion

- Chorioamnionitis is a serious obstetric problem, which if untreated can lead to significant maternal and neonatal morbidity and mortality.

- Chorioamnionitis is mostly diagnosed on the basis of clinical signs and symptoms.
- Once identified, prompt treatment with broad-spectrum antibiotics, antipyretics, supportive care and expedition of delivery reduce maternal and neonatal morbidity.
- Further research is needed to identify screening and predictive investigations.
- Further research is still needed to provide further information to help in the treatment and prevention of chorioamnionitis.

References

1. Callaghan WM, MacDorman MF, Rasmussen SA, Qin C, Lackritz EM. The contribution of preterm birth to infant mortality rates in the United States. *Pediatrics.* 2006; **118**(4).

2. American College of Obstetricians and Gynecologists. Preterm (Premature) Labor and Birth. 2016. www .acog.org/Patients/FAQs/Preterm-Premature-Labor-and-Birth?IsMobileSet=false.

3. Sato, TA, Keelan, JA, Mitchell, MD. Critical paracrine interactions between TNF-alpha and IL-10 regulate lipopolysaccharide-stimulated human choriodecidual cytokine and prostaglandin E2 production. *J Immunol.* 2003; **170**(1): 158–66.

4. Romero R, Sirtori M, Oyarzun E et al. Infection and labor. Prevalence, microbiology, and clinical significance of intraamniotic infection in women with preterm labor and intact membranes. *Am J Obstet Gynecol.* 1989; **161**(3): 817–24.

5. Agrawala V, Hirsch E. Intrauterine infection and preterm labor. *Semin Fetal Neonatal Med.* 2012; **17**(1): 12–19.

6. Cardenas I, Means RE, Aldo P, Koga K, Lang SM, Booth C. Viral infection of the placenta leads to fetal inflammation and sensitization to bacterial products predisposing to preterm labor. *J Immunol.* 2010; **185**(2): 1248–57.

7. Yudin MH, Money DM. Screening and management of bacterial vaginosis in pregnancy. SOGC Clinical Practice Guideline, No. 211, August 2008. https://sogc .org/wp-content/uploads/2013/01/gui211CPG0808 .pdf.

8. Rours GIJG, de Krijger RR, Ott A et al. Chlamydiatrachomatis and placental inflammation in early preterm delivery. *Eur J Epidemiol.* 2011; **26**(5): 421–8.

9. Rours GIJG, Duijts L, Moll HA et al. Chlamydia trachomatis infection associated with preterm delivery: a population-based prospective cohort study. In: Rours GIJG, Chlamydia trachomatis Infections during Pregnancy: Consequences for Pregnancy Outcome and Infants. Thesis, Erasmus University Medical Centre, Rotterdam; 2010: chapter 5. https://core.ac.uk/down load/pdf/18513246.pdf.

10. Varkha Agrawala, Emmet Hirsc. Intrauterine infection and preterm labor. *Semin Fetal Neonatal Med.* 2012; **17**(1): 12–19.

11. van de Laar R, van der Ham DP, Oei SG, Willekes C, Weiner CP, Mol BW. Accuracy of C-reactive protein determination in predicting chorioamnionitis and neonatal infection in pregnant women with premature rupture of membranes: a systematic review. *Eur J Obstet Gynecol Reprod Biol.* 2009; **147**(2): 124–9.

12. Aboyeji AP, Abdul IF, Ijaiya MA, Nwabuisi C, Ologe MO. The bacteriology of pre-labour rupture of membranes in a Nigerian teaching hospital. *J Obstet Gynaecol.* 2005; **25**(8): 761–4.

13. Venkatesh KK, Glover AV, Vladutiu CJ, Stamilio DM. Association of chorioamnionitis and its duration with adverse maternal outcomes by mode of delivery: a cohort study. *BJOG.* 2019; 1471-0528.15565.

14. Galinsky R, Polglase GR, Hooper SB, Black MJ, Moss TJM. The consequences of chorioamnionitis: preterm birth and effects on development. *J Pregnancy.* 2013; **2013**: 412831.

15. Kenyon S, Boulvain M, Neilson J. Antibiotics for preterm rupture of the membranes: a systematic review. *Obstet Gynecol.* 2004; **104**(5 Pt 1): 1051–7.

16. Kenyon SL, Taylor DJ, Tarnow-Mordi W. Broad-spectrum antibiotics for preterm, prelabour rupture of fetal membranes: the ORACLE I randomised trial. ORACLE collaborative group. *Lancet.* 2001; **357**: 979–88.

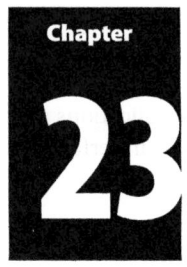

Appendicitis in Pregnancy

Christine Helmy Samuel Azer

Introduction

Appendicitis is the most common surgical emergency during pregnancy. It accounts for 25 per cent of surgeries for non-obstetric causes. The incidence is around 1/766 live births.[1,2]

Although it can occur at any time during pregnancy or postpartum period, it most commonly occurs in the second trimester.

Complication rate is higher if presented in the third trimester due to the delay in diagnosis and the decision on surgery which increases the rate of appendix rupture.

Clinical Presentation

A high level of suspicion is required as there is a wide range of symptoms and the laboratory tests cannot be used as diagnostic in pregnancy.

A new onset of abdominal pain in pregnancy should be alerting.

The most common instance is diffuse abdominal or periumbilical pain migrating to the right lower abdomen.

The gravid uterus will push the appendix cephalad, so the pain will be felt at the upper abdomen in 55 per cent of cases; sometimes it can be subcostal.

Pain may be felt in the right iliac fossa, in the right upper quadrant or mid-epigastric.

Rectal pain is common in the first trimester.

Anorexia, nausea and vomiting may start after the onset of pain.

Fever up to 101.0°F (38.3°C) may develop later.

Leucocytosis develops later[3] but it is inconclusive as up to 16 000 cells/mL is considered normal in pregnancy and up to 30 000 cells/mL is accepted during labour.

Non-specific symptoms like dysuria and diarrhoea are common. Tachycardia is common in pregnancy and cannot be used to favour the diagnosis of acute appendicitis.

C-reactive protein (CRP) is of no clinical significance in pregnancy.

On Clinical Examination

- Tender McBurney point
- Rebound tenderness
- Guarding
- Positive psoas or Rovsing's sign; if palpation of the left lower quadrant of the abdomen increases the pain felt in the right lower quadrant, the patient is said to have a positive Rovsing's sign and may have appendicitis[3]
- Rectal/pelvic tenderness
- Appendicular lump may be felt
- Decreased bowel sounds

Differential Diagnosis[4]

Gastrointestinal, e.g. gastroenteritis, mesenteric adenitis, pancreatitis, bowel obstruction and cholecystitis/

Urinary tract, e.g. infections, pyelonephritis and nephrolithiasis/

Gynaecological, e.g. ovarian cyst accidents, adnexal torsion, degenerated fibroid, ectopic pregnancy/

Obstetric, e.g. placental abruption and chorioamnionitis/

Musculoskeletal pain, e.g. rectus haematoma, usually has gradual onset/

Diagnostic Modalities

Early diagnosis is very important to avoid maternal and fetal risks. Surgical delay of more than 24 hours increases the risk of perforation. Appendicular perforation is associated with increased fetal loss and maternal morbidity, mainly sepsis and vulvo vaginitis.

MRI is the preferred diagnostic modality as it has a negative predictive value of 100 per cent and a positive predictive value of 83.3 per cent. It should be the first-line recommended imaging in patients with high clinical suspicion. It was helpful in excluding 88 per cent of unneeded surgery.

Ultrasound (US) is inconclusive in many cases, with weak positive predictive value, but it is helpful in excluding other causes of abdominal pain.[5,6]

The low yield of US, with a sensitivity and specificity of US alone as 12.5 and 99.2 per cent, respectively, versus MRI with 100 and 93.6 per cent, makes MRI the most accurate modality to diagnose appendicitis and avoid delay in its management.[7]

CT will expose the fetus to hazardous ionising radiation and it is not preferred in pregnancy.

Diagnostic laparoscopy is recommended in some studies when imaging modalities are inconclusive or not available. If appendicitis is diagnosed, then laparoscopic appendectomy can be performed immediately.

Fetal Implications

Untreated appendicitis or delay in treatment may lead to:

- Miscarriage
- Preterm labour
- Perinatal mortality

In a retrospective single-centre study of 102 cases of pregnant women who were diagnosed and managed for acute appendicitis, the fetal prognosis differed according to the delay in treatment and the occurrence of perforation with a significant difference. The rate of preterm labour was 5.1 per cent vs 1.3 per cent and the rate of fetal mortality was 25 per cent vs 1.7 per cent between patients with and without a perforated appendix.[8] [EL 2]

Maternal Implications

A large demographic UK study found that pregnant women are less likely to be diagnosed with acute appendicitis than non-pregnant women, with the lowest risk reported during the third trimester. Moreover, older women may be at increased risk of appendicitis in the postpartum period, suggesting that clinicians of all specialties should remain alert to the risk of acute appendicitis among postpartum older women presenting with lower abdominal pain.[9] [EL 2]

Maternal mortality from appendicitis is now almost zero and is nearly always associated with undiagnosed perforation and peritonitis.[10]

The overall reported maternal complications ranged around 5–8 per cent of peritonitis if perforation occurs.

Management

Appendicitis during pregnancy can cause significant morbidity and mortality if not promptly identified and treated.

Maternal and fetal prognosis relies on the interval between the beginning of symptoms and the onset and surgery. In a retrospective single-centre study, this symptom–surgery interval was the only predictive variable. A longer interval was associated with appendix perforation than with no appendix perforation. [EL 2]

Appendectomy is the main line of management; no maternal morbidities were related if treatment was carried out promptly.

Open Appendectomy

Open laparotomy is the basic surgical approach.

Laparoscopy

- Laparoscopic appendectomy is an accepted alternative in well-trained hands.
- It is not associated with increased maternal morbidity or mortality in pregnancy.
- In experienced hands, laparoscopic surgery decreases the operative time, hospital stay and reduces post-operative pain. It is also associated with early return of the gastrointestinal tract functions and better cosmetic appearance.
- Abdominal pressure should be kept between 12 and15 mm/Hg. Hasson open technique or Palmer's point entry is recommended.
- Cardiotocography electronic fetal monitoring (CTG) is recommended before and after surgery.
- Prophylactic tocolysis can be used to decrease the risk of preterm labour and fetal loss in cases with advanced gestation although there is no strong evidence for its efficacy.
- Steroids for lung maturity may be considered if preterm delivery is expected.
- Literature search suggests that laparoscopic appendectomy in pregnancy is associated with

a low rate of intraoperative complications in all trimesters.[11]

- In 2017 Mohammed M. Alkatary and Nagwan A. Bahgat reported their results for laparoscopic appendicectomy during pregnancy (six patients presented in the first trimester, seven patients in the second trimester and eight on the third trimester) and concluded that 'Laparoscopic appendectomy is safe for both the mother and the fetus during pregnancy irrespective of gestational age, and the procedure is associated with a low risk of post-operative complications.'[12]
- Other researchers reached the same conclusion.[13]

Medical Treatment

- Medical treatment has been successfully reported without severe maternal or fetal complications in selected cases, with 25 per cent failure rate.
- Broad-spectrum antibiotics with anaerobic coverage as second-generation cephalosporin are the treatment of choice.[14]
- In cases of perforated or gangrenous appendix, intravenous antibiotics can be used with metronidazole.
- It is most indicated when appendectomy is not accessible or when it is estimated a high-risk procedure.
- In a prospective study of 20 patients with ultrasonography-proven appendicitis, symptoms resolved in 95 per cent of patients receiving antibiotics alone, but 37 per cent of these patients had recurrent appendicitis within 14 months.[15] [EL 1]

Delivery

In the third trimester, caesarean section (CS) is rarely indicated at the time of appendicectomy.

Delivery and emptying the uterus will not change recovery from the surgery.

Opening the uterus when the abdominal cavity is infected with peritonitis increases the risk of intrauterine infection and adhesions, which may cause current and future problems and infertility.

If the patient is over 37 weeks of gestation with a plan of CS for obstetric indications and in suitable circumstances, appendectomy may be done simultaneously.

Conclusion

Inflammation and infection of the appendix is a common occurrence during pregnancy; if treated correctly and promptly it will not lead to fetal or maternal mortality or morbidity.

References

1. Andersen B, Nielsen TF. Appendicitis in pregnancy: diagnosis, management and complications. *Acta Obstet Gynecol Scand.* 1999; **78**(9): 758–62.

2. Choi JJ, Mustafa R, Lynn ET, Divino CMJ. Appendectomy during pregnancy. *Am Coll Surg.* 2011; **213**(5): 627.

3. Pastore PA, Loomis DM. Appendicitis in pregnancy. *Br J Surg.* 2012; **99**(11): 1470–8.

4. Basaran A, Basaran M. Diagnosis of acute appendicitis during pregnancy: a systematic review. *Obstet Gynecol Surv.* 2009; **64**(7): 481.

5. Meesa IR, Mammen L. MR imaging of pregnant women with abdominal pain and suspected appendicitis: diagnostic accuracy and o utcomes. *Int J Radiol Radiat Oncol.* 2016; **2**: 004–007.

6. Burns M, Hague CJ. Utility of magnetic resonance imaging for the diagnosis of appendicitis during pregnancy: a Canadian experience. *Can Assoc Radiol J.* 2017; **68**(4): 392–400.

7. Ramalingam V, LeBedis C, Kelly JR, Uyeda J, Soto JA, Anderson SW. Evaluation of a sequential multi-modality imaging algorithm for the diagnosis of acute appendicitis in the pregnant female. *Emerg Radiol.* 2015; **22**(2): 125–32.

8. Zhang Y, Zhao YY, Qiao J, Ye RH. Diagnosis of appendicitis during pregnancy and perinatal outcome in the late pregnancy. *Chi Med J.* 2009; **122**(5): 521–4.

9. Zingone F, Alyshah S, Humes, A, West DJ, Joe BMBS. Risk of acute appendicitis in and around pregnancy: a population-based cohort study from England. *Ann Surg.* 2015; **261**(2): 332–7.

10. Chawla S, Vardhan S, Jog SS. Appendicitis during pregnancy. *Med J Armed Forces India.* 2003; **59**(3): 212–15.

11. Machado NO, Grant CS. Laparoscopic appendicectomy in all trimesters of pregnancy. *JSLS.* 2009; **13**(3): 384–90.

12. Alkatary MM, Bahgat NA. Laparoscopic versus open appendectomy during pregnancy. *Int Surg J.* 2017; **4**(8): 2387–91.

13. Laustsen JF, Bjerring OS, Johannessen O, Qvist N. Laparoscopic appendectomy during pregnancy is safe for both the mother and the fetus. *Dan Med J.* 2016; **63**(8): A5259.

14. Young BC, Hamar BD, Levine D, Roqué H. Medical management of ruptured appendicitis in pregnancy. *Obstet Gynecol.* 2009; **114**(2 Pt 2): 453–6.

15. Eriksson S, Granström L. Randomized controlled trial of appendicectomy versus antibiotic therapy for acute appendicitis. *Br J Surg.* 1995; **82**(2): 166–9.

Complications Associated with Legal Termination of Pregnancy

Christine Helmy Samuel Azer

Introduction

Termination is ending of a pregnancy by removing a fetus or embryo before it can survive outside the uterus.

The legality of abortion/termination of pregnancy varies worldwide.

When allowed by law, it is considered as one of the safest procedures in medicine.[1,2]

The World Health Organization recommends safe and legal abortions be available to all women.[3]

In 95 per cent of cases, no complications develop; however, there is always a risk of infection. The risk is higher in surgical than medical terminations due to uterine instrumentation.

Today, about 50 million abortions are performed every year. The worldwide rate of abortion is 28 per 1000 women. With proper equipment and qualified medical personnel, legal abortion is one of the safest procedures.

Rates of upper genital tract infection in the setting of legal induced abortion in the United States are generally less than 1 per cent.

Infectious Complications

Risk Factors

The risk of infection has been estimated at up to 10 per cent.

Pre-existing sexually transmitted diseases like gonorrhoea or *Chlamydia* are the highest risk factor. Use of tampons, intercourse, vaginal douches, tub baths, bubble baths and swimming in the first two weeks after termination are also contributing risk factors.[4]

Clinical Picture

The commonest symptoms include
- Severe lower abdominal pain
- Heavy bleeding
- Fever > 38°C

- Tachycardia >90 bpm
- Tachypnea relative risk (RR) >20
- Systemic signs of sepsis as organ dysfunction (in cases of severe infection)
- Septic shock (tachycardia (>110), respiratory distress, oliguria, altered mental status and hypotension)

Diagnosis

Clinical Diagnosis

It is clinical diagnosis based on the clinical picture.

Laboratory Diagnosis

- Blood culture.
- Urine culture.
- Cervical cultures.
- Endometrial biopsy specimen or tissue obtained at uterine aspiration provides a better specimen for culture than does cervical discharge. Examination of the Gram-stained material can guide early management.
- Raised white blood cell count >12 000 or <4000, or >10 per cent immature forms.

Prevention

Primary Prevention

Prevention of unintended pregnancy is considered the primary method of preventing terminations and thus post-termination infections.

Secondary Prevention

There are two main strategies for the prevention of infection after termination of pregnancy:

Routine prophylaxis by giving antibiotics around the time of surgery for all women.

- Randomised controlled trials support the use of prophylactic antibiotics for surgical abortion in the first trimester.
- The current evidence supports pre-procedure but not post-procedure antibiotics for the purpose of prophylaxis.
- A Cochrane review concluded that 'Antibiotic prophylaxis at the time of first trimester surgical abortion is effective in preventing post-abortal upper genital tract infection.'[5] [EL 1]
- Perioperative oral doxycycline given up to 12 hours before a surgical abortion appears to effectively reduce infectious risk.
- A perioperative single-dose regime of nitroimidazole or tetracyclines seems to be safe and effective.[6]
- Azithromycin can be used for presumptive treatment of *Chlamydia* at the time of surgical abortion.

'Screen-and-treat', in which all women presenting for termination are screened for genital infections and those with positive results are treated.

In a study involving 1672 abortion cases, women managed by the screen-and-treat strategy had slightly higher rates of infective morbidity in the eight weeks after abortion than those managed by 'prophylaxis'. Prophylaxis appears to be more cost-effective than screen-and-treat policy.[7]

Treatment

Combination of broad-spectrum antibiotics. Randomised controlled trials (RCTs) and non-RCTs that compared different antibiotics concluded that there is no difference in efficacy between any of these regimens.

- Clindamycin (900 mg intravenously (IV) every eight hours)[8] [EL 1]
- Penicillin (5 million units IV every six hours) plus chloramphenicol
- Metronidazole (15 mg/kg initially followed by 7.5 mg/kg every eight hours) can also be used[9] [EL 1]
- Ampicillin (2 g IV every six hours) combined with gentamicin (2 mg/kg loading dose, followed by 1.5 mg/kg every eight hours or 5 mg/kg every 24 hours depending on blood levels and renal status)

Surgical Complications

Vacuum aspiration for surgical termination of pregnancy is less risky than the use of uterine instrumentation (curettage). According to studies, the death rate varies from 0 to 0.7 per 100 000 abortions, and is smaller when the procedure is done under local anaesthesia than general anaesthesia. The overall early complication rate (haemorrhage, uterine perforation, cervical injury) is between 0.01 and 1.16 per cent.[10]

In a Finnish study involving 42 619 patients, the overall incidence of adverse events was four-fold higher in the medical compared with surgical abortion cohort (20.0% compared with 5.6%, $p < 0.001$). Haemorrhage (15.6% compared with 2.1%, $p < 0.001$) and incomplete abortion (6.7% compared with 1.6%, $p < 0.001$) were more common after medical abortion. The rate of surgical (re-)evacuation was 5.9 per cent after medical abortion and 1.8 per cent after surgical abortion ($p < 0.001$).

Injuries requiring operative treatment or operative complications occurred more often with surgical termination of pregnancy (0.6% compared with 0.03%, $p < 0.001$). No differences were noted in the incidence of infections (1.7% compared with 1.7%, $p = 0.85$), thromboembolic disease, psychiatric morbidity, or death.[11] [EL 2] The study was a registry study cohort, not an RCT.

Another partially randomised trial concluded that side effects experienced were higher in women who underwent medical abortion compared with those who underwent surgery.

It also reported that 5.4 per cent of those who had medical termination required a second procedure, compared with 2.1 per cent who had surgery, although this difference was not statistically significant.[12]

Conclusion

Legal termination of pregnancy is a safe procedure; however there is a small risk of uterine infection which can progress to pelvic sepsis. Infection may cause secondary infertility.

Prevention by routine antibiotic prophylaxis or screen-and-treat is recommended. Prevention of surgical complications relies on avoiding instrumentation and the use of vacuum aspiration.

References

1. Grimes DA, Benson J, Singh S et al. Unsafe abortion: the preventable pandemic. *Lancet*. 2011; **368**(9550):1908–19.

2. Raymond EG, Grossman D, Weaver MA, Toti S, Winikoff B. Mortality of induced abortion, other outpatient surgical procedures and common activities in the United States. *Am Contraception.* 2014; **90**(5): 476–9.

3. Achilles SL, Reeves MF. Prevention of infection after induced abortion. *Contraception.* 2011: **83**(4): 295–309.

4. World Health Organization. *Safe Abortion: Technical and Policy Guidance for Health Systems.* Geneva: WHO; 2012.

5. Low N, Mueller M, Van Vliet HAAM, Kapp N. Perioperative antibiotics to prevent infection after first-trimester abortion. *Cochrane Database Sys Rev.* 2012. http://cochranelibrary-wiley.com/doi/10.1002/14651858.CD005217.pub2/full.

6. World Health Organization. *Perioperative Antibiotics to Prevent Infection after First-Trimester Abortion.* Geneva: WHO; 2013.

7. Stubblefield PG, Averbach SH. Septic Abortion: Prevention and Management. 2014. www.glowm.com.

8. Low N, Mueller M, Van Vliet HA, Kapp N. Perioperative antibiotics to prevent infection after first-trimester abortion. Cochrane Fertility Regulation Group 2012, Issue 1.

9. Atim U, Emmanuel E, Olabisi O, Babasola O, Obiamaka O. Antibiotics for treating septic abortion. Cochrane Fertility Regulation Group July 2016. No. CD011528. doi: 10.1002/14651858.CD011528.

10. Soulat C, Gelly MJ. Immediate complications of surgical abortion. *Gynecol Obstet Biol Reprod.* (Paris) 2006; **35**(2): 157–62.

11. Niinimäki M1, Pouta A, Bloigu A, Gissler M, Hemminki E, Suhonen S. Heikinheimo O. Immediate complications after medical compared with surgical termination of pregnancy. *Obstet Gynecol.* 2009; **114**(4): 795–804.

12. Ashok PW, Kidd A, Flett GM, Fitzmaurice A, Graham W, Templeton A. A randomized comparison of medical abortion and surgical vacuum aspiration at 10–13 weeks gestation. *Hum Reprod.* 2002; **17**(1): 92–8.

Chapter 25

Tuberculosis

Maimoona Ahmed

Introduction

Tuberculosis (TB) is one of the top 10 causes of death worldwide and is believed to be nearly as old as human history.[1] Tuberculosis remains the most common cause of death from infectious agents in child-bearing-age women (14–49 years) worldwide.

In 2017, TB caused an estimated 1.3 million deaths (range 1.2–1.4 million). The progress made in the diagnosis, treatment and control of TB has been offset by the HIV epidemic, the growing challenge of drug resistance and other epidemiological factors like population migration, poverty, overcrowding, poor sanitation and malnutrition in the developing countries.

Six countries, India, Indonesia, China, Nigeria, Pakistan and South Africa, account for 60 per cent of the total burden of new TB cases.

Microbiology and Etiopathogenesis

Tuberculosis (TB) is caused by bacteria called *Mycobacterium tuberculosis*, a contagious infection that usually attacks the lungs. It can also spread to other parts of the body, such as the brain and spine.[2]

The name *Mycobacterium* is derived from the Greek words *myk¯es*, meaning fungus, and *bakt¯erion* meaning 'little rod', which it resembles when grown on liquid culture media. It was discovered in 1882 by Robert Koch.

Mycobacterium tuberculosis (*M. tuberculosis*) is an obligate intracellular pathogen. It is an aerobic, non-motile, non-encapsulated spore-forming bacillus and is one of the five members of the *M. tuberculosis* complex (the others being *M. bovis*, *M. ulcerans*, *M. africanum* and *M. microti*). It is termed as acid-fast (25 per cent H_2SO_4) as it retains the colour of the stains (Ziehl–Neelsen and auramine-o) even after an acid-control wash.

Infection is caused mainly by:

- Inhalation of infectious particles aerosolised by coughing, sneezing, talking or manipulation of infected tissue
- Ingestion of unpasteurised milk
- Direct implantation through skin abrasion or the conjunctiva

Tuberculosis and Pregnancy

Incidence

- TB is a public health problem and a significant contributor to maternal mortality. It is among the three leading causes of death among women between 15 and 45 years of age. The exact incidence of TB during pregnancy is not readily available for low-resource countries; however, it is expected to be as high as that of the general population.
- The incidence of TB during pregnancy reported in the United States between 2003 and 2011 was 26.6 per 100 000 births.[3]
- As a cause of maternal mortality, in the UK, it accounted for 4.2 per 100 000 maternities in 2005–06.[4]

Effects of Pregnancy on TB

- Tuberculosis remains a significant worldwide concern among pregnant or postpartum women, with high maternal mortality rates. In 2008, an estimated 9.4 million new cases of TB occurred, with 1.7 million TB-related deaths, more than half among women.[5]
- Research has proved that pregnancy neither improves nor worsens the course of TB (sputum conversion, stabilisation of the disease and relapse rate), as long as it is diagnosed and treated appropriately and early.[6]

- Rather than pregnancy itself, the course and prognosis of the disease during pregnancy is associated with the current health status of the woman, the disease extent and radiographic pattern.
- The diagnosis of TB in pregnancy may be more challenging as the symptoms may initially be attributed to the pregnancy. The weight loss associated with the disease may temporarily be masked by the normal weight gain in pregnancy.
- Early postpartum women are twice as likely to develop TB as non-pregnant women, because of the suppression of T-helper 1 (Th1) pro-inflammatory response during pregnancy which reverses post-delivery, resulting in risk of exacerbation.[7]

Effects of TB on Pregnancy

The effects of TB on pregnancy depend on the severity of the disease, the presence of extrapulmonary spread, HIV co-infection and gestational age at the time of diagnosis. Poor prognosis is seen in cases of advanced disease diagnosed in puerperium and in those with HIV co-infection. Non-compliance with treatment also worsens the prognosis.[8,9]

Obstetric Outcomes

Obstetric complications of TB include miscarriage, intrauterine growth retardation, preterm labour, low birthweight and increased neonatal morbidity and mortality. Early start of anti-tuberculous treatment results in better outcomes comparable to that in non-pregnant patients.[10]

Late diagnosis and care is associated with increased maternal morbidity:[11]

- Pre-eclampsia
- Acute respiratory failure
- Poor weight gain in pregnancy
- Postpartum haemorrhage
- Difficult labour[11]

Advanced TB is associated with upregulation of pro-inflammatory cytokines such as tumour necrosis factor-alpha which could be the pathogenesis of increased rates of pre-eclampsia.

Poor nutritional state of the mother, hypo-proteinuria and anaemia predispose to TB infection in pregnancy and increase the morbidity and mortality.

Extrapulmonary TB is also associated with maternal morbidity in the form of recurrent admissions and disability as well as increased mortality with central nervous system complications.

Maternal Mortality

The risk of mortality is increased both during pregnancy and postpartum. Women co-infected with HIV are at higher risk of mortality. One post-mortem study in Africa on maternal deaths reported TB as a cause of death in 12.9 per cent of deaths overall and 27.7 per cent of deaths among HIV-infected women.[12] [EL 2]

Untreated, TB in pregnancy can have a mortality of up to 40 per cent.

Perinatal Outcomes

Preterm labour, low-birthweight babies and neonatal mortality are more prevalent in cases where diagnosis and treatment is delayed.[13]

Low birthweight is also seen in countries like the UK where TB during pregnancy is much less prevalent, i.e. 62/100 000 pregnancies. [EL 2]

In a recent systematic review and meta-analysis (2016):

- Perinatal death was four times more frequent
- Preterm birth was 1.6 times greater
- Low birthweight was 1.7 times greater
- Low APGAR score at 1 minute was five times greater
- Acute fetal distress was 2.3 times greater
- There was an odds ratio of 3.4 for congenital anomalies[14] [EL 1]

Mother-to-Child Transmission and Congenital Infection

Congenital TB is rare but associated with high perinatal mortality. Congenital infection by TB is caused by transplacental transmission via the umbilical vein to the fetal liver and lungs. In late pregnancy, aspiration and swallowing of infected amniotic fluid *in utero* or during labour causes primary infection of fetal lungs and gut.[15]

The primary focus develops in the liver with involvement of the periportal lymph nodes following haematogenous spread via umbilical vein. The fetal lungs are infected secondarily.

Dissemination to other systems is carried out via fetal circulation to other organ systems such as TB meningitis.

In a study by Pillay et al. in South Africa, vertical transmission of *Mycobacterium tuberculosis* was detected in 16 newborns (16 per cent) with no difference between HIV-infected and non-infected mothers.[15]

The risk of transmission from infected mother to neonate is greater in the first three weeks of life.

Cantwell et al. Modified Criteria for Diagnosis of Congenital Tuberculosis

- Lesion during the first week of life.
- A primary hepatic complex or caseating granuloma.
- Documented tuberculosis infection of placenta or endometrium.
- Exclusion of postnatal transmission through contact tracing.

Common clinical presentations of congenital TB include abdominal distension, hepato-splenomegaly, respiratory distress, failure to thrive, fever and lymphadenopathy usually presenting in the second or third week postnatal.

Radiographic abnormality is seen in almost all cases, with nearly half showing a miliary pattern. Overall mortality of congenital TB is 38 per cent in the untreated and 22 per cent in the treated newborns.[16]

Diagnosis of Congenital TB

Diagnosis is made based on clinical suspicion and culture.[17]

Acquired Newborn TB Infection

A newborn infant is at greater risk of acquiring TB postpartum than congenitally, especially if the mother is sputum-positive or if the maternal condition remains undiagnosed and untreated.

The newborn may acquire postnatal disease by contact:

- Droplet infection from the mother
- An infectious adult
- An infected family member, particularly if they are sputum-positive and not under treatment

Transmission of Tuberculosis through Breastmilk Does Not Occur [EL 2]

About 50 per cent of children born to mothers with active pulmonary TB develop the disease during the first year of life if chemoprophylaxis or Bacillus Calmette–Guérin (BCG) vaccine is not given.

Separation of mother and offspring is indicated only if the mother is non-adherent to medical treatment, needs to be hospitalised or if she has developed drug-resistant TB.

Clinically, signs of neonatal TB are non-specific but are usually marked by multiple organ involvement. The neonate may have fever, is lethargic or may look acutely or chronically ill with respiratory distress or non-responsive pneumonia, hepatosplenomegaly or failure to thrive.

Diagnosis can be confirmed by chest X-ray, culture of tracheal aspirate, gastric washings, urine, and cerebrospinal fluid or sometimes skin testing.

Evaluation and Diagnosis

Antenatal clinics present an opportunity for evaluation and management of TB among individuals with risk of TB who may not have previously presented for medical care.

Risk factors for TB infection during pregnancy include close contact with infectious cases, living in or travelling to places where TB is prevalent, having a condition associated with low immunity (HIV, diabetes or other medical disorders), substance and alcohol abuse, migrant worker and overcrowding.

Evaluation and treatment of TB in pregnancy depend on two types of presentations:

- **Latent Tuberculosis Infection (LTBI)**
- **Active Tuberculosis**

Latent Tuberculosis Infection (LTBI) in Pregnancy

M. tuberculosis infection is initially contained by host defences and remains latent in most cases. However, this latent infection has the potential to develop into active disease at any time. Identification and treatment of latent TB infection can reduce the risk of development of disease by as much as 90 per cent.[18]

In countries with low TB infection rates, immigrants from higher-incidence countries are the major pool of infected individuals.

Patients with LTBI are asymptomatic and are not contagious.

There is no risk for vertical transmission of LTBI.[19]

Screening

There is no role for routine LTBI testing in pregnant women with no risk factors for development of active TB. It is better to test for LTBI prior to pregnancy as this provides an opportunity for counselling about the risk of becoming pregnant while infected with LTBI.

In cohorts of pregnant women tested in the USA, the prevalence of latent infection varied from 14 to 48 per cent,[19] hence the antenatal period represents an opportunity for immigrant women to seek medical care. The Centers for Disease Control and Prevention recommend screening all high-risk pregnant women at the beginning of prenatal care. [EL 1]

Currently there does not seem to be any reliable incidence of conversion from latent to active TB during pregnancy.

Diagnosis of LTBI

Tools for LTBI testing include the tuberculin skin test (TST) and interferon-gamma release assays (IGRAs).

Tuberculin Skin Test (TST)/Mantoux Test

- Identifies individuals with prior sensitisation to mycobacterial antigens.
- Tuberculin material is injected intradermally, which stimulates a delayed-type hypersensitivity response mediated by T lymphocytes and causes induration within 48–72 hours.
- The transverse diameter of the induration (not erythema) should be demarcated, measured and recorded in millimetres.
- Sensitivity is 98 per cent using the 5 mm threshold, 90 per cent using the 10 mm threshold, but only 50–60 per cent using the 15 mm threshold. As the cutoff for mm of induration is increased, the sensitivity decreases and the specificity increases.[20]
- False-positive results can be seen in prior BCG vaccination. False-negative results may occur in immunocompromised patients, or due to improper injection of the tuberculin protein or inaccurate interpretation of the induration.

Interferon-Gamma Release Assays (IGRAs)

- In vitro blood tests that measure T-cell release of interferon (IFN)-gamma following stimulation by antigens specific to *M. tuberculosis*.[21]
- IGRA is preferred over TST in cases with low-to-intermediate risk of progression to active disease, for patients who are unlikely to return to have the TST read and for patients with a history of BCG vaccination.[21]
- IGRAs are more expensive than TST.

- These tests should not be used for diagnosis of active TB as they cannot distinguish between latent infection and active disease.[22]

Management of Established LTBI

- Patients with a positive TST or IGRA must undergo evaluation to rule out active tuberculosis. [*Grade A recommendation*]
- The role of treatment in latent TB infection, especially in pregnant women, is controversial, as pregnancy itself does not increase the risk of progression of the disease and pregnant and postpartum women are more vulnerable to isoniazid (INH) toxicity. There are no randomised controlled trials on the treatment of LTBI in pregnancy; consequently it is not possible to draw any firm conclusions about the safety of INH therapy antepartum.
- If there is no indication for prompt management, LTBI treatment should be deferred until three months after delivery, to minimise the risk of hepatitis. Women who were diagnosed with LTBI prior to pregnancy and started on treatment for an appropriate indication should continue LTBI treatment if they become pregnant. The prior treatment regimen should be modified to a regimen suitable for pregnancy. [*Grade B recommendation*]
- The preferred regimens for treatment of LTBI during pregnancy in non-HIV-infected women are [*Grade A recommendation*]
  - Isoniazid (5 mg/kg up to 300 mg daily) for nine months
  - Isoniazid (15 mg/kg up to 900 mg twice weekly) for nine months
  - Isoniazid should be administered together with pyridoxine supplementation, 25–50 mg daily. [*Grade A recommendation*]
- Pregnant women with HIV infection and LTBI should be treated with isoniazid with daily dosage schedule for nine months. [*Grade A recommendation*]

Active Tuberculosis in Pregnancy

Signs and Symptoms

Evaluation for active TB is indicated in cases positive for LTBI screening or in clinical suspicion for active disease.

Careful history taking and assessment of risk factors play a crucial role in establishing the diagnosis. Clinical features are the same in pregnant and non-pregnant women (persistent cough, localised wheeze, chest pain, breathlessness and/or haemoptysis).

The most common extrapulmonary site is the lymph node involvement (gradual, painless, enlargement, fluctuant swelling, superficial ulceration, sinus formation). The diagnosis of the central nervous system (headache, vomiting, altered behaviour and focal neurological signs) or bones and joints disease should not be overlooked.

Patients meeting clinical criteria on history taking should undergo chest radiography. If found suggestive of disease, three sputum specimens should be submitted for acid-fast bacillus (AFB) smear, mycobacterial culture and nucleic acid amplification testing (NAAT).

Diagnosis of Active TB Infection

Sputum AFB smear:
The most rapid and inexpensive diagnostic tool. The two common techniques are the older carbolfuchsin methods (including the Ziehl–Neelsen and the Kinyoun methods) and the more rapid, sensitive and preferred fluorochrome procedure (using auramine-O or auramine–rhodamine dyes with fluorescence microscopy).[23]

Sputum microscopy is cheap and quick but often unreliable (particularly for HIV-positive patients). The sensitivity of AFB smear microscopy is 45–80 per cent, and positive predictive value is 50–80 per cent. [EL 1]

Culture methods:
Definitive diagnosis is isolation of *M. tuberculosis* from body secretions (e.g. culture of sputum, bronchoalveolar lavage or pleural fluid) or tissue (pleural biopsy or lung biopsy). Conventional culture is the most sensitive tool for TB, detecting as few as 10 bacteria/mL. The sensitivity and specificity of sputum culture are about 80 and 98 per cent, respectively.

Culture is also required for drug susceptibility testing and for species identification.[24]

Identification of the species is done using nucleic acid hybridisation with a DNA/RNA probe, high-pressure liquid chromatography (HPLC), biochemical methods or mass spectrophotometry.

Drug susceptibility testing for at least isoniazid, rifampin, pyrazinamide and ethambutol should be performed. Patients at risk for drug-resistant disease should undergo routine testing for susceptibility to second-line agents.[25]

Rapid culture techniques are available.

The median turnaround time for the microscopic-observation drug susceptibility (MODS) is seven days.

Molecular tests:
There are two major types of molecular assays: probe-based (non-sequencing) tests and sequence-based assays.

- **Probe-based (NAAT) tests** – a specific nucleic acid sequence is amplified which is detected via a nucleic acid probe. They are used for rapid diagnosis (24–48 hours). Sputum or other tissue specimens can be tested. NAAT is more sensitive than smear but less sensitive than culture. However, culture is required for confirmation and for drug susceptibility testing.

- Gene Xpert MTB/rifampicin assay is a nucleic acid amplification test (molecular test) detecting the presence of TB bacteria. It also detects the genetic mutation (DNA of MTBC) associated with resistance to rifampicin) in less than two hours, whereas standard cultures can take two to six weeks for MTBC to grow and an additional three weeks for a conventional drug resistance test.

- **Sequence-based tests** – provide the genetic identity of a particular mutation and therefore can predict drug resistance with greater accuracy than probe-based assays.

The advantages of these molecular tests are their reliablility in comparison to sputum microscopy and speed of result compared with culture. It is a simple fully automated system, and minimum training is required to run the test

The availability of a quick test allows improved patient management and outcomes and avoids unnecessary treatment including isolation. Rapid diagnosis of rifampicin resistance allows effective treatment to be started sooner.

Imaging Modalities in Diagnosis of Tuberculosis

- Chest X-ray (with abdominal shield) is a simple, inexpensive and easily available tool. It gives important clues to the diagnosis but is not confirmatory. Focal infiltration of the upper lobe or the lower lobe may be unilateral or bilateral. Tissue destruction is by cavitation or fibrosis with traction. Enlarged hilar and mediastinal lymph nodes may be detected. High-resolution computed tomography (HRCT) is relatively more sensitive and shows randomly distributed miliary nodules. Miliary TB is a potentially fatal form of TB that results from massive lymphohaematogenous dissemination of *M. tuberculosis* bacilli. Atypical radiographic features such as lung mass (tuberculoma), small fibronodular lesions termed as 'miliary' lesions because they resemble scattered millet seeds, or pleural effusions may be seen more commonly among patients with advanced HIV disease.[26]

- Magnetic resonance imaging (MRI) can detect intrathoracic lymphadenopathy, pericardial thickening and pericardial and pleural effusions.[27]
- CT use in pregnancy is limited due to radiation exposure.

Role of serology: Enzyme-linked immunosorbent assay (ELISA) tests for tuberculosis (immunoglobulin M (IgM) and IgG antibodies in the serum for TB) are not of any value in diagnosing TB according to the World Health Organization (WHO).[28]

Treatment of Active Tuberculosis in Pregnancy

- Treatment must be initiated as early as possible as untreated active TB represents a greater hazard to the mother and fetus than anti-tuberculous therapy.[29] [*Grade A recommendation*] [EL 1]
- The management entails a multidisciplinary approach involving the obstetrician, chest physician, microbiologist, neonatologist, public health officials and nursing care.
- Directly Observed Therapy Short Course (DOTS) is best applied as a treatment option. It consists of an initial intensive phase, which aims to kill actively growing and semi-dormant bacilli, followed by a continuation phase, which eliminates most of the residual bacilli and reduces failures and relapses.
- Rifampicin, isoniazid and ethambutol are the first-line drugs, while pyrizinamide is growing more popular. Isoniazid preventive therapy (WHO recommendation) aims at the reduction of infection in HIV-positive pregnant women.
- Monthly review to evaluate for drug toxicity should be undertaken. Baseline liver function test before starting the treatment followed by monthly evaluation for symptoms of hepatitis, clinical examination and liver function testing should be done as pregnancy and puerperium confers increased risk for isoniazid-induced hepatotoxicity.[29]

- All four first-line drugs (isoniazid, rifampicin, ethambutol and pyrazinamide) have an excellent safety record in pregnancy and are not associated with congenital malformations.

Maternal Complications of Anti-TB Treatment

- Skin rash and fever, rarely hepatitis
- Peripheral neuropathy, optic retrobulbar neuritis
- Gastrointestinal reactions
- Thrombocytopenic purpura
- Ototoxicity and nephrotoxicity, arthralgia
- Giddiness, numbness and tinnitus
- Ataxia and deafness

Patients should be educated about symptoms like anorexia, nausea, vomiting, dark urine, icterus, rash, persistent paresthesia of the hands and feet, persistent fatigue, weakness or fever lasting three or more days, abdominal pain (particularly right upper quadrant discomfort), easy bruising or bleeding, or arthralgia and to report it at the earliest. [*Good practice point*]

Fetal Complications of Anti-TB Treatment

- Isoniazid (INH) is the safest treatment in pregnancy; there is no increase in malformations or growth restriction. It can cross placenta and cause demyelination, therefore pyridoxine supplementation is advised.
- Rifampicin: there is a theoretical risk of teratogenesis, central nervous system abnormalities, limb reduction defects, hypoprothrombinaemia and haemorrhagic disease of newborn. But the overall risk of congenital malformations remains low.
- Streptomycin should be avoided throughout the pregnancy.
- Ethambutol has a theoretical possibility of ocular toxicity. It readily crosses the placenta but there have been few reports of animal teratogenicity with its use.
- There were no significant animal teratogenicity studies or reports of malformations with pyrazinamide.
- Kanamycin, amikacin, capreomycin, ofloxacin, ciprofloxacin, ethionamide, prothionamide, cycloserine, para-aminosalicyclic acid are not

generally recommended, but inadvertent use is not an indication for termination of pregnancy.

- BCG vaccination should not be given during pregnancy. Even though no harmful effects of BCG vaccination on the fetus have been observed, further studies are needed to prove its safety.

Management in Labour

Obstetric management remains unchanged. Caesarean section is only done for obstetric indications. In a study by Schaefer et al., there was no significant difference between the three groups in the incidence of normal spontaneous delivery, instrumental delivery or caesarean section.

Management in Newborns

To reduce the risk of transmission to the newborn, the WHO recommends that newborns with a mother who has had less than two weeks of treatment and who is sputum-positive for AFB should be given prophylactic isoniazid preventive therapy (IPT). Recommended dose of 5 mg/kg, and pyridoxine (vitamin B6) 5–14 mg/kg, and have a tuberculin test at 6–12 weeks. If this is negative, then the treatment can be stopped and BCG vaccination can be given. [Grade A recommendation]

If the tuberculin test is positive, then treatment should be given for a total of six months.

Vaccination is recommended after completion of IPT as isoniazid inhibits vaccine efficacy the BCG vaccine is not recommended for babies of mothers who are HIV-positive until they have been shown to be HIV-negative.[30]

Vitamin K should be administered to an infant born to a mother taking rifampicin because of the risk of neonatal haemorrhage.[31] [Grade B recommendation]

In diagnosed or suspected TB, screening of household contacts should be carried out to help prevent infection of the newborn.

Breastfeeding in Tuberculosis

There have been no documented cases of TB transmission via breastmilk.[32]

WHO recommends breastfeeding in mothers on treatment for latent TB and in active TB once the mother is smear-negative.

Breastfeeding should be encouraged as it prevents other infections and malnutrition, especially in low-resource countries. [Grade A recommendation]

As part of prevention of mother-to-child transmission in HIV co-infection, women may be advised not to breastfeed.

Those affected with TB mastitis should breastfeed from the unaffected breast.

The amount of anti-tuberculous drugs secreted in breastmilk is too small for toxicity. In case the mother is on second-line therapy like para-aminosalicyclic acid (PAS) whose safety is unproven, taking medications immediately after the feed and substituting the next feed by formula feed reduces the adverse effects.

Pyridoxine should be supplemented in the neonate on isoniazid or if the mother is on isoniazid, as pyridoxine deficiency may cause seizures in the newborn. [Grade A recommendation]

A sputum-positive mother should wear a mask while breastfeeding her baby. If the mother is multi-drug-resistant (MDR TB) or extensively drug-resistant TB (XDR TB) positive, separation of the infant is warranted. Breastfeeding may have to be interrupted if the affected mother becomes acutely ill. In such cases, breastmilk should be expressed to prevent mastitis.

Multidrug-Resistant Tuberculosis (MDR TB)

This is caused by M. tuberculosis that is resistant to at least isoniazid and rifampicin. Extensively drug-resistant tuberculosis (XDR-TB) is caused by strains that are also resistant to any of the fluoroquinolones and one of the three injectable aminoglycosides: capreomycin, kanamycin and amikacin.[33]

General principles and selection of anti-tuberculous drugs are similar to those for non-pregnant patients. A study from Peru has demonstrated that the birth outcomes among pregnant women treated for MDR-TB are comparable with outcomes among non-pregnant women.

Long-term follow-up of six children with intrauterine exposure to second-line agents during treatment of MDR-TB in pregnancy documented no evidence of toxicity among the children (average age of follow-up 3.7 years), and one child was diagnosed with MDR-TB. However, as these drugs are known to cause fetal adverse effects, close follow-up of these children is indicated.

HIV and TB Co-infection

- HIV testing should be done for all patients with known or suspected TB. Over 50 per cent of the maternal mortality occurs in mothers with TB in pregnancy due to co-infection with HIV. Poor compliance with treatment, overlapping side effects and drug interactions of anti-TB and anti-retroviral drugs further add to the morbidity.
- Daily dosing is recommended in the intensive phase as opposed to thrice weekly in HIV-uninfected patients.[34] [*Grade A recommendation*]
- Drug susceptibility testing should be done at the start of TB therapy in all the patients. Rifabutin instead of rifampicin should be used as it has less effect on reduction in the serum concentration of efavirenz and nevirapine treatment for the HIV.

Prevention and Control

- Prevention plays a vital role in the control of tuberculosis. As TB is mainly a disease of poverty and overcrowding, intervention policies should concentrate on improving living conditions, ventilation and nutritional status, early diagnosis and treatment of disease, isolation of sputum-positive cases and contact tracing and treatment. Primary prevention of HIV/AIDS is another major step towards prevention of TB.
- The BCG vaccine is a part of the national tuberculosis programme in several countries and contains a live attenuated strain of the bacillus derived from *M. bovis*. It confers active immunity and is effective in preventing severe disease in infants and young children. BCG is not recommended for babies of mothers who are HIV-positive until they have been shown to be HIV-negative or if a member of the household has suspected or active TB. Non-immune women travelling to TB-endemic countries should also be vaccinated. As it is a live vaccine, it is contraindicated during pregnancy.[35]

Conclusion

Tuberculosis in pregnancy is associated with adverse maternal and fetal outcomes.

Early diagnosis and start of appropriate therapy is of utmost importance. Adherence to the treatment is essential to the cure while avoiding the emergence of drug resistance. Supervision and patient support remains the cornerstone of the management which should involve the patient's family, health care personnel and the community to achieve results. BCG vaccination confers active immunity and prevents severe TB disease in infants and young children. BCG vaccination is the mainstay in the prevention of TB infection.

Untreated TB in pregnancy poses a significant threat to the mother, fetus and family. Fear of complications of treatment may prevent many mothers from receiving proper and timely treatment. Therefore, support and supervision are suggested to improve compliance.

Successful control of TB demands improved living conditions, public education, primary prevention of HIV/AIDS and BCG vaccination.

References

1. World Health Organization. Global Tuberculosis 2018 Report. www.who.int/tb/publications/global_report/tb18_ExecSum_web_4Oct18.pdf?ua=1.

2. Grange J. Mycobacterium tuberculosis: the organism. In: Davies PDO, Barnes PF, Gordon SB, eds. *Clinical Tuberculosis*, 4th ed. Oxford: Oxford University Press; 2008: 66–8.

3. El-Messidi A, Czuzoj-Shulman N, Spence AR, Abenhaim HA. Medical and obstetric outcomes among pregnant women with tuberculosis: a population-based study of 7.8 million births. *Am J Obstet Gynecol*. 2016; **215**: 797.e1.

4. Knight M, Kurinczuk J, Nelson-Piercy C, Spark P, Brocklehurst P on behalf of UKOSS. Tuberculosis in pregnancy in the UK. *BJOG*. 2009; **116**: 584–8.

5. Kim JY, Shakow A, Castro A, Vande C, Farmer P. Tuberculosis control. World Health Organization. www.who.int/trade/gpgh/gpgh3/en/index1.html.

6. Zenner D, Kruijshaar ME, Andrews N, Abubakar I. Risk of tuberculosis in pregnancy: a national, primary care based cohort and self controlled case series study. *Am J Respir Crit Care Med*. 2012; **185**: 779–84.

7. Wallis RS, Amir-Tahmasseb M, Ellner JJ. Induction of interleukin 1 and tumor necrosis factor by mycobacterial proteins: the monocyte western blot. *Proc Natl Acad Sci USA*. 1990; **87**: 3348–52.

8. Ormerod P. Tuberculosis in pregnancy and the puerperium. *Thorax*. 2001; **56**(6): 494–9.

9. Vasishta JN, Saha SC, Ghosh K. Obstetrical outcomes among women with extra-pulmonary tuberculosis. *N Engl J Med*. 1999; **341**: 645–9.

10. Centers for Disease Control and Prevention (CDC). TB Treatment and Pregnancy. 2016. www.cdc.gov/tb/topic/treatment/pregnancy.htm.

11. Zumla A, Bates M, Mwaba P. The neglected global burden of tuberculosis in pregnancy. *Lancet*. 2014; **2**(12): e675–6.

12. Sugarman J, Colvin C, Moran AC, Oxlade O. Tuberculosis in pregnancy: an estimate of the global burden of diseases. *Lancet Glob Health*. 2014; **2**: e710–16.

13. Sobhy S, Babiker Z, Zamora, J, Khan KS, Kunst H. Maternal and perinatal mortality and morbidity associated with tuberculosis during pregnancy and the postpartum period: a systematic review and Zumla et al meta-analysis. *BJOG*. 2017; **124**: 727–33.

14. Mittal H, Das S, Faridi MMA. Management of newborn infant born to mother suffering from tuberculosis: current recommendations & gaps in knowledge. *Indian J Med Res*. 2014; **140**: 32–9.

15. Pillay T, Sturm AW, Khan M et al. Vertical transmission of Mycobacterium tuberculosis in KwaZulu Natal: impact of HIV-1 co-infection. *Int J Tuberc Lung Dis*. 2004; **8**(1): 59–69.

16. Adhikari M, Jeena P, Bobat R et al. HIV-associated tuberculosis in the newborn and young infant. *Int J Pediatr*. 2011; **2011**: 354208.

17. Mahendru A, Gajjar K, Eddy J. Review: diagnosis and management of tuberculosis in pregnancy. *The Obstetrician & Gynaecologist*. 2010; **12**: 163–71.

18. Pai M, Behr MA, Dowdy D et al. Tuberculosis. *Nat Rev Dis Primers*. 2016; **2**: 16076.

19. Malhamé I, Cormier M, Sugarman J, Schwartzman K. Latent tuberculosis in pregnancy: a systematic review. *PLoS ONE*. 2016; **11**(5):e0154825.

20. Centers for Disease Control and Prevention. Tuberculin Skin Testing, What is it? www.cdc.gov/tb/publications/factsheets/testing/skintesting.htm.

21. Lighter-Fisher J. Performance of an interferon-gamma release assay to diagnose latent tuberculosis infection during pregnancy. *Obstetrics & Gynecology*. 2012; **120**(2 Pt1): 398.

22. Pai M, Behr M. Latent Mycobacterium tuberculosis infection and interferon-gamma release assays. *Microbiol Spectr*. 2016; **4**(5).

23. Dheda K, Barry CE III, Maartens G. Tuberculosis. *Lancet*. 2016; **387**: 1211.

24. Steingart KR, Henry M, Ng V, Hopewell PC, Ramsay A, Cunningham J. Fluorescence versus conventional sputum smear microscopy for tuberculosis: a systematic review. *Lancet Infect Dis*. 2006; **6**: 570.

25. Iseman MD, Heifets LB. Rapid detection of tuberculosis and drug-resistant tuberculosis. *N Engl J Med*. 2006; **355**: 1606.

26. Bernardo J. 2017. Diagnosis of pulmonary tuberculosis in HIV-uninfected adults. In: Baron EL, ed., UpToDate. Retrieved 28 July 2017 from www.uptodate.com/contents/diagnosis of pulmonary tuberculosis in HIV-uninfected adults.

27. Restrepo CS, Katre R, Mumbower A. Imaging manifestations of thoracic tuberculosis. *Radiol Clin North Am*. 2016; **54**: 453.

28. Steingart KR, Henry M, Laal S et al. A systematic review of commercial serological antibody detection tests for the diagnosis of extrapulmonary tuberculosis. *Thorax*. 2007; **62**: 911.

29. World Health Organization. *Guidelines for Treatment of Tuberculosis*, 4th ed. Geneva: WHO; 2010. www.who.inj/eng.pdf?ua=1&ua=1.

30. Centers for Disease Control and Prevention. Guidelines for Vaccinating Pregnant Women. www.cdc.gov/vaccines/pregnancy/hcp/guidelines.html.

31. American Academy of Pediatrics. Tuberculosis. In: Kimberlin DW, Brady MT, Jackson MA, Long SS, eds. *Red Book: 2015 Report of the Committee on Infectious Diseases*, 30th ed. Elk Grove Village, IL: American Academy of Pediatrics; 2015: 805.

32. World Health Organization. Breastfeeding and maternal tuberculosis. 1998. www.who.int/maternal_child_adolescent/documents/breastfeeding_maternal_tb/.

33. Gandhi NR, Nunn P, Dheda K et al. Multi drug resistant and extensively drug resistant tuberculosis: a threat to global control of tuberculosis. *Lancet*. 2010; **375**: 1830–4.

34. World Health Organization. Tuberculosis and HIV. 2016. www.who.int/hiv/topics/tb/en/.

35. World Health Organization. BCG Vaccine. www.who.int/hiv/topics/tb/en/.

Vulvo Vaginitis, Candida (Yeast) Infection

Adel Elkady, Prabha Sinha and Soad Ali Zaki Hassan

Vulvitis and vaginitis is defined as a spectrum of conditions that cause vulval and/or vaginal symptoms. Candida is the most common cause of vulvovaginal complaints for which women seek medical advice, especially during pregnancy.

Vulvovaginal candidiasis (VVC) is an opportunistic mucosal mycosis, and one of the most common causes of vulvovaginal itching and discharge caused by *Candida* species (*C. albicans, C. glabrata. C. krusei, C. parapsilosis* and *C. tropicalis*).[1,2]

Candida albicans causes 80–90 per cent of vaginal fungal infection.[3,4]

Ten to twenty per cent of reproductive-age women who harbour *Candida* species are asymptomatic and do not require therapy.[5]

Vaginal candidiasis, commonly called 'yeast infection, or moniliasis', is relatively common during pregnancy (especially during the second trimester). with an estimated prevalence of 10–75 per cent.

Approximately 75 per cent of all pregnant women experience at least one episode of VVC during their lifetime, and 50 per cent of them suffer recurrent events.[7]

The *Candida* is harboured in the vagina as part of the body's beneficial flora. About 20 per cent of women have *Candida* in their vagina normally. That number goes up to 30 per cent during pregnancy. When the vaginal environment changes, it allows for the fungus to proliferate and cause problems.[6]

- Hormone fluctuations cause alteration in vaginal environment/pH.
- The causes of *Candida* colonisation during pregnancy are complex.
- Pregnancy causes increased levels of progesterone and oestrogen.
- Progesterone suppresses the ability of neutrophils to combat Candida.
- Oestrogen disrupts the integrity of vaginal epithelial cells against Candida and decreases immunoglobulins in vaginal secretions.

- Multiple recurrences of infection continue throughout the pregnancy.[7]

The increased glycogen content under the influence of reproductive hormones serves as a nutritional source for proliferating yeast.

Factors like gestational diabetes, frequent antibiotic therapy, HIV, contraceptives, reproductive hormones also predispose women to acute and chronic VVC. It is also common for women to get a yeast infection when they are taking antibiotics because they kill off a number of the other factors that keep the yeast in balance and control.

Candida infection is more likely to be associated with a retained intrauterine contraceptive device in early gestation, assisted reproduction techniques, history of amniocentesis, or cervical cerclage and preterm delivery.

Maternal Symptoms

May include one or more of the following:

- Increased discharge usually thin white/grey/greenish or yellowish, similar to cottage cheese and may smell like yeast/bread
- Redness, itching, or irritation of the lips of the vulva and vagina
- Burning sensation during urination or intercourse

Effect on Pregnancy

In pregnancy, yeast infections do not usually cause adverse effects for either the mother or her baby. However, they often cause significant discomfort which may be difficult to control.

The incidence of VVC is doubled in the third trimester of pregnancy, and multigravida suffer significantly more than primigravida.

Fetal Implication

Candida chorioamnionitis
Rarely the infection spreads into the bloodstream of the mother and therefore to the baby. This is a serious

condition which is sometimes fatal and can affect the heart, eyes, bones or brain.

It is often caused by using contaminated objects and by poor hygiene. These women are often immunocompromised, including HIV, presenting as chills and persistent fever.

Candida chorioamnionitis is rare but can lead to neonatal infection, high perinatal mortality and neurodevelopmental impairment.[8]

Despite the high incidence of vulvovaginal candidiasis during pregnancy (13–20 per cent), candidal chorioamnionitis is a rare occurrence. The prevalence of *C. chorioamnionitis* is 0.3–0.5 per cent of all pregnant women.

• Preterm birth and Stillbirth

Systematic review found two trials comparing the treatment of asymptomatic vaginal candidiasis in pregnancy for the outcome of preterm birth. These trials suggested Candida infection may manifest as preterm labour, preterm rupture of membranes (PROM) without fever or even stillbirth.[9] [EL 1]

The exact mechanism of premature labour is unknown. It is thought that the acid pH of the vagina has some effect on the hormones that trigger labour. In a recent study, it was shown that 25 per cent of women with preterm labour were suffering from a yeast infection.

• Growth Restriction

In a literature search of 14 eligible studies, the Johns Hopkins study investigators found a significant association between growth restriction and *Candida albicans* colonisation (odds ratio 1.9).

Therefore, constant check-ups regarding Candida infection and immediate treatment are advised for any mother-to-be.[10]

Urinary tract yeast infection during postpartum period occurs in 6.8 per cent of patients, and risk increases in patients with compromised immune system, catheterisation and the use of antibiotics.

Neonatal Implications

Congenital Candidiasis

Transmission of Candida may be vertical (from maternal vaginal infection) or nosocomial.[11]

Two forms of neonatal infection have been described:

Congenital cutaneous candidiasis in which an extensive skin rash presents within 12 hours of birth.

A macular erythema that may evolve from a pustular, papular or vesicular phase finally results in extensive desquamation. Rash appears shortly after birth and it is essentially benign and self-limiting.

Congenital systemic candidiasis is a serious and common cause of late-onset sepsis, with a high mortality rate (25–35 per cent), especially in very low-birthweight (VLBW) infants. At least 50 per cent of babies present with a cutaneous rash, pneumonia (most common), meningitis, candiduria and/or candidemia. *C. albicans* and *C. parapsilosis* are the most common species found in neonates.

The usual therapeutic agents are amphotericin and fluconazole. Amphotericin B is recommended as the first-line treatment in cases of invasive candidiasis in pregnant women and neonatal candidiasis. It crosses the placenta but has no reported adverse effects in humans.

Neonatal thrush is not life-threatening but it can make swallowing uncomfortable and hinder feed if present inside the mouth of the baby. If the mother breastfeeds, infected breasts can easily pass the infection on to the child or vice versa.

Diagnosis

Culture is the most sensitive method for the diagnosis of VVC.

Gram-stain smear offers an immediate diagnosis; however, its low sensitivity (30–50 per cent) has restricted its use in routine practice.[12]

Therefore, a reliable diagnosis cannot be made based on Gram stain/KOH mount alone without the collaborative evidence of a culture report.

Treatment

- Systemic absorption of azoles or nystatin from the vagina is so limited that both can be safely used during all trimesters of pregnancy. Boric acid, fluconazole, itraconazole and ketoconazole should not be used during pregnancy.
- Candidiasis in pregnancy is more resistant to treatment, is more likely to relapse, and responds better to 7- or even 14-day therapy compared with 1- to 3-day therapy in the non-pregnant.
- Treatment in pregnant women is primarily indicated for relief of symptoms, as vaginal candidiasis is not associated with adverse pregnancy outcomes.
- For symptomatic pregnant women, topical imidazole (clotrimazole or miconazole) vaginally

is most commonly recommended for seven days and is a preferred choice.

- Topical imidazole appears to be more effective than nystatin in pregnancy.[13]
- Oral treatment with azole has potential risks in pregnancy, and therefore should be avoided, particularly during the first trimester. Its impact on miscarriage risk is unclear, and high doses appear to increase the risk of birth defects. Since topical therapy is an effective alternative, it is preferred to oral dose.
- A cohort study of over 3300 women who received 150–300 mg oral fluconazole between 7 and 22 weeks of pregnancy reported an approximately 50 per cent increased risk of miscarriage in exposed women compared with vaginal azole therapy.[14,15] [EL 2]
- In the largest study, which included 7352 pregnancies, there was no overall risk of embryopathy associated with exposure to cumulative fluconazole doses during the first trimester nor with exposure to oral itraconazole or ketoconazole.
- Overall, these data appear reassuring for women who took low-dose fluconazole before realising that they were pregnant, although an increased risk of specific anomalies cannot be definitively excluded.

Breastfeeding Women

- Nystatin does not enter breastmilk, and therefore can be used by breastfeeding mothers.
- Fluconazole is excreted in human milk, but the American Academy of Pediatrics considers fluconazole safe in breastfeeding, as no adverse effects have been reported in breastfed infants.
- Systemic absorption of vaginal administration is minimal, therefore topical use in breastfeeding mothers is not contraindicated.

Treatments for Recurrent Vulvovaginal Candidiasis

- Vaginal candidiasis is more difficult to eradicate during pregnancy, therefore prolonged durations of treatment for 7–14 days are recommended.
- Multiple formulations and strengths of topical imidazoles are available; however, during

pregnancy, only the dosage forms designed for prolonged-duration therapy should be used.

- Miconazole and clotrimazole are the preferred topical agents in pregnancy. Miconazole 100 mg vaginal suppository or the 2 per cent vaginal cream should be applied for a seven-day course. Clotrimazole 2 per cent vaginal cream should be used for seven days. Recurrent infections should be treated for 14 days.
- Miconazole is classified by the US Food and Drug Administration (FDA) as pregnancy risk category C; however, the topical vaginal formulation achieves minimal systemic absorption. In clinical trials that included patients in the first trimester, no harm was demonstrated to the mother or fetus.[16]
- Clotrimazole vaginal formulations are classified pregnancy risk category B. Studies in the second and third trimesters have not demonstrated adverse outcomes on the mother or fetus. Data are inadequate to categorise risk in the first trimester.
- Use of oral fluconazole in pregnancy has been controversial.[17]
- Animal data suggest that high-dose fluconazole is associated with craniofacial malformations.
- Results from a significantly larger Danish cohort suggested that patients who receive even low doses of fluconazole have a 48 per cent greater risk for spontaneous abortion. Women who received fluconazole had a 62 per cent greater risk for spontaneous abortion than women treated with topical azoles. This study prompted the FDA to issue a safety alert for the prescribing of oral fluconazole during pregnancy.

In summary, treatment of vaginal candidiasis in pregnancy should only be undertaken with guidance from a health care provider. Topical imidazoles (miconazole and clotrimazole) have the largest body of evidence regarding safety for both the mother and the fetus during pregnancy. Therapy should be continued for a total of 7–14 days.

Treatment of Newborn

Smear 1 mL of miconazole oral gel round the mouth and gums with a finger after feeds four times a day.

After seven days, change to nystatin suspension if no response to miconazole gel.

Complementary therapy: there is no evidence from randomised trials that garlic, tea tree oil, yogurt (or other products containing live *Lactobacillus* species) or douching is effective for treatment or prevention of vulvovaginal candidiasis due to *C. albicans*.

Prevention

Most yeast infections can usually be avoided by doing the following:

- Wear loose, breathable cotton clothing and cotton underwear.
- After thorough regular washing with unscented, hypoallergenic or gentle soap, use blow dryer on a low, cool setting to help dry the outside of the genital area.
- Always wipe from front to back after using the toilet.
- Shower immediately after swimming.
- Limit sugar intake, as sugar promotes the growth of yeast.

Do *Not*

- Douche
- Use feminine hygiene sprays
- Use sanitary pads and tampons that contain deodorant
- Take a bubble bath/use scented soaps
- Use coloured or perfumed toilet paper

Do

- Include yogurt with 'lactobacillus acidophilus' in diet.
- Get plenty of rest to make it easier for your body to fight infections.

References

1. Eschenbach, DA Chronic vulvovaginal candidiasis. *New Eng J Med.* 2004; **351**: 851–2.

2. Omar, AA. Gram stain versus culture in the diagnosis of vulvovaginal candidiasis. *East Mediter Health J.* 2001; **7**(6): 925–34.

3. British Association for Sexual Health and HIV. *Management of vulvovaginal candidiasis.* 2007.

4. Holland J, Young ML, Lee O, Chen C-A. Vulvovaginal carriage of yeasts other than Candida albicans. *Sex Transm Infect.* 2003; **79**(3): 249–50.

5. Clinical Effectiveness Group (Association of Genitourinary Medicine and the Medical Society for the Study of Venereal Diseases). National Guideline for the Management of Vulvovaginal Candidiasis. *Sex Transm Infect.* 1999; **75**(suppl 1): S19.

6. Sobel JD. Vulvovaginal candidosis. *Lancet.* 2007; **369**: 1961–71.

7. Xu DJ, Sobel JD. Candida vulvovaginitis in pregnancy *Curr Infect Dis Rep.* 2004; **6**: 56–9.

8. Maki Y, Fujisaki M, Sato Y, Sameshima H. Candida chorioamnionitis leads to preterm birth and adverse fetal-neonatal outcome. *Can J Infect Dis Obstet Gynecol.* 2017.

9. Roberts CL, Algert CS, Rickard KL, Morris JM. Treatment of vaginal candidiasis for the prevention of preterm birth: a systematic review and meta-analysis. *Syst Rev.* 2015; **4**: 31.

10. Vedmedovska N, Rezeberga N, Donder GGG. Is abnormal vaginal microflora a risk factor for intrauterine fetal growth restriction? *Asian Pac J Reprod.* 2015; **4**(4): 313–16.

11. Chintaginjala A, Seetharam K. Congenital candidiasis. *Indian Dermatol Online J.* 2014; **5**(suppl 1): S44–7.

12. Pappas PG, Kauffman CA, Andes DR et al. Clinical Practice Guideline for the Management of Candidiasis: 2016 Update by the Infectious Diseases Society of America. *Clin Infect Dis.* 2016; **62**(4): e1-50.

13. Mølgaard-Nielsen D, Svanström H, Melbye M et al. Association between use of oral fluconazole during pregnancy and risk of spontaneous abortion and stillbirth. *JAMA.* 2016; **315**: 58.

14. Czeizel AE, Kazy Z, Puhó E. Population-based case-control teratologic study of topical miconazole. *Congenit Anom.* (Kyoto) 2004; **44**: 41–5. Abstract.

15. Menegola E, Broccia ML, Di Renzo F, Giavini E. Antifungal triazoles induce malformations in vitro. *Reprod Toxicol.* 2011; **15**: 421–7.

16. Fluconazole (Diflucan): Drug Safety Communication – FDA evaluating study examining use of oral fluconazole (Diflucan) in pregnancy. www.fda.gov /Safety/MedWatch/SafetyInformation/Safety AlertsforHumanMedicalProducts/ucm 497656.htm.

Chapter 27

Malaria

Bhavya Balasubramanya

Background and Epidemiology

Malaria is a life-threatening disease caused by the bite of the female *Anopheles* mosquito, which results in infection of the red blood cell. Malaria is a protozoal disease caused by infection with the parasites of genus *Plasmodium* (species *falciparum, vivax, ovale, malariae and knowlesi*). *P. falciparum* is associated with a greater maternal and fetal mortality/morbidity (low birthweight and anaemia) than non-*falciparum* infections.[1]

In 2016, there were an estimated 216 million cases of malaria in 91 countries, an increase of 5 million cases over 2015. Malaria deaths reached 445 000 in 2016, with most malarial cases and deaths occurring in sub-Saharan Africa.

In 2008, there were six deaths reported in the UK from malaria.[2]

Specific risk groups more vulnerable to malaria are young children, non-immune pregnant women, semi-immune pregnant women, semi-immune HIV-infected pregnant women, individuals with HIV/AIDS, travellers from non-endemic areas and immigrants.

Life Cycle

The female anopheline mosquito, while taking her blood meal, injects 'sporozoites' into the bloodstream of the intermediate host (man or woman). These sporozoites reach the liver and develop into 'schizonts'. This stage is known as tissue schizogony. A few of these schizonts become dormant forms in the liver, known as 'hypnozoites' (seen in *P. vivax* and *P. ovale* infections). Hypnozoites are responsible for relapse of malaria. The schizonts burst to release 'merozoites', merozoites develop into trophozoites or immature sexual forms which are then taken up during the mosquito's blood meal. The sexual cycle of the parasite takes place in the definitive host (female anopheline mosquito).[3]

It has been observed that pregnant women are at two times higher risk of being bitten by a mosquito than their non-pregnant counterparts. This is probably due to physiological phenomena during pregnancy: increased exhalation leading to release of volatile substances which attract mosquitoes, and the higher temperature of the abdominal surface temperature, increasing blood flow to the skin.[2] [EL 2]

Signs and Symptoms of Malaria

Malaria is an acute febrile illness.

- Fever and chills
- Headache may be mild but it is not specific enough to recognise as malaria
- Myalgia
- Cough
- Neurological signs and symptoms (confusion, disorientation, dizziness or coma)
- Gastrointestinal (nausea, vomiting, diarrhoea)

If malaria is not treated within 24 hours, *P. falciparum* malaria can progress to severe illness, often leading to death.

Asymptomatic pregnant women can become severely anaemic, with poor fetal outcome due to placental sequestration.

Classification of Malaria

Uncomplicated Malaria

Fewer than 2 per cent parasitised red blood cells in a woman with no signs of severity and no complicating features.

Severe and Complicated Malaria

The parasitaemia of severe malaria can be less than 2 per cent. Pregnant women with 2 per cent or more parasitised red blood cells are at higher risk of developing severe malaria and should be treated with the extensive malaria protocol.

Malaria is classified as being severe malaria if any of the following are present:

- Impaired consciousness or coma
- Repeated generalised convulsions
- Jaundice
- Renal failure
- Acute respiratory distress syndrome, pulmonary oedema
- Hypotension, circulatory collapse
- Haemoglobinuria
- Spontaneous bleeding disseminated intravascular coagulation
- Severe anaemia (Hb < 8g %)
- Thrombocytopenia
- Hypoglycaemia (<2.2 mmol/L)
- Acidosis (pH < 7.3)
- Hyperlactaemia
- Parasitaemia > 2%

Congenital Malaria

Congenital malaria in the newborn is caused by the passage of parasites or infected red blood cells from the mother to the newborn while *in utero* or during delivery.

Diagnosis[4]

Treatment for malaria should not be initiated until there is a laboratory confirmation, except in cases where there is a strong clinical suspicion.

The following tests are available to diagnose malaria from blood samples:

- Gold standard test: thick and thin peripheral smears
- Rapid diagnostic tests (RDT)
- Polymerase chain reaction (PCR)

Microscopic Examination of a Peripheral Smear

The diagnosis of malaria relies on microscopic examination (the current gold standard) of thick and thin blood films for parasites.

Thick smears help pick up the presence of malarial parasite whereas a thin smear helps identify the species and quantify parasite density. A series of three blood smears should ideally be examined by a qualified laboratory technician.[4] [*Grade A recommendation*]

Rapid Diagnostic Test (RDT)

A rapid diagnostic test is an alternative way of quickly establishing the diagnosis of malaria infection by detecting specific malaria antigens in the blood and is available in the form of dipsticks or cassettes.

RDTs permit a reliable detection of malaria infections, particularly in remote areas with limited access to good-quality microscopy service. The test determines within 15 minutes whether patients are infected with malaria.

Invalid results mean RDT kits are damaged. If the RDT is negative, no treatment for malaria is required; however, if the symptoms persist, a repeat test should be carried out after a couple of days as the test might miss early malaria infection.

Nucleic Acid Amplification-Based Diagnostics

A nucleic acid amplification test can detect low-density malaria infections. It is more sensitive and specific than microscopy as it detects the parasite nucleic acid. It can also detect resistance patterns. The test is more expensive and requires a reference laboratory to run the test.

Maternal Implications

Malaria during pregnancy has an adverse effect not only on the mother but also on the fetus and newborn, posing a huge public health problem.

Maternal Mortality: worldwide, in 2016, the World Health Organization (WHO) reported 216 million malaria cases with 445 000 deaths. Malaria accounts for over 10 000 maternal deaths per year.[5]

The mortality rate from severe disease approaches 50 per cent.

Severe Life-Threatening Complications

- Profound hypoglycaemia
- Pulmonary oedema
- Respiratory distress
- Secondary bacterial infection
- Convulsions
- Renal failure
- Severe anaemia
- Thrombocytopenia
- Obstetric haemorrhage

Fetal Implications[6,7]

- Globally, malaria accounts for 200 000 neonatal deaths per year.
- Pregnant women with malaria are at risk of miscarriage, stillbirth, low-birthweight baby, congenital infection of the neonate and perinatal mortality.
- Children born to mothers with malaria during pregnancy may be low-birthweight and carry subsequent risks into adulthood.
- The exact mechanism is not known; malarial parasites sequester the placenta and replicate; also immune status of women during pregnancy is low, thus making them vulnerable to a plethora of infections. Vertical transmission rarely occurs at the time of birth.
- All neonates whose mothers developed malaria in pregnancy should be screened for malaria with standard microscopy of thick and thin blood films at birth, and subsequent weekly tests until 28 days.

Preventive Measures

The WHO recommends the following package of interventions as effective prevention strategies for malaria in pregnant women.

- Long-lasting insecticide treated nets (LLIN)
- Intermittent Preventive Treatment in Pregnancy (IPTp) – to be initiated in all areas with medium to high malaria transmission
- Prompt diagnosis and effective treatment of malaria infections

Prevention of Mosquito Bites

- Long-sleeved clothing and trousers
- LLIN are the mainstay in preventing mosquito bites. LLIN are made of insecticides such as permethrin/deltamethrin or cypermethrin embedded in the fibres of the net, can withstand up to 20 washes and must be replaced once in three years
- Skin repellents should include 50 per cent diethyl-meta-toluamide (DEET) [EL 1]
- Knock-down mosquito sprays [EL 2]
- Electrically heated bed mats that vaporise pyrethroids

Intermittent Preventive Treatment in Pregnancy (IPTp) [EL 1]

The WHO recommends that *all* pregnant women in medium- to high-transmission areas, irrespective of whether they are infected with malaria, should receive IPTp. This involves offering antenatal women three doses of sulfamethoxazole–pyrimethamine (SP), initiated early in the second trimester. The three-monthly doses are each given one month apart. IPTp reduces maternal malaria episodes, maternal and fetal anaemia, placental parasitaemia, low birthweight and neonatal mortality.

Chemoprophylaxis[8]

The choice of drug for chemoprophylaxis depends on the trimester of pregnancy and drug resistance pattern in the area. It is also suitable for lactating women. There are two types of chemoprophylaxis:

- Causal chemoprophylaxis – directed against the liver schizonts, and must be continued for one week after leaving the malarious area. Drug of choice is atovaquone–proguanil.
- Suppressive chemoprophylaxis – directed against the red blood cell stages of the parasite and is continued for four weeks after leaving the malarious area.
- Drug of choice is mefloquine.

Doxycycline and primaquine are contraindicated in pregnancy.

Treatment of Malaria in Pregnancy[9]

Malaria in pregnancy is an emergency.

The following four factors must be kept in mind when treating a confirmed case of malaria:

- Infecting species
- Whether it is uncomplicated or severe malaria
- Parasite drug resistance
- Trimester of pregnancy

Treatment Modalities

Supportive Management

- Antipyretics
- Antiemetics if patient is vomiting. Metoclopramide is safe in all trimesters
- Iron and folic acid should be used to treat anaemia

Hospital Admission

- Women with uncomplicated malaria to be admitted in the ward and started on oral anti-malarials. [*B recommendation*]
- Chloroquine is the drug of choice in *P. vivax*, *P. malariae* and *P. ovale* infections.
- In uncomplicated *P. falciparum* or mixed infections, quinine and clindamycin are the drugs of choice. [*B recommendation*]

Intensive Care Admission

- Severe life-threatening complications require intensive supportive care.
- Women with severe malaria to be treated in intensive care units [*A recommendation*] and started on intravenous artesunate. [*A recommendation*]
- Severe anaemia, hypoglycaemia and acidosis to be corrected.
- Primaquine is contraindicated in pregnancy. [*D recommendation*]

Medications

- **Any species**
  - Artesunate IV 2.4 mg/kg at 0, 12 and 24 hours, then daily thereafter. When the patient is well enough to take oral medication she can be switched to oral artesunate 2 mg/kg (or IM artesunate 2.4 mg/kg) once daily, plus clindamycin.
  - A three-day course of Riamet® (GSK) or Atovaquone-Proguanil (Malarone®, Novartis) or a seven-day course of quinine and clindamycin at 450 mg three times a day for seven days, if oral artesunate is not available.

    or
  - Intravenous quinine IV 20 mg/kg loading dose in 5 per cent dextrose over four hours and then 10 mg/kg IV over four hours every eight hours plus clindamycin IV 450 mg every eight hours (max. dose quinine 1.4 g), then continue oral quinine 600 mg three times a day to complete five to seven days and oral clindamycin 450 mg three times a day for seven days.

- *P. falciparum*
  - Oral quinine 600 mg eight-hourly and oral clindamycin 450 mg eight-hourly for seven days (can be given together) or Riamet® four tablets/dose for weight > 35 kg, twice daily for three days, or atovaquone–proguanil (Malarone®) four standard tablets daily for three days.

- *P. vivax, P. ovale, P. malariae*
  - Oral chloroquine (base) 600 mg followed by 300 mg 68 hours later, then 300 mg on day 2 and again on day 3.

Obstetric Management

- Uncomplicated malaria is not a reason for induction of labour unless indicated for obstetric reasons.
- Prompt effective antimalarial treatment can prevent stillbirth and preterm labour.
- Regular antenatal care including fetal growth assessment should be carried out for women who recover from an episode of malaria.

Breastfeeding

- Newborn babies do not get malaria infections from breastmilk.
- Breastfeeding mothers travelling to malaria-endemic regions can continue their antimalarial medications.
- The breastfeeding infant should still continue with antimalarial medications.[10]

Exclusive breastfeeding (EBF) protects against fever among infants with malaria infection, and EBF reduces the odds of clinical malaria. [EL 2] This reduction in malaria susceptibility among EBF infants may be related to the immunodulatory effects of breastmilk.[11]

Treatment of Malaria in Neonates/Infants

Infants with suspected malaria should have prompt parasitological confirmation of the diagnosis before treatment begins.

Artemisinin-based combination therapy (ACT) is the recommended treatment for uncomplicated malaria in infants. Artemisinin derivatives are safe and well tolerated by young children, so the choice of ACT will be determined largely by the safety and tolerability of the partner drug.

For infants weighing less than 5 kg with uncomplicated *P. falciparum*, WHO recommends treatment with an ACT at the same mg/kg body weight dose as for children weighing 5 kg.

In cases of suspected severe malaria, rectal artesunate should be administered as pre-referral treatment and the infant should then immediately be transferred to a facility where comprehensive care for severe malaria can be provided.

A single dose of rectal artesunate as pre-referral treatment reduces the risk of death in children under six years of age. [EL 2]

Malaria Vaccine

Until today we do not have any commercially available malaria vaccine. Currently around 20 candidate vaccines are undergoing clinical trials. Phase 3 trial has been completed for the RTS and S/A S01 vaccines. [EL 1].

In 2019, the first childhood anti-malarial vaccine RTS,S has been rolled out for pilot testing in select areas of three countries, namely Ghana, Kenya and Malawi.

References

1. World Health Organization. Malaria. Fact sheet. Updated November 2017. www.who.int/mediacentre/factsheets/fs094/en/.

2. Royal College of Obstetricians and Gynaecologists. The prevention of malaria in pregnancy. Green-top Guideline No. 54. April 2010.

3. Malaria in pregnancy. Infectious diseases. Series from the *Lancet* journals. Published 30 January 2018. www.thelancet.com/series/malaria-pregnancy.

4. World Health Organization. Malaria. Diagnostic testing. www.who.int/malaria/areas/diagnosis/en.

5. World Health Organization. Global Malaria Programme: pregnant women and infants. http://apps.who.int/malaria/pregnantwomenandinfants.html.

6. Soma-Pillay P, Macdonald AP. Malaria in pregnancy. *Obstet Med.* 2012; **5**(1): 2–5.

7. Schantz-Dunn J, Nour NM. Malaria and pregnancy: a global health perspective. *Rev Obstet Gynecol.* 2009; **2**(3): 186–92.

8. Schwartz E. Prophylaxis of malaria. *Mediterr J Hematol Infect Dis.* 2012; **4**(1): e2012045.

9. World Health Organization. Malaria. Guidelines for the treatment of malaria. Third edition April 2015. www.who.int/malaria/publications/atoz/9789241549127/en/]10-.

10. Centers for Disease Control and Prevention. Breast feeding. Malaria. www.cdc.gov/breastfeeding/disease/malaria.htm.

11. Brazeau NF, Tabala M, Kiketa L et al. Exclusive breastfeeding and clinical malaria risk in 6-month-old infants: a cross-sectional study from Kinshasa, Democratic Republic of the Congo. *Am J Trop Med Hyg.* 2016; **95**(4): 827–30.

12. World Health Organization. What the first malaria vaccine means to a mother and child. https://www.who.int/immunization/diseases/malaria/malaria_vaccine_implementation_programme/en/.

Chapter 28

Parasitic Infestation: Protozoa

Mithila B. Prasad

Introduction

The name 'proto-zoa' literally means 'first animals', and early classification systems grouped the protozoa as basal members of the animal kingdom. However, they were recognised as a discrete assemblage on the basis of their unicellularlity and were assigned to the taxon Protozoa (but still invariably figured as the trunk of the animal tree of life).

Protozoa is a parasitic single-celled organism that can divide only within a host organism. Parasites are a diverse group of organisms that account for the majority of human infections.[1]

According to a World Health Organization (WHO) study in 2010, the prevalence was as high as 48.5 million, with 59 724 deaths annually and 8.78 million Disability Adjusted Life Years. The disability-adjusted life year (DALY) is a measure of overall disease burden, expressed as the number of years lost due to ill-health, disability or early death).[2] [EL 1]

Diagnosis may initially be difficult and is based largely on travel history and a variety of tests required (stool, blood tests and imaging) depending on presenting signs and symptoms.

The sequel on maternal and fetal health relies on type of infection, gestational age at presentation, patient's own natural immunity, early diagnosis, prompt treatment and the prevention of complications.

The decision to treat parasitic infection in pregnancy should be based on risk–benefit ratio. The women should be informed of all potential risks on the fetus and should be allowed to make an informed choice.

Withholding treatment may be appropriate when infection does not pose immediate threat to the life of the mother or fetus in the presence of normal maternal haemoglobin and normal fetal growth.

Use of praziquantel (Biltricide®) medication for helminthic infections, during pregnancy and lactation was historically withheld due to concerns in 1994 of effects on the fetus. However, WHO informal consultation recommended that use of the drug would result in reduced maternal anaemia and perinatal morbidity. [EL 2]

General Features of Protozoa

Protozoa are single-celled micro-organisms which represent the earliest form of animal life. They have a typical tri-laminar unit membrane which encloses the cytoplasm. Various organelles present in cytoplasm play a vital role in respiration, nourishment, reproduction and regulation of osmotic pressure.

They have been classified into four groups or phyla: *Sarcomastigophora*, *Apicomplexa*, *Microspora* and *Ciliophora*.

The species traditionally collectively termed 'protozoa' are not closely related to each other, and have only superficial similarities (eukaryotic, unicellular and motile).

In this chapter, we will be dealing with four main protozoa that affect humans: *Giardia*, Trichomonas, Amoeba and *Toxoplasma*.

GIARDIA LAMBLIA

Introduction

Giardia intestinalis is a flagellated protozoan parasite caused by flagellate *Giardia lamblia*. It is the most common pathogen causing intestinal infection which may be asymptomatic or cause diarrhoea.[3]

Epidemiology

Giardiasis is found worldwide, with its prevalence being more common in areas of poor sanitation. Infection is more common in children due to their poor natural immunity and lack of adequate intestinal immunoglobulin A (IgA).

While ingestion of contaminated food and water is a more common mode of transmission, direct person-to-person transmission may also occur in children and homosexual men.[3]

Morphology and Life Cycle

Giardia lives in the duodenum and upper jejunum and is the only protozoa found in the lumen of the human small intestine.[1] It occurs in vegetative and cystic forms. Infections occur by ingestion of cysts in contaminated food and water. As few as 10 cysts are capable of initiating an infection. Within an hour of ingestion, the cyst hatches out into two trophozoites which multiply by binary fission and colonise the duodenum.

Pathogenesis and Clinical Features

The incubation period is about one to two weeks. The organisms are typically seen in the crypts of the duodenum or the ileum.[1,2] The villous architecture is damaged, causing atrophy resulting in malabrption of fat, nutrients and vitamins particularly A and B12. The mechanism causing alteration of mucosal architecture is possibly immune-mediated.[6]

Occasionally, *Giardia* may colonise the gall bladder, causing biliary colic and jaundice.

The acute stage lasts for three to four days and is characterised by sudden onset of watery diarrhoea, abdominal distension, flatulence, nausea, anorexia and abdominal cramps. The stools are malodorous and loose, but with no blood. If untreated, it may progress to chronic infection resulting in malabrption and steatorrhoea. Bacterial overgrowth is responsible for fat malabsorption.

Maternal Implications

Complications and Symptoms

- Chronic intestinal upset, flatulence, diarrhoea, reflux acidity
- Malnutrition, signs of anaemia
- Poor weight gain
- Pregnant women may also suffer from an exaggerated form of hyperemesis gravidarum

The effects in pregnancy are mainly related to associated diarrhoea, malabsorption, fluid and electrolyte disturbances.

Maternal-to-fetal transmission has not been documented.

Fetal Implications

Fetal implications are usually secondary to maternal anaemia rather than a direct effect on the fetus.

- Low birthweight.
- Intrauterine growth restriction (IUGR). Late-onset IUGR is more frequently seen in women presenting with symptoms of *Giardia* infection and subsequent anaemia. [EL 1]
- Preterm deliveries. Preterm delivery more frequently occurs in second and third trimesters. [EL 2]
- Fetal anaemia.

Diagnosis[4]

Stool examination (microscopy) commonly reveals cysts and occasionally trophozoites.

Concentration, centrifugal and flotation is useful when cysts are sparse. The stools usually do not show any red blood cells or pus cells.

Duodenal aspiration, when stool samples have negative results and there is strong suspicion of the disease, may be done to confirm diagnosis.

Immunodiagnostic tests such as enzyme-linked immunoassay (ELISA) and immunochromatographic strip tests have also been developed for detection of *Giardia* antigens in faeces, but not for routine use. Antibody demonstration is not useful in diagnosis.

Treatment[5]

The pregnant woman should be treated only if symptomatic, and the mainstay of the treatment is maintaining adequate hydration.

Metronidazole (pregnancy category B) with a cure rate of 85–90 per cent is the most commonly prescribed first-line antibiotic used in the treatment.

The recommended dose is 250 mg orally three times a day for five to seven days. However, its use has been associated with significant failure rates in clearing parasites from the gut and is associated with poor compliance.

Tinidazole (TNZ) either as an oral single dose of 2 g or 500 mg twice daily for three to five days. It causes minor side effects of bitter or metallic taste. Major side effects may include change in consciousness, difficult or noisy breathing, wheezing or tightness in chest.

In countries such as the United States where tinidazole is not licensed for use in pregnant women (pregnancy category C), metronidazole 250 mg three times daily for five days can be used.

Breastfeeding

In breastfeeding women, it is advisable to stop breastfeeding for 12–24 hours after metronidazole therapy, especially after single high dose has been used.

Metronidazole is FDA pregnancy category B. (Animal reproduction studies have failed to demonstrate a risk to the fetus and there are no adequate and well-controlled studies in pregnant women.) It is best avoided in the first trimester.

The US Food and Drug Administration does not recommend furazolidone use in pregnancy. It is recommended only if benefits outweigh the risks and no other alternative is available (category C).

Prevention

Better personal hygiene and prevention of intake of contaminated food and water is by far the best protection available for all faecal–oral infections.

It is a self-limiting disease in most healthy immunocompetent individuals.

TRICHOMONAS VAGINALIS (TV)

Introduction and Epidemiology[6]

- *Trichomonas vaginalis* is an anaerobic, flagellated protozoan parasite.
- *Trichomonas* is a facultative anaerobe, unable to survive outside the body, therefore infection is transmitted directly from person to person.
- It is a sexually transmitted infection commonly found in the human genitourinary tract.
- *T. vaginalis* selectively infects the squamous epithelium.[6]
- Approximately more than 250 million people get infected by this parasite annually.
- The incidence is more than 3.5 million in the United States, whereas in the UK it is relatively uncommon, and tends to be clustered in specific urban areas among black ethnic minorities.
- The incidence ranges from 5 to 10 per cent in healthy women to as high as 50–70 per cent

amongst sex workers and female prison inmates.
- The peak incidence is about 16–35 years. *Trichomonas vaginalis* lives in the vagina and cervix and may also be found in the Bartholin's gland, urethra and urinary bladder.
- Trichomonas often coexists with other sexually transmitted infections (candidiasis, gonorrhoea, syphilis and HIV). The pH of the vagina is a critical growth-limiting factor, and the favourable pH is usually 5.5–7.

Signs and Symptoms

- The incubation period may vary from four days to four weeks.
- Symptoms of severe vulvo vaginitis, irritation of the genital area, itching, an increased, strong-smelling frothy vaginal discharge, discomfort while urinating and or dyspareunia.
- The vulva may be erythematous, with the presence of fresh red spots and excoriations.
- The cervix and vagina may demonstrate characteristic red punctuate haemorrhages, giving it a classical 'strawberry cervix' appearance.
- Regional lymphadenopathy and endometritis and pyosalpinx are infrequent complications due to early diagnosis and treatment.

Fetal Implications

Colonisation of the lower genital tract with trichomonas has been shown to increase the risk of:
- Premature rupture of membranes (PROM)
- Preterm labour
- Small for gestational age

Evidence that treatment of colonised patients prevents PROM is lacking.

Neonatal Implications

Neonatal effects occur due to contact with the organism during the process of childbirth. [EL 2]
- Rarely, neonatal pneumonia and conjunctivitis have been reported in infants born to infected mothers.[9]
- Vaginal infection in the female neonate incidence is 2–17 per cent. The infection site is vaginal epithelium as neonatal vaginal epithelium is relatively mature due to maternal oestrogen making it susceptible to trichomonas.

- Within three to four weeks the maternal oestrogen is metabolised and thus the epithelium becomes resistant to trichomonas.

Diagnosis

Trichomonas may be isolated from urine sediment and vaginal secretions by

Wet mount preparations of the vaginal discharge (placing a small amount of vaginal discharge on a microscope slide and mixing with a few drops of saline solution). *T. vaginalis* can be identified by its characteristic jerky movements. The sensitivity ranges between 38 and 82 per cent). It is a reliable and simple method and treatment can thus be initiated immediately.

Cultures – trichomonas can be grown in a variety of solid and liquid media, in tissue culture and in egg cysteine, peptone, liver, maltose (CPLM).

Papanicolaou test smears and special stains. High vaginal swab (HVS) collected on cotton swabs left for some time in a tube containing 5 per cent glucose saline shows better shape and motility of the organism.

Serological tests like indirect haemagglutin and gel diffusion are available for antibody detection.

Nucleic acid amplification tests (NAATs) to offer the highest sensitivity, up to 75–90 per cent for detection of *T. vaginalis*.

A combination of wet mount and culture increases the sensitivity of detecting trichomonas to 98 per cent, as reported by several studies.

Screening

Evidence does not support routine screening for trichomoniasis in asymptomatic pregnant women.

Treatment[7,8]

Metronidazole is the drug of choice. [EL 1]

- More than 98 per cent of the strains are sensitive to the drug, although some resistance has been demonstrated both in vivo and in vitro studies.
- The recommended dose for initial treatment is 2 g orally, although in pregnancy a five-day course is recommended. Both the partners should be treated simultaneously, and sexual intercourse should be avoided until the completion of treatment.
- Meta-analyses and more recent studies have concluded that there is no evidence of teratogenicity from the use of metronidazole [EL 1] and it can be used in all stages of pregnancy and during breastfeeding.
- The British National Formulary advises against high-dose regimens in pregnancy, i.e. 2 g stat dose, and instead low-dose regimen 400 mg eight-hourly for five to seven days is recommended.

Tinidazole is an alternative drug of choice.

- In the United States, tinidazole in pregnancy is category C and its safety in pregnant women has not been well evaluated. The manufacturer states that the use of tinidazole in the first trimester is contraindicated.

Failed Treatment

- Failure of treatment may be due to inadequate therapy, resistance, reinfection, or low patient compliance.
- A history should be taken to try to find any of the above reasons for failure of treatment.
- In case of non-response, initial regime should be repeated with a higher-dose course of metronidazole (800 mg three times daily for seven days. [EL 3]
- If there is further failing, of this third regime, resistance testing should be performed (if available).

Breastfeeding and metronidazole: metronidazole is secreted in breastmilk and may affect its taste. The manufacturers recommend avoiding high doses if breastfeeding, or if using a single dose of metronidazole, breastfeeding should be discontinued for 12–24 hours to reduce infant exposure.

Prevention

As it is a sexually transmitted infection, the best prevention is to practise safe sex.

Follow-Up

Follow-up tests of cure are only recommended if the patient remains symptomatic following treatment, or if symptoms recur. [EL 4]

ENTAMOEBA HISTOLYTICA

Epidemiology

Entamoeba is prevalent worldwide; the infection ranges from 1 to 40 per cent in Central America, Asia and Africa and 0.2 to 10.8 per cent in endemic areas of the developed world such as the USA. It is the third leading parasitic cause of mortality, after malaria and schistosomiasis.

Prevalence is greater in areas of poor sanitation, and the majority of the infected are asymptomatic.

Invasive illness causing disabling illness is often seen in Africa, Asia and Latin America.[9]

Morphology and Transmission

Entamoeba histolytica is an anaerobic parasitic amoebozoa, part of the genus *Entamoeba*.

The active (trophozoite) stage exists only in the host and in fresh loose faeces; cysts survive outside the host in water, in soils and on foods.

The infection can occur through the ingestion of any contaminated objects (water, food or touch with contaminated fingers) that may have touched the faeces of an infected person.[9]

Pathogenesis

Not all strains are pathogenic, and factors such as stress, malnutrition, alcoholism and immunodeficiency influence the outcome of infection.

The trophozoites penetrate the epithelial cells in the colon to produce discrete ulcers. Some amoebae may penetrate the radicles of the portal vein where they are lodged in the hepatic lobules. This stage is called amoebic hepatitis and is characterised by the formation of hepatic abscesses commonly seen in the upper right lobe of the liver.

Involvement of the distant organs is usually by haematogenous spread. Sexual transmission can also occur, leading to infection of the penis following anal intercourse. Cutaneous involvement is by direct spread, from rectum to perianal area and from sinuses draining from liver abscesses.

Clinical Features

The incubation period may vary from four days to four months. The organ affected, and the extent of damage determines the course of illness. The clinical course is characterised by prolonged latency, relapses and intermissions. The patient is usually afebrile and non-toxic.

Symptoms

- Colicky abdominal pain, with or without diarrhoea.
- The stools are large, foul-smelling and brownish-black in colour.
- Fulminant colitis due to ulceration and necrosis of the colon; the patient may become febrile and septic.
- Chronic involvement may simulate a picture of appendicitis.

Maternal Implications

- In pregnancy, amoebic disease is usually associated with acute exacerbations and prominent symptoms. Infected women may have bloody dysenteric stools with abdominal pain and tenderness.
- Electrolyte imbalance and dehydration may adversely affect the outcome of pregnancy.
- Hepatic involvement is the most common extra-intestinal complication of the disease; it is not a frequent complication in pregnancy. Affected women present with heaviness and pain in the right hypochondria and referred pain around the right shoulder. Fever with chills can occur. Jaundice is a common complication when the hepatic abscesses compress on the gall bladder.
- Cutaneous amoebiasis results in abscesses that occur on the vulva, vaginal wall or the cervix and the lesion can resemble carcinoma.

Fetal Implications

There is no clear evidence of placental transmission of the parasite to the fetus.

Prematurity, oligohydramnios and growth restrictions are the commonly occurring complications. In a retrospective cross-sectional study in Tanzania involving 30 797 births, pregnant women who were recorded to have amoebiasis had 79 per cent increased odds of having a preterm delivery.

Diagnosis

Microscopy: the diagnosis is based on demonstration of *E. histolytica* trophozoites or its cysts in stools, tissues or exudates from the lesions. Examination of multiple stool samples becomes necessary as excretion of the cysts and trophozoites is variable.

Culture and serology are usually negative in the early stage of the illness.

Immunological tests such as ELISA, radio-immunoassay and DNA probes can detect amoeba antigens in blood and faeces, but they are very expensive and cannot be used as a routine.

CT scan and ultrasonography, if there is hepatic involvement, are useful in hepatic amoebiasis, as stool samples are usually negative for amoebae.

Invasive methods such as sigmoidoscopy and pus aspiration are not generally recommended in pregnancy due to increased risk of bleeding and risk of introducing secondary infections. They are usually delayed until after delivery.

Treatment[10]

Symptomatic relief and eradication of the organism forms the mainstay of treatment in amoebiasis. The drugs for treatment can be classified into two main groups: luminal amoebicides that act in the intestinal luminal, and tissue amoebicides that act at a systemic level.

The luminal amoebicides include diloxanide furoate, paromomycin and iodoquinol.

Tetracyclines are absolutely contraindicated in pregnant and breastfeeding women.

The tissue amoebicides include emetine and chloroquine.

Metronidazole, 750 mg, three times daily for 7–10 days is the most commonly adopted regimen.

Many amoebicides are unsafe in pregnancy and thus the treatment of amoebiasis in pregnancy should be tailored to the severity of symptoms. Treatment, if not urgent, should be delayed until 12 weeks of gestation or until after delivery.

Paromomycin, 25–30 mg/kg per day can be added to treat systemic infections. The use of metronidazole alone has a high cure rate of 90 per cent, which with the additional drug paromomycin increases to nearly 100 per cent.

Chloroquine for liver abscess since it has been used safely (at lower doses) in pregnant women for malaria prophylaxis.

- Surgical intervention is only recommended for acute abdomen pain that may arise due to perforated amoebic abscess, massive gastrointestinal bleeding or due to toxic megacolon.

- In hepatic abscesses that are less than 10 cm in diameter, metronidazole for 10 days is the drug of choice.

- Needle aspiration may be useful in diagnosis and treatment, but is generally contraindicated in pregnancy as it increases the rate of secondary bacterial infections. Failure to respond to medical treatment in established hepatic abscess is an indication for ultrasound-guided drainage. Broad-spectrum antibiotics can be used in case of superimposed bacterial infections.

However, in pregnancy surgical intervention should be done as a last resort when no response to medical treatment has been demonstrated.

TOXOPLASMA

Introduction

Toxoplasmosis is caused by the protozoan parasite *Toxoplasma gondi*. The name Toxoplasma is derived from the Greek word toxon meaning arc or bow, referring to the crescentic shape of the trophozoite.

It is now recognised as the most common protozoan parasite globally, with highest infection rates being in areas with hot, humid climates and low altitudes.

Epidemiology

The infection is prevalent worldwide, with seropositive rates ranging from 10 to over 90 per cent (WHO), but more common in places where cats are domesticated as pet animals. It is estimated that nearly 400–4000 infants born in the USA every year are congenitally infected with toxoplasmosis. Most of these infants are asymptomatic during the neonatal period, but the manifestations may become apparent in the second or third decade of life. In France, the infection is highly prevalent and is attributed to the habit of eating raw meat. It is estimated that 1.1–1.3 per cent of women seroconvert each year.[11]

The full natural cycle is maintained predominantly by cats and mice. Toxoplasmosis is not passed from person to person, except in instances of mother-to-child transmission (MTCT) and blood transfusion or organ transplantation. People become infected by three principal routes of transmission.

- Food-borne
- Animal-borne
- Congenital

Humans can become infected by any of these routes: eating undercooked meat of animals harbouring tissue cysts, consuming food or water contaminated with cat faeces or by contaminated environmental samples (such as faecal-contaminated soil or changing the litter box of a pet cat).

The freshly passed oocysts are not infectious. It takes five days for the oocyte to mature and become infective. It is resistant to environmental conditions and can remain infective in soil for more than a year and, when ingested, the sporozoites are released in the intestine, which initiates infection.

Clinical Features of Infections during Pregnancy

Most human infections are asymptomatic.

Maternal Infection

Most pregnant women (>90 per cent) do not experience obvious signs and symptoms, and spontaneous recovery is the rule.

The most common clinical signs are:

- Fatigue with flu-like symptoms.
- Fever with pneumonitis, myocarditis .and encephalitis which can be fatal.
- Adenopathy (cervical, suboccipital, supraclavicular, axillary and inguinal). Retroperitoneal and mesenteric lymph nodes along with the liver and spleen may also be involved.
- Chorioretinitis is a late manifestation of the disease and is often seen in immunocompromised pregnancy states such as those with AIDS.

Congenital Infection[12]

- Congenital infection occurs predominantly after primary infection in a pregnant woman.
- Other possible causes of transmission may include from women who were infected shortly before pregnancy, from immunosuppressed women undergoing reactivation, and from women previously infected with one serotype developing a new infection with a second serotype during pregnancy.
- For untreated women, the rate of MTCT depends on the stage of pregnancy when infection occurs:

25 per cent in the first trimester

54 per cent in the second trimester

65 per cent in the third trimester.

- Infants affected with congenital toxoplasmosis may be stillborn or affected at birth.
- Most newborns are asymptomatic and may remain so throughout.
- Some develop clinical manifestations of the disease in weeks, months or years after birth.
- Congenital toxoplasmosis has a wide spectrum of clinical manifestations, but it is subclinical in approximately 75 per cent of infected newborns.

The classic triad of congenital toxoplasmosis includes:

- Hydrocephalus,
- Chorioretinitis
- Intracranial calcifications

Other signs and symptoms:

- Fever
- Jaundice
- Diarrhoea
- Petechial rashes
- Lymphadenitis
- Pneumonitis
- Myocarditis
- Hepatosplenomegaly

Newborns affected at birth have a poor prognosis (85 per cent being mentally retarded later in life), with a high percentage of them developing visual and hearing impairment at some point in life.

Diagnosis of Maternal Infection

Maternal serological findings:

- Is the most commonly used method for the diagnosis.
- IgG and IgM antibodies appear within one to two weeks after initial infection. The standard test used now is ELISA.
- Rising IgM titres indicate a recent infection.
- Presence of IgG antibody in the absence of IgM indicates past infection. Positive IgM and negative IgG denotes current infection.
- Positive IgM and IgG tests make it difficult to determine when the infection occurred.
- Serial ELISA tests give better information.

IgG avidity is another important test because the strength of antibody binding to the parasite increases approximately five months after the primary infection.

In cases of positive IgG and IgM antibodies and unknown timing of infection, avidity can distinguish between acute and chronic toxoplasmosis.

- High avidity (avidity index (AI) ≥ 60%) means that *Toxoplasma* infection was acquired before three months ago.
- Borderline avidity (50% < AI < 60%) means infection at an indeterminate period.[20]
- Low avidity (AI ≤ 50%) means that the infection was acquired within the last three months.

The *Toxoplasma* serological profile is useful in counselling infected pregnant women and has been shown to decrease the rate of unnecessary terminations by 50 per cent.

Microscopic demonstration of the parasites in the Giemsa-stained smear. Tissue sections show the cystic forms in body fluids obtained within 7–10 days of the infection.

Fetal Implications

- Maternal–fetal transmission occurs between one and four months following placental colonisation by tachyzoites.
- Without treatment, the overall risk of congenital infection from acute *Toxoplasma gondii* infection during pregnancy ranges from 20 to 50 per cent.
- Congenital transmission to the fetus occurs mainly if women acquire their primary infection during pregnancy.
- Congenital transmission has rarely been reported in chronically infected pregnant women unless infection was reactivated because the woman was immunocompromised.
- Infection remains in the placenta for the duration of the pregnancy, and therefore may act as a reservoir supplying viable organisms to the fetus throughout pregnancy.
- Historically, before the use of anti-*Toxoplasma* medication, studies showed that the risk of vertical transmission increases with gestational age, with the highest rates (60–81 per cent) in the third trimester.
- Disease severity, however, decreases with gestational age, with first-trimester infection resulting in fetal loss or major sequelae.
- Classic congenital toxoplasmosis is characterised by chorioretinitis, hydrocephalus, intracranial calcification, growth restriction and convulsion.

Diagnosis of Fetal Congenital Infections

Ultrasound Features of Congenital Toxoplasma Infection

- Intracranial calcifications
- Microcephaly
- Hydrocephalus
- Ventricular dilations
- Hepatosplenomegaly
- Ascites
- Severe IUGR

Quantitative Polymerase Chain Reaction (PCR) Detection in Amniotic Fluid

If primary infection during pregnancy is suggested, the next step would be to check for fetal congenital infection. The most sensitive test for congenital toxoplasmosis is quantitative DNA polymerase chain reaction (PCR) detection in amniotic fluid. It has a sensitivity of 87 per cent and specificity of 99 per cent when performed up to five weeks after maternal diagnosis. [EL 1]

A high DNA load and infection prior to 20 weeks indicate poor fetal/neonatal outcome.

Mouse Inoculation with Fetal Blood or Immunofluorescence

The specificity of antenatal diagnosis can be increased to 90 per cent, in mothers with positive serology. As per the National Institute for Health and Care Excellence (NICE) recommendation, amniocentesis should not be offered for the identification of infection at less than 18 weeks and should be offered after four weeks of suspected acute maternal infection to minimise the false-negative results. [EL 2]

Treatment

Treatment of Maternal Infection[13]

Spiramycin

- The main aim of the treatment during pregnancy is to reduce the severity of congenital infection.
- If maternal infection has occurred without fetal infection, spiramycin is used for fetal prophylaxis

to minimise placental transmission of infection. [EL 1]

- Evidence from a Systematic Review on Congenital Toxoplasmosis (SYROCOT) international consortium showed the odds of MTCT were 52 per cent lower if antepartum treatment was promptly initiated within three weeks after maternal seroconversion as compared with ≥eight weeks. [EL 1]

- Spiramycin does not readily cross the placenta, and therefore is not reliable for the treatment of fetal infection. Use is aimed at preventing vertical transmission of the parasite to the fetus, and it is indicated only before fetal infection.

- It is given at a dose of 1 g (3 million U) orally every eight hours. It should be prescribed for the duration of the pregnancy if the amniotic fluid PCR is reported negative for *T. gondii*.

Treatment of Fetal Infection

If fetal infection has been confirmed or is highly suspected:

Pyrimethamine (2 mg/kg per day, orally, divided twice per day for the first two days; then from day 3 to two months or to six months in symptomatic congenital toxoplasmosis.[22] [EL 1] Pyrimethamine is a folic acid antagonist that acts synergistically with sulfonamides. This drug should not be used in the first trimester because it is potentially teratogenic.

Sulfadiazine: 100 mg/kg per day, orally, divided twice per day.

Folinic acid, olinic acid (leucovorin): 10 mg, three times per week, to prevent the reversible, dose-related depression of the bone marrow of the pyrimethamine.

The combination of pyrimethamine and sulfadiazine results in a significant decrease in disease severity.

Neonatal Infection

Neonatal congenital toxoplasmosis is suspected in babies who are born to mothers exposed to primary *T. gondii* infection during pregnancy, or babies who have clinical findings indicating infection (intracranial calcifications, chorioretinitis, inexplicable mononuclear cerebrospinal fluid pleocytosis or increased cerebrospinal fluid protein).

The baby's blood should be tested for immunoglobulin M (IgM) and immunoglobulin G (IgG).

Follow-Up and Treatment of Neonatal Congenital Toxoplasmosis[13]

Clinical Follow-Up

Clinical evaluation of infants with suspected congenital toxoplasmosis (CT) should include:

- Detailed physical examination
- Neurologic evaluation
- Ophthalmologic examination (preferably by a retinal specialist)
- Brainstem auditory evoked responses

Serological Evaluation

Serial IgG antibody titres every four to six weeks after birth until complete disappearance of *Toxoplasma* IgG antibodies

Imaging Evaluation

- CT of the head (or head ultrasonography)
- Abdominal ultrasonography, serial IgG antibody titres every four to six weeks after birth until complete disappearance of *Toxoplasma* IgG antibodies

Treatment

A combination of:

- Pyrimethamine: 2 mg/kg per day, orally, divided twice per day for the first two days; then from day 3 to two months depending on symptoms and CT finding, 1 mg/kg per day, orally, every day; and after that, 1 mg/kg per day, orally, three times per week
- Sulfadiazine: 100 mg/kg per day, orally, divided twice per day
- Folinic acid (leucovorin): 10 mg, three times per week
- Corticosteroids may be considered (after 72 hours of anti-*Toxoplasma* therapy), if there is severe chorioretinitis or elevated CSF protein concentration ≥1 g/dL

Breastfeeding

- Mother with toxoplasmosis can continue to breastfeed her infant, but should be cautious if her nipples are cracked or bleeding.[14]
- There are no studies documenting transmission of *T. gondii* in humans through breastmilk.
- It is advisable to stop breastfeeding for 12–24 hours after metronidazole therapy, especially after single high doses have been used.
- Metronidazole is FDA pregnancy category B. (Animal reproduction studies have failed to demonstrate a risk to the fetus and there are no adequate and well-controlled studies in pregnant women.) It is best avoided in the first trimester.
- The US Food and Drug Administration does not recommend furazolidone use in pregnancy because of the complication of occurrence of mammary tumours in pregnant rats. It is recommended only if benefits outweigh the risks and no other alternative is available.

Screening

According to NICE, routine screening of women at low risk should not be performed. [EL 2]

Screening poses challenges, and it is important to consider the cost, risk factors, and availability of appropriate tests, relatively low incidence of acute infection, low sensitivity of screening (false-positive test results) and treatment effectiveness during gestation.

Screening is recommended for high-risk women who are immunosuppressed or HIV-positive, with ultrasound findings of hydrocephalus, intracranial calcifications, microcephaly, fetal growth restriction, ascites or hepatosplenomegaly. [EL 1]

Among Western European countries, France, Italy, Slovenia and Austria have implemented long-standing free national routine antepartum toxoplasmosis screening programmes.

Prevention

Primary prevention of infection should include advice to only eat well-cooked meat or poultry, thoroughly washed fruits and vegetables, washing and cleaning hands and cooking utensils adequately.

Pregnant women should avoid cleaning cat litter, wear gloves when gardening, during any contact with soil or sand, and wash hands afterwards.

Cats should feed only on canned or dried commercial food or well-cooked table food.

References

1. Centers for Disease Control and Prevention. Protozoan Parasites. parasite.org.au/para-site/contents/protozoa-intoduction.html.

2. Pullan RL, Smith JL, Jasrasaria R, Brooker SJ. Global numbers of infection and disease burden of soil transmitted helminth infections in 2010. *Parasites & Vectors*. 2014; 7: 37.

3. Centers for Disease Control and Prevention. Parasites – Giardia. www.cdc.gov/parasites/giardia/index.html.

4. Behr MA, Kokoskin E, Gyorkos TW, Cédilotte L, Faubert GM, MacLean JD. Laboratory diagnosis for Giardia lamblia infection: a comparison of microscopy, coprodiagnosis and serology. *Can J Infect Dis*. 1997; 8(1): 33–8.

5. Centers for Disease Control and Prevention. Parasites – Giardia. Treatment. www.cdc.gov/parasites/giardia/treatment.html.

6. Kissenger P. *Trichomonas vaginalis*: a review of epidemiologic, clinical and treatment issues. *BMC Infectious Diseases*. 2015; 15: 307 NCBI.

7. Sherrard J, Ison C, Moody J et al. *United Kingdom National Guideline on the Management of Trichomonas vaginalis, NICE guideline. Int J STD AIDS*. 2014; 25: 541.

8. Clinical Effectiveness Group (Association for Genitourinary Medicine and the Medical Society for the Study of Venereal Diseases). 2001 National Guideline on the Management of Trichomonas vaginalis.

9. Showler AJ, Boggild AK. Entamoeba histolytica. *CMAJ*. 2013; 185(12): 1064.

10. Blessmann J, Tannich E. Treatment of asymptomatic intestinal Entamoeba histolytica infection. *N Engl J Med*. 2002; 347: 1384.

11. Centers for Disease Control and Prevention. *Toxoplasmosis*. https://www.cdc.gov/parasites/toxoplasmosis/index.html.

12. McAuley JB. Congenital toxoplasmosis. *J Pediatric Infect Dis Soc*. 2014; 3(suppl 1): S30–5.

13. Paquet C, Yudin MH. Toxoplasmosis in pregnancy: prevention, screening, and treatment. *J Obstet Gynaecol Can*. 2013; 35(1): 78–81.

14. Centers for Disease Control and Prevention. Toxoplasmosis. Breastfeeding. www.cdc.gov/breastfeeding/breastfeeding-special-circumstances/maternal-or-infant-illnesses/toxoplasmosis.html.

Chapter

29

Puerperal Sepsis

Christine Helmy Samuel Azer

Introduction

The World Health Organization defines puerperal sepsis as 'infection of the genital tract occurring at any time between the onset of the rupture of membranes or labor and the 42nd day postpartum'.

Sepsis in the puerperium is still an important cause of maternal morbidity and mortality.

In the UK, according to the 2012–14 maternal mortality report, it accounts for 10 deaths per year.[1]

Globally, puerperal sepsis is a major cause of maternal death and accounts for 15 per cent of all maternal deaths in developing countries. It is also a major cause of morbidity (long-term health problems, e.g. chronic pelvic pain, chronic pelvic inflammatory disease (PID) and infertility.[2]

Severe sepsis with acute organ dysfunction has a mortality rate of 20–40 per cent, rising to around 60 per cent if septicaemic shock develops.

In the UK, 2012–14 maternal mortality report, direct sepsis (genital tract sepsis and other pregnancy-related infections) and indirect sepsis (influenza, pneumonia, others) accounted for seven maternal deaths, being the second cause of maternal mortality after cardiac disease.

Definitions

SEPSIS: infection plus systemic manifestations of infection.

SEVERE SEPSIS: sepsis plus sepsis-induced organ dysfunction or tissue hypo perfusion.

SEPTIC SHOCK: the persistence of hypoperfusion despite adequate fluid replacement therapy.[3]

Risk Factors

General and Community Risk Factors

- Poor standards of hygiene
- Poor aseptic technique
- Use of unclean hand or non-sterile instrument
- Pre-existing anaemia and malnutrition
- Pre-existing sexually transmitted infections
- Inadequate or no immunisation with tetanus toxoid
- Impaired glucose tolerance/diabetes
- Obesity
- History of pelvic infection
- Black or minority ethnic group origin
- Group A beta-haemolytic *Streptococci* (GAS) in close contacts/family members
- MRSA carriage and infection

Obstetric Risk Factors

- Prolonged/obstructed labour
- Prolonged rupture of membranes
- Frequent vaginal examinations
- Caesarean section and instrumental deliveries
- Retained products of conception
- Unrepaired cervical or large vaginal lacerations
- Amniocentesis
- Fetal scalp electrode or intrauterine pressure measurement during tocography
- Cervical cerclage
- Postpartum haemorrhage

Signs and Symptoms

- Fever (temperature of 38°C or more), rigours
- Chills
- General malaise
- Lower abdominal pain, pelvic tenderness
- Tender sub-involuted uterus
- Purulent, foul-smelling lochia

- Light vaginal bleeding
- Diarrhoea or vomiting – may indicate exotoxin production (early toxic shock)
- Wound infection – spreading cellulitis or discharge
- General – non-specific signs such as lethargy
- Reduced appetite
- Shock

Differential Diagnosis

- Urinary tract infection (acute pyelonephritis)
- Surgical site infection
- Mastitis or breast abscess
- Thromboembolic disorders, e.g. thrombophlebitis or deep vein thrombosis
- Respiratory tract infections (pneumonia)
- Extragenital infections: gastroenteritis, pharyngitis, bacterial meningitis
- Other infections, such as malaria and typhoid
- HIV-related infections

Infecting Organisms

- *Streptococci*
- *Staphylococci*
- *Escherichia coli* (E. coli)
- *Clostridium tetani*
- *Clostridium welchii*
- *Chlamydia*
- Gonococci
- Tetanus

Warning Signs and Symptoms of Puerperal Sepsis

Warning signs and symptoms should prompt need for early medical attention and urgent referral for hospital assessment:

- Woman appears seriously unwell, by emergency ambulance
- Pyrexia more than 38°C
- Sustained tachycardia more than 90 beats/minute
- Breathlessness (respiratory rate more than 20 breaths/minute; a serious symptom)
- Abdominal or chest pain
- Diarrhoea and/or vomiting

- Uterine pain and tenderness
- Woman is generally unwell or seems unduly anxious or distressed

Indications for Intensive Care Unit (ICU) Admissions[4]

- Cardiovascular: hypotension or raised serum lactate persisting despite fluid resuscitation, suggesting the need for inotrope (agents to increase the strength of muscular contraction) support
- Respiratory: pulmonary oedema
- Neurological: significantly decreased conscious level
- Miscellaneous multiple organ failure
- Uncorrected acidosis
- Hypothermia

Diagnosis and Investigations

Blood Culture

Blood cultures are essential first-line investigation. Bloods should be sent to the lab before antibiotic therapy, but empirical antibiotic treatment should be started immediately after taking the blood sample.

Serum Lactate

Serum lactate indicates the level of tissue perfusion; levels $\geq$ 4 mmol/L indicate tissue hypoperfusion. Sample should be taken within six hours of hospital or ICU admission. [EL 2]

Routine Blood Tests

Routine blood tests are full blood count, urea, electrolytes and C-reactive protein (CRP). Thrombocytosis, a rising CRP and a swinging pyrexia usually indicate a collection of pus or an infected haematoma in the woman.

Swabs and Cultures

Swabs for culture and sensitivity requests are guided by the clinical situations and suspicion of focus of infection. These may include high cervico-vaginal swabs, urine for culture and sensitivity or throat swabs, sputum, cerebrospinal fluid, epidural site swab, caesarean section or episiotomy site wound swabs and expressed breastmilk.

If the MRSA is unknown, a pre-moistened nose swab may be sent for rapid MRSA screening if a facility for this testing is available. Swabs should be taken before start of any antibiotics.

If there is a history of diarrhoea, a stool sample should be sent for *C. difficile* toxin testing and routine culture (e.g. *Salmonella*, *Campylobacter*).[5]

Imaging Studies

- Chest X-ray
- Pelvic ultrasound scan
- CT scans if pelvic abscess is suspected
- MRI may show an enlarged uterus or retained products of conception, or any pelvic haematomas or abcesses[6]

Management

Medical Management

Antibiotics

- Administration of high-dose broad-spectrum intravenous antibiotics as soon as a diagnosis of puerperal sepsis is made may be life-saving.
- Initial empirical administration of a broad-spectrum antibiotic regimen should be started immediately without waiting for the different culture and sensitivity results.
- A combination of either piperacillin/tazobactam or a carbapenem plus clindamycin provides one of the strongest regimens of treatment for severe sepsis.
- Clindamycin (900 mg clindamycin phosphate every eight hours) is not nephrotoxic and may be given in combination with ZOSYN (US Food and Drug Administration (FDA) pregnancy category B) which is a piperacillin/tazobactam combination. Each vial of ZOSYN contains 4 g piperacillin (as sodium salt) and 0.5 g tazobactam (as sodium salt given as 4.5 g intravenously (IV) every six hours, for 7–10 days). A second option is a combination of clindamycin and carbapenem (500 mg IV infusion every eight hours for 5–14 days). Carbapenem is FDA pregnancy category B (animal studies have failed to reveal evidence of fetal harm, although slight changes in fetal body weight were noted.

There are no controlled data in human pregnancy).

- MRSA is usually resistant to clindamycin; therefore a glycopeptide such as vancomycin or teicoplanin may be added until sensitivity is available.
- Cefuroxime and metronidazole for sepsis in the puerperium do not provide any protection against MRSA, *Pseudomonas* or extended spectrum beta-lactamases (ESBL).[7]
- Side effects of antibiotics include vomiting, severe watery diarrhoea and abdominal cramps, allergic reaction (shortness of breath, hives, swelling of lips, face or tongue, fainting), rash, vaginal itching or discharge, white patches on the tongue.
- A prospective, placebo-controlled, double-blinded study by Livingston et al., 2003, showed that gentamicin 5 mg/kg and clindamycin phosphate 2700 mg administered as a single-daily dose has a similar success rate to the standard eight-hourly dosing schedule. [EL 2]

Intravenous Immunoglobulin (IVIG)

- IVIG is the recommended therapy for severe invasive streptococcal or staphylococcal infection if other therapies have failed.
- IVIG has an immunodulatory effect.
- In staphylococcal and streptococcal sepsis, it also neutralises the super-antigen effect of exotoxins and inhibits production of tumour necrosis factor and interleukins.
- IVIG is contraindicated in congenital deficiency of immunoglobulin A.[8]

Fluid Replacement Therapy

- If there is hypotension and oliguria, fluid replacement therapy is essential.
- However, postpartum women are more susceptible to develop pulmonary oedema.
- Achieving the correct balance requires central venous pressure monitoring and vasopressor treatment, most probably better achieved in ICU under the care of the anaesthetist and the critical care team.[3]

Pain Relief Therapy

Paracetamol

- Paracetamol is an effective pain relief medication.

- Regular dosing prevents pain from developing, and if pain occurs it is usually less severe and requires smaller doses of adjuvant stronger pain medicines to provide relief.
- Paracetamol has been safely used to treat pain after birth for more than 50 years.
  The adult dose of paracetamol is two 500 mg tablets four times a day, up to a maximum daily dose of 4000 mg (4 g) –
  e.g. eight 500 mg tablets.
- Paracetamol is also used as an antipyretic.

Non-steroidal anti-inflammatory drugs (NSAIDs)

- NSAIDs should be avoided for pain relief in puerperal sepsis because they impede the ability of polymorphs to fight GAS infections.

Opioids

- Opioids are a wide range of strong pain relievers including codeine, morphine, pethidine, tramadol and oxycodone.
- They are effective pain relievers and are used for moderate to severe pain.
- Common side effects include nausea, vomiting, itch, confusion or mental clouding, headache and dizziness, sweating and constipation.
- However, these side effects are more common with high doses and continued use.
- The doses used after birth are usually fairly small.
- Use of opioids for long durations may cause addiction.

Anticoagulants

Septic Pelvic Phlebitis Treatment

The main treatments are a combination of antibiotics and anticoagulants.

Broad-spectrum antibiotics should be administered. Initial choice of antibiotics should cover gram-positive, gram-negative and anaerobic organisms. Ampicillin and gentamicin with metronidazole or clindamycin is a common regimen.

Anticoagulation may be indicated. There is no universal guideline or recommendation for anticoagulation therapy in septic pelvic thrombosis. Liaison with a haematologist is advisable.

- Unfractionated heparin in an initial bolus of 60 units/kg (4000 units maximum) followed by 12 units/kg/h (maximum of 1000 units/h) is recommended. The activated partial thromboplastin time (aPTT) is monitored for two to three times the normal value.
- Alternatively, low molecular-weight heparin may be used with a dose of 1 mg/kg.[9]

Infection Control

- The infected woman should be isolated in a single room to reduce the risk of transmission of infection.
- Health care workers should wear personal protective equipment including facemasks, disposable gloves and aprons when in contact with the patients.[10]
- Women with previously documented carriage of or infection with multiresistant organisms (e.g. extended spectrum beta lactamases (ESBL)-producing organisms, MRSA, GAS or a result for Panton–Valentine leukocidin (pvl) infection) should prompt notification of the infection control team.

Surgical Management

- Removal of any retained products of conception
- Emptying any haematoma
- Incision and drainage of any abscess or pelvic collection
- Incision and drainage of any breast abscess

Breastfeeding

- The mother is usually too ill to breastfeed.
- Mother should also be isolated from her baby for fear of transfer of infection.

Neonatal Infections in Puerperal Sepsis

Babies are at a special risk of streptococcal and staphylococcal infection during birth and during breastfeeding.

The paediatrician should be consulted in the event of maternal puerperal sepsis, and the baby managed accordingly.

Prevention

- Advise all women to avoid contamination of the perineum by washing hands before and after using the lavatory or changing sanitary towels.

It is equally important to avoid any contact with any member of her family or close contact who may have a sore throat or upper respiratory tract infection.

- Proper immediate treatment of any infections during pregnancy.
- Avoidance and observation of the above community and obstetric risk factors.
- Early hospital discharge once the patient is well to help prevent or reduce nosocomial infections.
- Antibiotic administration is recommended for women with preterm, prelabour rupture of membranes.
- Prevention of postpartum tetanus infections. The World Health Organization (WHO) recommends all women in pregnancy should have their immunisation status checked and be given a course of tetanus toxoid, if not fully immunised.[11]

Conclusion

Postpartum maternal sepsis may cause serious morbidity and mortality. Postpartum is an indication for prompt aggressive in-hospital treatment. Aggressive use of a combination antibiotic is the main management modality.

References

1. Knight M, Nair M, Tuffnell D et al., eds. on behalf of MBRRACE-UK. *Saving Lives, Improving Mothers' Care – Surveillance of Maternal Deaths in the UK 2012–14 and Lessons Learned to Inform Maternity Care from the UK and Ireland Confidential Enquiries into Maternal Deaths and Morbidity 2009–14*. Oxford: National Perinatal Epidemiology Unit, University of Oxford; 2016. www.npeu.ox.ac.uk/downloads/files/mbrrace-uk/reports/MBRRACEUK%20Maternal%20Report%202016%20-%20website.pdf.

2. World Health Organization. Managing Puerperal Sepsis. 2008. http://apps.who.int/iris/bitstream/handle/10665/44145/9789241546669_6_eng.pdf;jsessionid=D4313296EF43A070BD28E1149EED35FF?sequence=6.

3. Royal College of Obstetricians and Gynaecologists. Bacterial Sepsis following Pregnancy. Green–top Guideline No. 64b. April 2012. www.rcog.org.uk/globalassets/documents/guidelines/gtg_64b.pdf.

4. Plaat F, Wray S. Role of the anaesthetist in obstetric critical care. *Best Pract Res Clin Obstet Gynaecol*. 2008; **22**(5): 917–35.

5. Rouphael NG, O'Donnell JA, Bhatnagar J et al. Clostridium difficile-associated diarrhea: an emerging threat to pregnant women. *Am J Obstet Gynecol*. 2008; **198**: 625.e1–6.

6. Plunk M, Lee JH, Kani K, Dighe M. Imaging of postpartum complications: a multimodality review. *Am J Roentgenology*. 2013; **200**: W143–54. 10.2214/AJR.12.9637.

7. Sibhghatulla S, Jamale F, Shazi S, Mohd S, Rizvi D, Kamal MA. Antibiotic resistance and extended spectrum beta-lactamases: types, epidemiology and treatment.*Saudi J Biol Sci*. 2015; **22**(1): 90–101.

8. Soares MO, Welton NJ, Harrison DA et al. Intravenous immunoglobulin for severe sepsis and septic shock: clinical effectiveness, cost-effectiveness and value of a further randomised controlled trial. *Crit Care*. 2014; **18**(6): 649.

9. Garcia J, Aboujaoude R, Apuzzio J, Alvarez J. Septic pelvic thrombophlebitis: diagnosis and management. *Infect Dis Obstet Gynecol*. 2006; **2006**: 15614.

10. Gould IM. Alexander Gordon, puerperal sepsis, and modern theories of infection control – Semmelweis in perspective. *Lancet Infect Dis*. 2010; **10**(4): 275–8.

11. World Health Organization. WHO recommendations for prevention and treatment of maternal peripartum infections. http://apps.who.int/iris/bitstream/handle/10665/186171/9789241549363_eng.pdf;jsessionid=13937978B38749A835FD57FC274858CD?sequence=1.

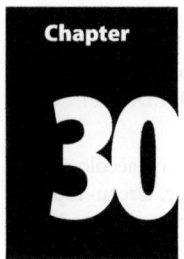

Chapter

30

Puerperal Endometritis

Christine Helmy Samuel Azer

Introduction

Endometritis refers to infection of the decidua (endometrium). The infection may also extend into the myometrium (endomyometritis) or involve the parametrium (parametritis).[1,2]

Commonly isolated organisms include *Ureaplasma urealyticum*, *Peptostreptococcus*, *Gardnerella vaginalis*, *Bacteroides bivius* and group B *Streptococcus*.

Chlamydia has been associated with late-onset postpartum endometritis.

Enterococcus is identified in up to 25 per cent of women with puerperal endometritis.

Ascending infection from the vagina is the main mechanism.

The highest incidence is during childbirth: 1–3 per cent of vaginal births, and up to 27 per cent of caesarean births. In the USA the incidence after caesarean section ranges from 13 to 90 per cent, depending on the risk factors present and whether perioperative antibiotic prophylaxis had been given.

Signs and Symptoms

Infection may appear up to six weeks postpartum.[3] [EL 1]

- Fever
- Lower abdominal and pelvic pain
- Foul-smelling lochia
- Abnormal vaginal discharge
- Abnormal postpartum vaginal bleeding
- Dyspareunia
- Dysuria (may be present in patients with pelvic inflammatory disease)
- Subfertility (long-term sequelae)

Sometimes the only symptom is a low-grade fever which usually appears within the first 24–72 hours postpartum.[4]

On Examination

- The uterus is soft, large and sub-involuted.
- The uterus is tender.
- Induration at the base of the broad ligaments, extending to the pelvic walls or posterior cul-de-sac.

When the parametrium is affected, pain and fever are severe.

Predisposition and Risk Factors

- Prolonged rupture of the membranes
- Internal fetal monitoring
- Prolonged labour
- Caesarean delivery
- Multiple repeated digital examination
- Retention of placental fragments
- Group B *Streptococcus* infections
- Postpartum haemorrhage
- Colonisation of the lower genital tract
- Anaemia
- Bacterial vaginosis
- Young maternal age (higher incidence of sexually transmitted infection)
- Low socioeconomic status

Complications

- Peritonitis
- Pelvic abscess
- Pelvic thrombophlebitis (with risk of pulmonary embolism)
- Pelvic haematoma
- Septic pelvic thrombophlebitis
- Rarely, septic shock and its sequelae which becomes a life-threatening condition
- Long-term disabilities: chronic pelvic pain

- Secondary infertility because of fallopian tube blockage
- Unexplained repeated implantation failure (RIF) in IVF cycles. Chronic endometritis was identified in 30.3 per cent of patients with repeated implantation failure at IVF. Antibiotic treatment significantly improves the reproductive outcome at a subsequent IVF cycle.[5] [EL 2]

Diagnosis

Clinical Diagnosis

Clinical diagnosis depends on the above clinical picture.

A temperature of 38°C or higher within the first 10 days postpartum is diagnostic of postpartum endometritis.

Laboratory Diagnosis

- Microbial cultures:
  - High vaginal and cervical swabs culture and sensitivity result guide towards the treatment
  - Blood culture (positive in 10–30 per cent of cases)
- Endometrial tissue samples can confirm the diagnosis
- Urine analyses and urine culture should be done to exclude urinary tract infections

Imaging Studies

Imaging is useful on patients who do not respond to adequate antimicrobial therapy in 48–72 hours.

Pelvic ultrasound is usually a readily available diagnostic modality. Ultrasonography of the abdomen and pelvis may yield normal findings in patients with a clinical diagnosis of endometritis. Abnormal findings may show retained products of conception, intrauterine haematoma or adnexal masses.

CT scanning of the abdomen and pelvis may be helpful for excluding broad ligament masses, septic pelvic thrombophlebitis, ovarian vein thrombosis and phlegmon.

Differential Diagnosis

- Urinary tract infection
- Wound infection
- Septic pelvic thrombophlebitis
- Perineal wound infection

Treatment

Medical Therapy

Intravenous clindamycin plus gentamicin, with or without ampicillin.[6] (EL 1)

The first-line choice is clindamycin 900 mg q 8 h plus gentamicin 1.5 mg/kg q 8 h or 5 mg/kg once/day.

Ampicillin 1 g q 6 h is added if enterococcal infection is suspected or if no improvement occurs by 48 hours.

Severe cases of endometritis should be treated as an inpatient setting.

For mild cases following vaginal delivery, oral antibiotics in an outpatient setting may be adequate

Surgical Management

Surgical management is not usually necessary in acute endometritis in the obstetric population.

Dilation, evacuation of retained products of conception and curettage may be indicated for any retained products of conception.

Hysterectomy may be necessary as a life-saving intervention in rare instances of overwhelming infection non-responsive to conservative therapy.

Prevention

Summary list of World Health Organization (WHO) recommendations for prevention and treatment of maternal peripartum infections:[7]

- Routine perineal/pubic shaving prior to giving vaginal birth is not recommended.
- Digital vaginal examination at intervals of four hours is recommended for routine assessment of active first stage of labour in low-risk women.
- Routine vaginal cleansing with chlorhexidine during labour for the purpose of preventing infectious morbidities is not recommended.
- Routine vaginal cleansing with chlorhexidine during labour in women with group B Streptococcus (GBS) colonisation is not

recommended for prevention of early neonatal GBS.

- Intrapartum antibiotic administration to women with GBS colonisation is recommended for prevention of early neonatal GBS infection.
- Routine antibiotic prophylaxis during the second or third trimester for all women with the aim of reducing infectious morbidity is not recommended.
- Routine antibiotic administration is not recommended for women in preterm labour with intact amniotic membranes.
- Routine antibiotic administration is not recommended for women with prelabour rupture of membranes at or near term.
- Routine antibiotic administration is not recommended for women with meconium-stained amniotic fluid.
- Routine antibiotic prophylaxis is recommended for women undergoing manual removal of the placenta.
- Routine antibiotic prophylaxis is not recommended for women undergoing operative vaginal birth.
- Routine antibiotic prophylaxis is recommended for women with a third- or fourth-degree perineal tear.
- Routine antibiotic prophylaxis is not recommended for women with episiotomy.
- Routine antibiotic prophylaxis is not recommended for women with uncomplicated vaginal birth.
- Vaginal cleansing with povidone-iodine immediately before caesarean section is recommended.
- The choice of an antiseptic agent and its method of application for skin preparation prior to caesarean section should be based primarily on the clinician's experience with that particular antiseptic agent and method of application, its cost and local availability.
- Routine antibiotic prophylaxis is recommended for women undergoing elective or emergency caesarean section.

- For caesarean section, prophylactic antibiotics should be given prior to skin incision, rather than intraoperatively after umbilical cord clamping. (EL 2)
- For antibiotic prophylaxis for caesarean section, a single dose of first-generation cephalosporin or penicillin should be used in preference to other classes of antibiotics.
- A simple regimen such as ampicillin and once-daily gentamicin is recommended as first-line antibiotics for the treatment of chorioamnionitis.
- A combination of clindamycin and gentamicin is recommended as first-line antibiotics for the treatment of postpartum endometritis.

References

1. 'Endometritis' at *Dorland's Medical Dictionary*.

2. Chen KT. Postpartum endometritis. UpToDate. www .uptodate.com/contents/postpartum-endometritis.

3. Rivlin ME, Alderman E, Chandran L, Simmons GT. Endometritis. Medscape. Updated 1 December 2017. https://emedicine.medscape.com/article/254169-overview.

4. Moldenhauer JS. Puerperal Endometritis. MSD manual. www.msdmanuals.com/professional/gynecology-andobstetrics/postpartum-care-and-associated-disorders/puerperal-endometritis.

5. Cicinelli E, Matteo M, Tinelli R et al. Prevalence of chronic endometritis in repeated unexplained implantation failure and the IVF success rate after antibiotic therapy. *Human Reproduction*. 2015; **30**(2): 323–30,

6. Mackeen A, Packard RE, Ota E, Speer L. Antibiotic regimens for postpartum endometritis. *Cochrane Database Sys Rev*. 2015: **2**: CD001067. doi: 10.1002/14651858.CD001067.

7. World Health Organization. Recommendations for Prevention and Treatment of Maternal Peripartum Infection. Geneva. 2015. http://apps.who.int/iris/bit stream/10665/186171/1/9789241549363_eng.pdf?ua=1.

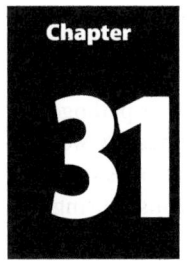

Puerperal Mastitis

Christine Helmy Samuel Azer

Introduction and Epidemiology

Mastitis is an infection in the tissue of one or both mammary glands inside the breasts.

It is rare during pregnancy, but more common during breastfeeding.

It is also known as lactation mastitis.

The incidence according to the World Health Organization (WHO) is between 5 and 33 per cent of breastfeeding mothers.[1]

It usually presents during the first few weeks after delivery or at the time of weaning.

Between 10 and 33 per cent of breastfeeding women develop lactation mastitis. The incidence is highest in the first few weeks postpartum, decreasing gradually after that. However, cases may occur as long as the woman is breastfeeding.

In a retrospective study involving 136 459 deliveries in a US teaching hospital, the incidence of mastitis was 6.7 per 10 000 deliveries, and the incidence of mastitis with breast abscess was 2.6 per 10 000 deliveries. In the same study, the incidence of puerperal mastitis requiring hospital admission was seen most commonly with community-acquired MRSA ($n = 18$, 67%).[2] [EL 2]

Severe cases are common in young primiparous women; just 23.7 per cent of the cases weaned their infants during the first six months after birth, due to mastitis.

The bacteria most commonly involved are *Staphylococcus aureus* (31 per cent) and *Streptococci* (10 per cent), through skin lesions of the nipple or through the opening of the nipple.

Staphylococcus infections tend to be more invasive and localised, leading to earlier abscess formation; while *Streptococcus* infections tend to present as diffuse mastitis with focal abscess formation in advanced stages. Gram-negative bacilli such as E. coli, *Salmonella* spp., mycobacteria, *Candida* and *Cryptococcus* have been identified in rare instances.

Risk Factors

- Damaged nipple, especially if colonised with *Staphylococcus aureus*
- Infrequent feedings or scheduled frequency
- Missed feedings
- Weak or uncoordinated suckling leading to inefficient removal of milk
- Illness in mother or baby
- Breast engorgement and milk stasis
- Blocked lactiferous ducts
- Sore and cracked nipple
- Pressure on the breast (e.g. tight bra)
- History of mastitis after a previous pregnancy
- Maternal stress and fatigue
- Infant mouth anomalies such as cleft palate

Clinical Picture

- The onset is typically rapid. It usually affects one breast
- Fever (38.3°C or greater)
- Flu-like symptoms at first (fatigue, chills, anxiety or stressed), followed by the local symptoms
- Local pain (may be continuous or only during breastfeeding)
- Redness (in a wedge-shaped pattern)
- General soreness
- Abnormal nipple discharge (may be white or contain streaks of blood)

On examination the breast appears swollen, red, lumpy, tender to touch and warm; 0.4–5 per cent will present with breast abscess.

There is segmental erythema usually in the upper, outer quadrant, with variable degrees of induration.

Breast abscess will present with a palpable, fluctuant mass which may be indurated at the beginning of the infective process.

Severe cases may present by septicaemia and may require hospitalisation.

Complications

If a woman fails to clinically improve with first-line therapy over 48 hours of treatment, she should be considered to have a complicated mastitis.

Concerns are:

- Resistant organism or MRSA-related mastitis
- The development of an abscess
- An underlying cancer

Physical examination, cultures of the affected skin area and of the milk, possibly an ultrasound, and a change in antibiotics are indicated.

Prognosis and Outcome

Most cases of mastitis are self-limited.

A 10- to 14-day course of antibiotics and continuous breastfeeding is expected to produce good results.

Women with mastitis are more inclined to discontinue breastfeeding and should be offered additional support and encouragement.

Continued breastfeeding, even while on antibiotics, does not pose a risk to the infant.

Diagnosis

On clinical examination: it is mainly a clinical diagnosis, although investigations may be needed in some cases.

Ultrasound: used mainly to distinguish simple mastitis from breast abscess.

If there is an abscess: irregular, hypo-echoic to anechoic mass with fluid and debris and posterior acoustic enhancement.

If it is mastitis: ill-defined, hypo-echoic region with periductal inflammation.

Mammograms: are rarely used. Mammogram shows skin and trabecular thickening due to breast oedema; abscess may be seen as ill-defined mass.

Breast biopsies: normally performed on women who do not respond to treatment for five weeks or on non-breastfeeding women, to distinguish mastitis from inflammatory breast cancer (IBC) as it may coincide with mastitis or develop shortly afterwards and has a very similar clinical picture. IBC is the most aggressive type of breast cancer, with high mortality rate.

Culture of the nipple discharge: although this is not helpful in the diagnosis of mastitis as pathogenic, bacteria detected in the breastmilk of healthy women can be used to aid the choice of antibiotics in some cases by detecting the specific organisms causing the infection.[3]

Prevention

Proper breastfeeding technique is the main protective method.

- Avoiding suddenly going longer between feeds or cutting down suddenly
- Instruction in hand washing
- Encourage early unrestricted feeding
- Expression and breast massage
- Identification of mothers with increased risk of nipple trauma
- Purified lanolin cream or ointment to help the healing process for sore cracked nipple[4]

Treatment

Treatment should start as soon as possible, mainly before 48 hours, to avoid the formation of breast abscess, chronic or recurrent mastitis.

First-Line Treatment

Reassurance

The pain of puerperal mastitis should not be allowed to interfere with ability to continue breastfeeding or affect the long-term appearance of the breast.

Women should be encouraged to continue breastfeeding. They must be assured that to continue breastfeeding will not cause any harm to the baby.

If breastfeeding is too painful, women should consider feeding via expressing milk until symptoms improve.

Good hydration of mother and baby is key.

Non-Pharmacological Therapies
Hot and Cold Compress

In a randomised controlled study of 60 mothers, cold cabbage leaves and hot and cold compress were both equally effective in decreasing breast engorgement and in relieving pain due to puerperal mastitis.

It is advised that hot compresses be used before breastfeeding and cold cabbage compresses after breastfeeding.[5] [EL 1–]

Improve Milk Removal

- Manual expression of milk to empty the breast after feeding.
- Self-massage of the breast before feeding or expression, or application of heat by warm compresses, shower or heat packs.
- Increase feeding frequency.
- Feeding on the affected side first while symptoms persist so this breast is emptied most effectively.
- Advise not wearing a bra at night.
- Women may require emotional support.

Analgesia

Paracetamol or ibuprofen may be used for pain and inflammation where appropriate.

Be aware that many women may require emotional support.

Antibiotics

A Cochrane Reviews study comparing no treatment, breast emptying and antibiotic therapy with breast emptying suggested more rapid symptom relief with antibiotics.[6] [EL 1]

Guidelines by the World Health Organization (WHO) and the Academy of Breastfeeding Medicine suggest first-line measures for 24 hours before starting antibiotics unless the woman is acutely unwell or has an infected nipple injury.[7]

Treatment should be in accordance with local prescribing guidelines; 15 per cent will need antibiotic treatment.

Dicloxacillin or cephalexin are first choice. Flucloxacillin or erythromycin may also be used. There is no significant difference detected when comparing these antibiotics. [EL 2]

Cephalexin is usually safe in women with suspected penicillin allergy, but clindamycin is suggested for cases of severe penicillin hypersensitivity. 16 (III) dicloxacillin appears to have a lower rate of adverse hepatic events than flucloxacillin. Many authorities recommend a 10–14-day course of antibiotics.

Surgical Management

Surgical management (incision and drainage) is indicated for breast abscesses.

Parenteral antibiotics should be administered. Pus from the abscess should be sent for culture and sensitivity, to give proper antibiotic treatment.

Needle aspiration of the abscess has been suggested as an alternative to open drainage (repeated every other day until the pus is no longer present).

Any persisting mass will need further investigation to exclude sinister causes.

In conclusion, puerperal mastitis is a preventable condition, is easily amenable to correct and timely management and should not lead to any long-term consequences.

References

1. World Health Organization. Geneva. 2000. Mastitis, Causes and Management. https://apps.who.int/iris/bit stream/handle/10665/66230/WHO_FCH_CAH_00.13_ eng.pdf;jsessionid=9B75CA94DEDE197C164AC47A1 D5CA2C1?sequence=1.

2. Stafford I, Hernandez J, Laibl V, Sheffield J, Roberts S, Wendel G Jr. Community-acquired methicillin-resistant Staphylococcus aureus among patients with puerperal mastitis requiring hospitalization. *Obstetrics & Gynecology.* 2008; **112**(3): 533–7.

3. American College of Obstetricians and Gynecologists. Benign Breast Problems and Conditions. March 2017. www.acog.org/Patients/FAQs/Benign-Breast-Problems -and-Conditions?IsMobileSet=false.

4. Abou-Dakn M, Richardt A, Schaefer-GU, Wöckel A. Inflammatory breast diseases during lactation: milk stasis, puerperal mastitis, abscesses of the breast, and malignant tumors – current and evidence-based strategies for diagnosis and therapy. *Breast Care.* 2010; **5**: 33–7.

5. Arora S, Vatsa M, Dadhwal V. A comparison of cabbage leaves vs. hot and cold compresses in the treatment of breast engorgement. *Indian J Community Med.* 2008; **33** (3): 160–2.

6. Antibiotics for mastitis in breastfeeding women. *Cochrane Database Syst Rev.* 2013; **2**: CD005458.

7. The Academy of Breastfeeding Medicine. Reece-Stremtan S, Marinelli, KA. ABM Clinical Protocol #21: Guidelines for Breastfeeding and Substance Use or Substance Use Disorder, Revised 2015. *Breastfeed Med.* 2015; **10**(3): 135–41. www.ncbi.nlm.nih.gov/pmc/arti cles/PMC4378642/.

Chapter

32

Breast Abscess

Christine Helmy Samuel Azer

Introduction and Epidemiology

Most breast abscesses develop as a complication of lactation mastitis. The incidence ranges from 0.4 to 11 per cent of all lactating mothers. Lactational breast abscesses are most often caused by *Staphylococcus aureus* and streptococcal species, Methicillin-resistant *S. aureus* is becoming increasingly common.[1]

Risk Factors

- Primiparity
- Birth after 41 weeks' gestation
- Age >30 years
- Recent mastitis
- Previous history of mastitis or breast abscess[2]

Clinical Picture

Patients may provide lactation history. You need to ask about any history of prior breast infections and the previous treatment. It is also important to ask about the patient's medical history, including diabetes, especially in recurrent or chronic cases.

Signs and Symptoms

- Severe breast pain
- Breast erythema, warmth and possibly oedema are the most common
- Tender on palpation
- Induration
- Fever and rigours
- Nausea, vomiting
- Palpable mass or area of fluctuance
- Purulent discharge at the nipple or site of fluctuance
- Reactive axillary adenopathy may be present
- In a large breast or if the abscess is deeply located, a mass may not be felt

Diagnosis

Clinical Diagnosis

It is a clinical diagnosis, based on the clinical picture.

Laboratory Diagnosis

- Full blood count may show leucocytosis but this is not specific
- Culture and sensitivity of any breast discharge
- Breast ultrasound

Breast ultrasound scan is used to differentiate abscess from mastitis, also to exclude breast cancer.

Abscess appears as ill-defined mass with very stiff outer rim due to oedema and inflammation. There are internal septations and very soft central area.

Treatment

Incision and drainage (I&D) of the abscess under coverage of antibiotics is the standard care for breast abscess.

- Many antibiotics are secreted in milk, but penicillin, cephalosporins and erythromycin are considered safe.
- A course of antibiotics may be given before or following drainage of breast abscesses.
- Cultures should be obtained to guide antibiotic therapy, especially in recurrent breast abscesses.
- Surgical I&D should be considered for first-line therapy in large (>5 cm), multiloculated or long-standing abscesses, or if percutaneous drainage is unsuccessful.[3]
- If there is a large cavity after I&D, packing of the cavity may be done to promote further drainage and prevent the skin incision from healing before drainage is complete.
- Incision and drainage have lower recurrence rates, but they are more invasive than needle aspiration

and may lead to prolonged healing time, regular dressings, difficulty in breastfeeding due to scarring, and the possibility of milk fistula with unsatisfactory cosmetic outcome.

- If the cause of the abscess is an obstructed or ectatic lactiferous duct, surgical excision may be necessary.

Ultrasound (US)-assisted drainage of the abscess may be an effective first-line alternative in small breast abscesses <3 cm. Multiple aspiration sessions may be required for cure.

US-guided percutaneous catheter placement

- May be considered as an alternative approach for treatment of abscess >3 cm, chronic or recurrent abscesses.
- A catheter can be inserted using the Seldinger technique under US guide and connected to a three-stop way to allow drainage and irrigation of the cavity until its resolution.
- This approach has the potential benefits of superior cosmoses, shorter healing time, safe, well-tolerated, cost-effective procedure, avoidance of general anaesthesia and preserving breastfeeding.[4]

Signs of sepsis should be considered for admission to the hospital.

Pain can be controlled by prescribing non-steroidal anti-inflammatory drugs (NSAIDs) and/or narcotics according to the severity of pain.

However, in a Cochrane study, there is insufficient evidence to determine whether needle aspiration is a more effective option than I&D for lactational breast abscesses.[5]

Suppression of Lactation

- Lactation should be continued, allowing for proper drainage of the ductolobular system of the breast.
- Continuing breastfeeding does not present any risk to the nursing infant.
- Drug-induced suppression of lactation may cause nausea, vomiting and bad general feeling.
- Drug-induced suppression of lactation is contraindicated because of its negative impact on the immune system as well as physical and mental development of the suckling baby.
- If suppression of lactation is indicated, the most effective suppressant currently available is cabergolamine, which is effective as a single dose and preferable to bromocriptine.
- The engorged breast should be emptied.
- Fluid restriction and firm binding seem unnecessary.[6]

References

1. Kataria K, Srivastava A, Dhar A. Management of lactational mastitis and breast abscesses: review of current knowledge and practice. *Indian J Surg.* 2013; 75(6): 430–5.

2. Martin JG. Breast Abscess in Lactation. Medscape OBGYN and Women's Health. https://www .medscape.com/viewarticle/589139_2.

3. Fahrni M, Schwarz EI, Stadlmann S, Singer G, Hauser N, Kubik-Hucha RA. Breast abscesses: diagnosis, treatment and outcome. *Breast Care.* (Basel) 2012; 7(1): 32–8.

4. Ulitzsch D, Nyman MK, Carlson RA. Breast abscesses in lactating women: US-guided treatment. *Radiology.* 2004; **232**: 904–9.

5. Irusen H, Rohwer AC, Steyn D, Young T. Treatments for breast abscesses in breastfeeding women. The Cochrane Library. 17 August 2015. www.cochrane.org/ CD010490/PREG_treatments-breastabscesses-breastfeeding-women.

6. Rolland R, Goeij W. Single dose cabergoline versus bromocriptine in inhibition of puerperal lactation: randomized double blind multicentre study. *BMJ.* 1991; **302**: 1367–71.

Chapter

33

Pelvic Inflammatory Disease

Ahmed Khalil

Definition

Pelvic inflammatory disease (PID) is a clinical syndrome caused by ascending spread of infection from the vagina and/or endocervix into the pelvis causing endometritis, salpingitis, parametritis, oophritis, tubovarian abscess and even peritonitis in severe cases.[1]

Aetiology

- PID is almost always a sexually transmitted infection disease.
- The most common micro-organisms that have been implicated are *Neisseria gonorrhoeae* and *Chlamydia trachomatis*. Other organisms including vaginal anaerobes, *Mycoplasma genitalium* and *Gardnerella vaginalis* have also been implicated.
- A large study of 315 123 Western Australian women found that gonorrhoeal infection conferred a higher risk than chlamydia for hospitalisation or presentation with PID. The emergence of gonorrhoea antimicrobial resistance may have a serious impact on rates of PID and its sequelae.[2] [EL 2]

Incidence

- The incidence of PID is unknown, mainly due to the difficulty in making a diagnosis.
- First attack of PID is often unrecognised if it has atypical presentation or is asymptomatic.
- In a large cohort historical follow-up study of women tested for *Chlamydia trachomatis*, Bakken et al. showed that PID was diagnosed in 1.7 per cent of primary care physician attendances by women 16–46 years of age.[3]
- Approximately 125 000–150 000 hospitalisations occur yearly in the United States because of PID.

- PID is a clinical syndrome and diagnosis is mainly clinical.
- Expert opinion from the British Association for Sexual Health and HIV (BASHH) recommends making the diagnosis of PID based on history and clinical examination alone and having a low threshold for initiating treatment.[4]

Symptoms

- PID can be asymptomatic
- Lower abdominal pain (which is usually bilateral)
- Abnormal vaginal discharge
- Deep dyspareunia
- Menorrhagia
- Intermenstrual bleeding
- Post-coital bleeding

Signs

- Lower abdominal tenderness which is usually bilateral
- Adnexal tenderness on bimanual vaginal examination
- Cervical motion tenderness on bimanual vaginal examination
- Fever (>38°C)

Risk Factors

- Age less than 20 years poses a greater risk for development of PID
- High number of sexual partners
- Previously treated sexually transmitted infections (STIs) increase the risk of PID significantly
- Commercial sex workers
- Women who do not use condom contraception
- Women in areas with a high prevalence of STIs

- Young age at first intercourse is also a risk factor for PID
- An intrauterine device (IUD) for contraception confers a relative risk of 2.0–3.0 for the first four weeks following insertion; this risk subsequently decreases to baseline. This risk is usually associated with sexually transmitted infection. However, the best evidence suggests that the risk of PID among IUD users is very low.[5]

Differential Diagnosis

- Ectopic pregnancy is the most important differential diagnosis to exclude in young women presenting with acute abdominal pain.
- Ovarian cyst accidents (ovarian cyst torsion or rupture or bleeding inside an ovarian cyst).
- Appendicitis.
- Urinary tract infection.
- Mittelschmerz pain (painful ovulation, pain occurs during ovulation in the midpoint between menstrual periods, about two weeks before a period may begin. The discomfort can appear on either side of the lower abdomen depending on which ovary is producing the ovum.
- Endometriosis.
- Functional pain (that is of unknown physical origin).

Complications

Chronic Pelvic Pain

Chronic pelvic pain occurs in approximately 25 per cent of patients with a history of PID. The pain may be the result of adhesions or hydrosalpinx.

Infertility

According to one study, the risk of tubal infertility was 0.6 per cent after mild infection, and 21.4 per cent after severe infection.

Ectopic Pregnancy

The risk of ectopic pregnancy is increased 15–50 per cent in women with a history of PID.

Tubo-ovarian Abscess (TOA)

- TOA can manifest as an adnexal mass, fever, elevated white blood cell count, lower abdominal–pelvic pain, and/or vaginal discharge.
- PID may cause TOA and extend to produce pelvic peritonitis and Fitz-Hugh–Curtis syndrome (perihepatitis).
- TOA occurred in as many as one-third of women hospitalised for PID.[6]
- Acute rupture of a TOA with resultant diffuse peritonitis is a rare but life-threatening event that calls for urgent abdominal surgery.
- MRI is superior in evaluating the extent of disease, the characteristics of the lesion and to make the diagnosis of a TOA. However, due to high cost and more limited availability, MRI is not usually the first-line imaging used.

Pelvic Abscess

- An abscess occurs when pus from the fallopian tube spills onto the ovary and infects it at the site of follicular rupture or by direct penetration.
- Symptoms include abdominal and pelvic pain that may be bilateral and is aggravated by motion and intercourse. Fever with leucocytosis, tachycardia and prostration are the common symptoms of pelvic abscess.
- Abdominal and pelvic examination may reveal a fluctuant mass, although the degree of pain and guarding may mask the diagnosis.
- Rectal examination may provide a clue.
- Imaging modalities (US, CT and MRI) help diagnoses and may elicit other causes of pain.

Pregnancy-Related Factors

- PID rarely occurs in pregnancy.
- Chorioamnionitis can occur in the first 12 weeks of gestation, before the mucous plug solidifies and seals off the uterus from ascending bacteria.
- Fetal loss may result if chorioamnionitis occurs.
- Pregnancy influences the choice of antibiotic therapy for PID.

- Uterine infection is usually limited to the endometrium but may be more invasive in a gravid or postpartum uterus.
- Pregnant women with suspected PID should be admitted to hospital, as intravenous (IV) antibiotics are required due to the increased risk of maternal and fetal morbidity and preterm delivery.

Neonatal Implications

Neonatal complications can occur as a result of perinatal transmission of, and may include ophthalmia neonatorum (due to *Chlamydia trachomatis* or *Neisseria gonorrhoeae* infection) and chlamydial pneumonitis.

Diagnosis and Work-Up

History of Risk Factors and Clinical Presentation

Pregnancy should be excluded in women of childbearing age who present with lower abdominal pain.

Laboratory Diagnosis

High vaginal and endocervical swabs for identification of the infecting organisms and antimicrobial culture. The swab should be inserted inside the cervical os and firmly rotated against the endocervix.

Wet-mount microscopy of the vaginal or endocervical secretions to diagnose bacterial vaginosis and other common vaginal infections.[7]

Nucleic acid amplification (NAAT) for DNA probe testing for *Chlamydia* and gonorrhoea.

An elevated C-reactive protein or erythrocyte sedimentation rate or leucocyte count may support a diagnosis of PID but is not specific.

Laparoscopy is helpful in the diagnosis of PID or other conditions, e.g. ovarian cyst accidents, dermoid cysts or endometriosis.[8]

Imaging modalities. Transvaginal ultrasound and MRI play an important diagnostic role in PID.

Transvaginal ultrasonography has a sensitivity rate of 81 per cent, a specificity rate of 78 per cent and accuracy of 80 per cent. MRI had a sensitivity of 95 per cent, a specificity of 89 per cent and an accuracy of 93 per cent in the diagnosis of PID.[9]

Management

General Considerations

- Treatment of PID should aim to eradicate the current infection, to relieve acute symptoms, and minimise the risk of long-term sequelae.
- Early diagnosis and treatment appear to be critical in the preservation of fertility.
- In view of the diagnostic difficulties and the serious complications of PID, current guidelines suggest that empirical treatment should be started in at-risk women who have lower abdominal pain, adnexal tenderness and cervical motion tenderness.
- Physicians should maintain a low threshold for aggressive treatment. Immediate overtreatment has more advantages than delayed treatment.[10] [EL 2]

Antibiotic Treatment

Antibiotics should cover *N. gonorrhea, C. trachomatis* and a variety of aerobic and anaerobic bacteria commonly isolated from the upper genital tract in women with PID.

Some of the best evidence for the effectiveness of antibiotic treatment in preventing the long-term complications of PID comes from the PID Evaluation and Clinical Health (PEACH) study where women were treated with cefoxitin followed by doxycycline. Pregnancy rates after three years were similar to or higher than in the general population.[11] [EL 1]

Outpatient regimes include:

- Intramuscular ceftriaxone 500 mg as single dose with 14 days of oral doxycycline 100 mg twice daily and metronidazole 400 mg twice daily.
- Oral ofloxacin 400 mg twice daily plus oral metronidazole 400 mg twice daily for 14 days.

Inpatient regimes include:

- IV ceftriaxone 2 g daily plus oral doxycycline 100 mg twice daily. This is followed by oral doxycycline 100 mg twice daily plus oral metronidazole 400 mg twice daily for a total of 14 days.
- IV clindamycin 900 mg three times daily plus intravenous gentamicin (2 mg/kg) loading dose followed by 1.5 mg/kg three times daily (or a single dose of gentamicin 7 mg/kg). This is followed by oral

clindamycin 450 mg four times daily (or oral doxycycline 100 mg twice daily) plus oral metronidazole 400 mg twice daily to complete 14 days.
- Microbiology advice should be requested for pregnant patients and those who are known to have particular allergies.
- Indications for hospital admission include pyrexia of more than 38°C, TOA, pelvic abscess and pelvic peritonitis.

Oral cefixime as an alternative to intramuscular ceftriaxone:

- Ceftriaxone primarily covers gonorrhoea.
- A single dose of oral cefixime 400 mg (off-label use) is recommended by the Health Protection Agency as an alternative to the intramuscular ceftriaxone component of the regimens for practical issues of administration in primary care.

Drug choice during very early pregnancy:

The BASHH states that the risk of giving any of the recommended antibiotic regimens in very early pregnancy is justified by the need to provide effective therapy and the low risk to the fetus.

- Ceftriaxone crosses the placental barrier, but has not been associated with adverse events on fetal development in laboratory animals. The risk associated with use of cephalosporins during pregnancy is thought to be low. The cephalosporins as a class are considered to be an appropriate choice during pregnancy.
- Metronidazole has been in clinical use for a long time, and experience suggests that it is not teratogenic in humans.
- Ofloxacin has only limited pregnancy-exposure data.
- Quinolones have caused arthroplasty in animal studies.
- Azithromycin and erythromycin are macrolides. Azithromycin is considered by many to be the treatment of choice for *C. trachomatis* genitourinary infection because it may be administered as a single dose.

Follow-up and management of sexual contacts:

- Review of patients is advised at 72 hours, to ensure symptoms are resolving.

- Persisting or worsening symptoms warrant a review of the diagnosis and further investigation and treatment.
- Patients should avoid sexual contact until treatment is complete.[12]
- All recent sexual partners within the previous six months should be offered screening and treatment.
- If partners are unwilling to be screened, they should be offered empirical treatment to avoid potential prolonged infectivity and its complications.
- Referral to a genitourinary medicine (GUM) clinic should be considered, to ensure further counselling and complete sexual health screen including blood-borne viruses such as hepatitis and HIV.

Treatment of Complications

Tubo-Ovarian Abscess

Surgery is indicated if there are serious vital threats (generalised peritonitis, toxic shock).

In uncomplicated TOA, the evacuation of abscesses (by draining under imaging or laparoscopy) with the antibiotic treatment gives better rates of cure than the antibiotic treatment alone.

Laparoscopy allows a shorter hospitalisation with fewer complications and a faster resolution of the fever than the laparotomy. The radical surgery, by laparotomy, has high rates of complications.

Transvaginal ultrasound-guided aspiration can drain the abscess with identical success to laparoscopy.

Summary

PID is defined as an infection ascending from the female lower genital tract which can be caused by STIs as well as vagina flora.

A pregnancy test should be performed to exclude ectopic pregnancy as a differential diagnosis.

Antibiotic therapy should be given early if there is a high index of suspicion based on the symptoms and risk factors.

Untreated or repeated PID infections can lead to infertility, pelvic abscesses and adhesions, and may add to chronic pelvic pain.

Those testing positive for STIs should be offered treatment. GUM clinic referral should be considered to screen for blood-borne viruses such as HIV and hepatitis.

References

1. Centers for Disease Control and Prevention. Self-Study STD Modules for Clinicians. Pelvic Inflammatory Disease (PID). 2017. www2a.cdc.gov/stdtraining/self-study/pid/pid_clinical_self_study_from_cdc.html.

2. Reekie J, Donovan B, Guy R et al. Risk of pelvic inflammatory disease in relation to chlamydia and gonorrhea testing, repeat testing, and positivity: a population-based cohort study. *Clin Infect Dis.* 2018; **66**(3): 437–43.

3. Bakken IJ, Ghaderi S. Incidence of pelvic inflammatory disease in a large cohort of women tested for Chlamydia trachomatis: a historical follow-up study. Clinical presentation and risk assessment. *BMC Infect Dis.* 2009; **9**: 130. doi: 10.1186/1471-2334-9-130.

4. British Association for Sexual Health and HIV. UK National Guideline for the Management of Pelvic Inflammatory Disease. 2011. www.bashh.org/documents/3572.pdf.

5. Hubacher D. Intrauterine devices & infection: review of the literature. *Indian J Med Res.* 2014; **140**(suppl 1): S53–7.

6. Kim HY, Yang JI, Moon CS. Comparison of severe pelvic inflammatory disease, pyosalpinx and tubo-ovarian abscess. *J Obstet Gynaecol Res.* 2015; **41**(5): 742–6.

7. Benigno BB. Medical and surgical management of the pelvic abscess. *Clin Obstet Gynecol.* 1981; **24**(4): 1187–97.

8. Mylonas I, Bergauer F. Diagnosis of vaginal discharge by wet mount microscopy: a simple and underrated method. *Obstet Gynecol Surv.* 2011; **66**(6): 359–68.

9. American Family Physician. Diagnosing PID: Comparing Ultrasound, MRI, Laparoscopy. www.aafp.org/afp/191999/0315/p1656.html.

10. Liu B, Donovan B, Hocking JS, Knox J, Silver B, Guy R. Improving adherence to guidelines for the diagnosis and management of pelvic inflammatory disease: a systematic review. *Infect Dis Obstet Gynecol.* 2012; **2012**: 325108.

11. Ness RB, Soper DE, Peipert J et al. Design of the PID Evaluation and Clinical Health (PEACH) study. *Control Clin Trials.* 1998; **19**(5): 499–514.

12. Centers for Disease Control and Prevention. 2015 Sexually Transmitted Diseases Treatment Guidelines. www.cdc.gov/std/tg2015/pid.htm.

Index

Tables appear in **bold**